DETECTION AND TREATMENT OF
EARLY BREAST CANCER

DETECTION AND TREATMENT OF EARLY BREAST CANCER

Ian S Fentiman

MD, FRCS
Consultant Surgeon and Deputy Director
ICRF Clinical Oncology Unit, Guy's Hospital
London

MARTIN DUNITZ

First published in the United Kingdom in 1990
by Martin Dunitz Ltd, London

British Library Cataloguing in Publication Data

Fentiman, Ian, *1945–*
    Detection and treatment of early breast cancer.
    1. Women. Breasts. Cancer. Diagnosis
    I. Title
    616.99449075

    ISBN 1-85317-010-0

Phototypeset by Scribe Design, Gillingham, Kent
Printed in Great Britain by The University Press, Cambridge

CONTENTS

To Elizabeth, Nina, Alan and John

PREFACE

It was with some hesitation that I accepted the invitation to write a book on early breast cancer. My rationalization was that it was time an attempt was made to write a cohesive account of the present problems, in a different style from that usually encountered. In this I enlisted the help of Amanda Ramirez, who gallantly reviewed the enormous body of psychological research to contribute Chapter 8.

I would also like to acknowledge gratefully the enormous help given to me by colleagues who read drafts and were able to suggest multiple improvements. These included Michael Richards, Murid Chaudary, Max Rendall, Rosemary Millis, Janice Wilkins, Huw Gravelle, David Tong and Dennis Wang. I thank Kim Bullock, my secretary who cheerfully accepted multiple revisions and produced an impeccably typed manuscript.

I do not anticipate that anyone will be in total agreement with what has been written, but I trust that some will find subjects for further consideration.

CHAPTER 1

THE CAUSES OF BREAST CANCER

Sir, I have found you an argument;
but I am not obliged to find you an understanding.

Samuel Johnson

How paradoxical it is that the external symbol of life and womanhood should be responsible for the deaths of half a million women every year. For reasons that are not understood the mammary epithelial cells, whose differentiated function is to provide succour for the neonate, behave in an aberrant manner. At the junction of the duct and lobule the well-ordered structure of luminal and basal epithelial cells becomes disturbed and local control mechanisms fail to operate so that there is an increase in number followed by derangement of both structure and function.

In parallel, intercellular communication is either blocked or becomes unconstrained so that previously non-communicating cells exchange signals. At the same time, inappropriate synthesis and secretion of proteases leads to dissolution of the basement membrane, enabling entry of the transformed epithelial cells into the stromal domain. Once the breakout from the constraints of the basement membrane and the negative feedback of the surrounding cells has been achieved any human barrier can be overcome by the malignant cells. The invasive cancer may be small but it is armed and ready to kill.

Searches for causes

Prodigious efforts and enormous expenditure have characterized breast-cancer research. At the level of looking for causes, work has been largely epidemiological, recently aided by work from both cellular and molecular biologists. Much of the original investigation, particularly relating to endocrinology, was derived from rodent model systems, the relevance of which is debatable. Until recently it would have been possible to be equally dismissive about the role of tumour virology which had provided work for scientists but no feedback of value to clinicians. Applications of basic science can be unpredictable. With the discovery of the roles of oncogenes and growth factors and receptors in real tumours, results derived from work on retroviruses have come to be regarded as very important in relation to human cancer.

After study of the descriptive epidemiological literature on breast cancer it is hard to escape the conclusion that much of this has been re-invention of the wheel, namely, confirming that the human breast is an endocrine-sensitive organ. Luckily, more recent analytical epidemiology has divulged important clues as to the aetiology of breast cancer. However, despite identification of high-risk groups and risk factors, three-quarters of breast-cancer cases have no identifiable cause. Thus the main aetiological factors still elude the epidemiologist. Closer cooperation between clinicians, basic scientists and epidemiologists may lead to the framing of more appropriate questions for epidemiological study.

Age incidence

For the majority of cancers there is a direct relationship between incidence and age so that if plotted on a log/log scale, the rising curve becomes a linear slope. Breast cancer behaves atypically. On a semi-logarithmic scale, there is an inflexion of the line around age 50 so that the incidence, although continuing to rise, does so at a reduced rate. Similar results were derived from all Western countries, but the Japanese data appeared to be different, with a postmenopausal downward turn in incidence. However, it was found that, after adjustment for birth cohort (birth decade) and year of diagnosis, the Japanese incidence curve was superimposable upon the Western data.[1] Thus worldwide, breast-cancer incidence increases with age.

It is likely that this increase is due, not to any inherent instability of aging cells, but to an increase in probability of mutagenic events with time. If lung cancer can be taken as an analogy, the percentage rate of increase is greater for smokers than non-smokers when measured from birth.[2] However, when the starting time is birth for non-smokers and the commencement of smoking for smokers, the rate of increase is similar for both groups, suggesting that length of exposure to carcinogens determines the risk rather than the age of cells. This is further supported by the observation that incidence of lung cancer remains constant after cessation of smoking.

Cairns has argued that the increasing risk of cancer with age is the result of the emergence of 'fitter' variants with a survival advantage.[3] These cells represent intermediate stages. Whereas normally DNA replication is semi-conservative, this could mean that the immortal DNA strand remains in the daughter cell that remains in situ, whereas the daughter cell that will be shed contains the newly synthesized DNA. Thus a mutagenic hit would normally have no consequence since the stem-cell lineage would retain the original DNA. Local changes in cell/cell orientation could lead to loss of this defence mechanism and an accumulation of mutant DNA.

Basing themselves upon data concerning smoking and lung cancer, Armitage and Doll proposed a multistage theory of carcinogenesis with a series of discrete steps, culminating in the emergence of a malignant clone.[4] Breast cancer may represent a further level of complexity because of the endocrine influence on both normal and malignant mammary epithelium.

Moolgavkar has suggested a two-stage process of mammary carcinogenesis, with the normal cell undergoing mutation to an intermediate cell which may then undergo a second mutation.[5] The estimated human somatic mutation rate was one per 10^7 cells/year per locus. The probability of two such mutations would be the product, that is 10^{-14} (a very rare event). According to Moolgavkar, tissue kinetics are the major determinant of risk: hormones exerting their influence on carcinogenesis via effects on cell growth rather than any direct mutational activity. Population risks were determined by transition times between normal and intermediate states and from intermediate to malignant expression.

Pike proposed a mathematical model which took into account breast-tissue age, starting at menarche and ending at the menopause.[6] Incorporation of the first full-term pregnancy, age at menarche and age at menopause achieved a good fit for the model's prediction when tested on the age-incidence data for the third National Cancer Survey.

Menstruation

Normal ovulatory cycles produce a proliferation of mammary epithelium which attains its zenith in the luteal phase.[7] This has been taken as a response to progesterone but might be the delayed consequence of a mid-cycle oestrogen surge. For whatever reason, menstrual cycles imply cell division, thereby increasing the probability of mutagenic change and progression from normality to any intermediate stage, or from an intermediate change to malignancy. This being so, the greater the number of menstrual cycles, the greater the risk of breast cancer.

Such are the findings. Early menarche increases risk so that Polish girls who started menstruating before the age of 16 carried a 1.8-fold increase compared with those whose menarche was later than age 16.[8] At the other extreme of the reproductive spectrum, late menopause also increases risk. Trichopoulos et al reported a doubling of risk for women who continued menstruating beyond the age of 55 compared with those whose natural menopause was before the age of 45 years.[9]

An artificial menopause had been shown to protect women against subsequent breast cancer. MacMahon reported that 7 per cent of 28 breast cancer patients had a prior artificial menopause compared with 16 per cent of 55 controls.[10] Feinlieb conducted a cohort study of 6908 women who had undergone gynaecological surgery, including bilateral oöphorectomy, and 1479 women whose ovaries were conserved.[11] Among those who underwent hysterectomy and bilateral oöphorectomy before age 40, the observed/expected (O/E) ratio was 0.25, that is a four-fold reduction in incidence of breast cancer. For those who underwent similar surgery, but had stopped menstruating prior to this, the O/E ratio was 0.79 for those aged 40–44, and 0.99 for those aged 45–55. Thus the earlier the artificial menopause, the greater the protection.

A similar effect was shown by Trichopoulos, whose data are presented in Table 1.1.[9] There was a gradual increase in relative risk so that those who had an induced menopause before age 35 had a relative risk of 0.3 compared with a relative risk of one for those who had a natural menopause between

Table 1.1 Effect of artificial menopause on incidence of breast cancer.[9]

Age at artificial menopause	Observed	Expected	Relative risk
<35	73	184	0.36
35–39	106	141	0.68
40–44	141	197	0.65
45–49	132	165	0.73
>50	72	67	0.98

the ages of 45 and 54, and a relative risk of 0.98 for those who had an artificial menopause after age 50. This is compelling evidence of a role for the ovaries in the development of breast cancer. Of the gang of ovarian hormones the prime suspect is oestradiol. However, the likelihood is that oestrogens act in physiological concentrations and that in the majority of patients with breast cancer, no major abnormality of ovarian function is present.

Endogenous oestrogens

The study of ovarian hormones and their role in breast cancer may be likened to a walk across a treeless plain, criss-crossed by ditches. On arrival at the other side it is apparent that little of interest has been achieved but the walk was constantly enlivened by the relief of getting out of the ditches.

Because of the restraints of technology, original studies concentrated on measurement of urinary hormones. Almost invariably no abnormalities of oestrogen excretion were found, but this is not surprising since the production of oestrogen and its metabolic clearance is unrelated to levels of oestrone (E_1), oestradiol (E_2) and oestriol (E_3) in the urine.[12] However, when urinary androgens were measured it was found that androsterone and aetiocholanolone were significantly reduced in women who subsequently developed breast cancer.[13] Progesterone excretion as measured by urinary levels of pregnanediol was found to be elevated in breast-cancer cases, but others found no differences between cases and controls.[14,15]

It was hoped that these confusing data might be explained once radio-immune assays were developed so that blood levels of hormones could be determined accurately. Such hope was in vain. For every study which showed an abnormality of oestradiol in the blood of breast-cancer patients,[14] there was another showing no difference.[15] Similarly, for those at risk of breast cancer by virtue of family history, no consistent abnormalities were found.[16,17]

Again, expectations were raised when it became appreciated that most of the oestrogen in blood was protein-bound. Of the total oestrogen in blood, 40–50 per cent binds tightly to sex hormone binding globulin (SHBG), 50–60 per cent loosely to albumin and only 1–2 per cent is free and therefore biologically available.[18] Siiteri reported that women with breast cancer had significantly higher proportions of free oestradiol (free E_2).[19] However, as with work on urinary and blood total oestradiol, subsequent case-control studies have both confirmed and refuted this finding.[20,21]

This increase in percentage of free E_2 was largely the result of a reduction in SHBG binding capacity rather than a fall in absolute levels of SHBG.[19,20] Bruning and Hart reported that oestradiol could be displaced from SHBG in vitro by increasing concentrations of polyunsaturated free fatty acids.[22] In addition, it was found that the increase in free fatty acids resulting from overnight fasting caused an increase in the percentage of free E^2.

In a study of normal women from Guernsey it was found that those who subsequently developed breast cancer had higher proportions of free E_2 and lower concentrations of SHBG than controls who remained disease-free.[23] Despite this apparent link between free E_2 and breast cancer, Siiteri was unable to confirm his original findings and suggested that changes in the proportion of free E_2 might have been related to the storage time of samples.[24] Thus it is likely that levels of free oestradiol within the physiological range are present in the majority of patients with breast cancer. Nevertheless, reduction of those levels may lead to significant reductions in the risk of breast cancer, and pharmacological increases with oral contraceptives and hormone replacement therapy may increase the transition through the multistages in the development of breast cancer.

Pregnancy

The effect of age at first full-term pregnancy on breast cancer risk still remains one of the most puzzling epidemiological phenomena. It has been suggested that, rather than being protective, early abortion may increase the risk of breast cancer. Pike reported that a first trimester spontaneous or induced abortion before first full-term pregnancy (FFTP) carried a relative risk of 2.4.[25] In contrast, there was a three-fold increase in risk for women who had their first baby when aged over 30 years, compared with those who delivered before the age of 18.[26] When nulliparous women were compared with parous women whose first pregnancy occurred after the age of 30, the latter group have a higher risk.[27] This implies that pregnancy after a relatively few years of menstruation induces changes of differentiation which protect the breast. After a longer duration of menstruation (possibly more than 15 years) pregnancy may promote intermediate cells to undergo terminal transformation into malignancy.

Not only does early pregnancy protect, but in addition further pregnancies even after the age of 30 provide extra reduction in risk.[28] Furthermore, the age at which a parous woman has her last baby also determines risk—the later the pregnancy the less the chance of breast cancer developing subsequently.[29] Thus present-day customs of delayed pregnancy and small families may exert a deleterious effect on breast-cancer risk.

One possible explanation of these findings is that they are mediated by long-term changes in prolactin secretion.

Prolactin

A considerable body of circumstantial evidence links prolactin with the development of breast cancer. However, many of these data are derived from rodent model systems which may have overemphasized the role of prolactin in terms of human disease.[30] There are specific receptors for this polypeptide hormone on the cell membranes of the mammary epithelium. Prolactin is required for the growth and differentiation of the breast, together with the maintenance of lactation. It is not altogether surprising that some properties of normal cells are maintained in others with a malignant phenotype. Thus the presence of prolactin receptors in human breast cancers is not synonymous with causality.[31]

Studies of individuals with hyperprolactinaemia as a result of reserpine administration have shown a minimal effect on breast-cancer risk.[32,33] Ross measured prolactin levels in 15 postmenopausal patients who had been taking reserpine for more than 5 years and for comparison used age-matched controls taking other anti-hypertensive agents and others receiving no medication.[34] The reserpine-treated group had prolactin levels which were 50 per cent higher than those in the other two groups. Using the Pike model of breast-cancer incidence, it was calculated that this increase in prolactin would lead to a relative risk of 1.2, a figure consistent with that reported in case-control studies. Subsequently Stanford re-examined duration of reserpine usage and breast cancer.[35] It was found that prolonged use, greater than 10 years, led to a significantly increased relative risk of 4.5.

Malarkey measured hourly blood samples in 23 breast-cancer patients and 41 controls and found that premenopausal cases had a higher nocturnal secretion of prolactin.[36] Postmenopausal cases had a significantly diminished night-time release of prolactin. Although Henderson reported elevated levels of prolactin in daughters of breast-cancer patients, this was not confirmed by Boffard.[16,17]

To examine the relationship between parity and prolactin, Wang performed assays on two cohorts of normal women of 5000 each, and examined the data in a multivariate analysis.[37,38] There was a significant decrease in prolactin levels with increase in parity among both premenopausal and postmenopausal women. This suggested that this endocrine sequel of parity was a permanent effect. This could explain the benefits of multiparity, and the protection given by late age at final pregnancy.

Bulbrook examined the relationship between age and prolactin level, and calculated that this fitted a cubic equation.[39] This was consistent with the observed age-incidence curves, and was in favour of prolactin being a promoter rather than an inducer of mammary carcinogenesis.

Lactation

Lactation is a plausible candidate for protection against breast cancer. This could occur as a result of shedding of transformed cells or release of retained carcinogens. Alternatively, the process of differentiation resulting in milk production might lead to the growth inhibition of premalignant cells or clones. However, until recently the received epidemiological wisdom was that lactation had no effect on risk of breast cancer, which in relation to pregnancy was dependent upon age at first full-term pregnancy. Almost all the negative or neutral results were derived from studies of postmenopausal women, without consideration of the total duration of lactation.

Byers reported that there was a protective effect of prolonged lactation but that this only manifested itself in relation to premenopausal women.[40] On review of the literature,

Table 1.2 Relative risk of breast cancer in relation to lactation.[45]

Lactation history	Relative risk	
	Premenopausal	*Postmenopausal*
Ever lactated	0.49	1.0
Total duration		
Never	1.0	1.0
1–3 months	0.66	1.0
4–12 months	0.45	0.98
13+ months	0.45	0.38
Duration of first nursing		
Never	1.0	1.0
1–2 months	0.67	1.3
3–5 months	0.56	1.8
6+ months	0.54	0.66

evidence of similar benefit could be culled from several other studies.[41–4]

McTiernan and Thomas conducted a case-control study in which 329 breast-cancer cases were compared with 332 neighbourhood controls, derived by random-digit dialling.[45] The results are shown in Table 1.2. For the premenopausal women there was a significant decrease in relative risk for those who had ever lactated. When examined in relation to length of lactation, a protective effect was seen in premenopausal women who had breast-fed for 3 months, but the postmenopausal benefit was seen only in those who lactated for more than one year. Similar protection was seen in relation to length of lactation after the first full-term pregnancy.

By use of a logistic regression model it was found that the protective effect of lactation was unconfounded by age, number of pregnancies or age at first full-term pregnancy. Thus lactation can be recognized as a protective factor in relation to breast cancer—another reason for recommending breast-feeding as being of benefit to both baby and mother.

Diet

Several interconnecting strands of evidence have been used to construct the belief that dietary components, in particular animal fats, play a role in the development of breast cancer. At a clinical level, surgeons have noted that they perform mastectomies more frequently on fat rather than thin women. Secondly, international comparisons of incidence figures for breast cancer have shown significant correlations with national consumption of animal fats. Thirdly, animal experiments using the rodent model systems have indicated an increase in breast tumours in those given high-fat diets. In rodents, animal fat acts as a promoter rather than an initiator of carcinogenesis.

At the same time, good evidence has emerged concerning the relationship of animal-derived saturated fatty acids and risk of coronary heart disease. Thus sensible dietary modifications have been proposed to reduce the incidence of deaths from heart attacks. It has also been suggested that there might be a protective effect on breast cancer with this type of diet. This is wishful thinking. Indeed, there is evidence suggesting that a shift from animal-derived fats towards a vegetarian diet could increase the risk of breast cancer.

It is of course highly likely that the majority of carcinogens acting upon mammary epithelium and stroma are dietary in origin. Many of these agents will be fat-soluble and thus the greater the consumption of fats, the more likely the occurrence of first, second or third events in a carcinogenic cascade. This, however, is at variance with animal evidence suggesting a promotional role for fat.

Weight

De Waard found that obesity carried a greater risk of breast cancer in postmenopausal women and postulated that the disease might have two variants, separated by the menopause.[46] According to this theory the ovaries provide the major promotional drive in the premenopausal but this role is taken over by the adrenal cortex in the postmenopausal, with amplification by peripheral aromatization by adipose tissue. The American Cancer Society followed 419 060 women to examine weight and mortality from cancers.[47] After subdivision into seven weight categories, as shown in Table 1.3, there was a highly significant correlation between obesity and risk of death from breast cancer ($r = 0.96$). Among the

Table 1.3 Mortality ratio for breast cancer in relation to percentage of average weight for all ages.[47]

	Weight index (%)					
	<80	80–89	90–109	120–129	130–139	140+
Mortality ratio	0.8	0.9	1.0	1.2	1.2	1.5

heaviest women there was a 50 per cent increase in breast-cancer mortality. Information on menopausal status at the time of diagnosis was unavailable.

A recent Swedish study confirmed the findings of De Waard.[48] For women aged less than 50 years, the relative risk of development of breast cancer associated with a 10 kg increase in weight was 0.91 (that is a reduction), whereas for women over 50 years the same weight increase was associated with a relative risk of 1.1, a significant elevation.

What does this imply? The increased risk in the postmenopausal obese women may be due to peripherally synthesized oestrogens which promote the growth of transformed epithelium. This is plausible, but what of the premenopausal? Is peripheral fat acting as a sump in which ovarian-derived steroids collect and are thereby rendered less effective at the level of mammary epithelium? Does obesity within the relatively low-risk premenopausal group protect or does leanness endanger? Tornberg found that beta-lipoprotein, cholesterol and Quetelet's index (weight/height^2) emerged from a Cox regression analysis as the significant variables of risk in the premenopausal. Both cholesterol and Quetelet were negatively associated but beta-lipoprotein was positively associated with development of breast cancer. Since beta-lipoprotein is a measure of low-density lipoprotein (LDL), and as levels of LDL receptor are related to proliferation rates of tumour cells, this could explain the risk to the lean.[49] In these thinner women, levels of beta-lipoprotein tend to be higher, so that this could promote tumour growth in the susceptible.

International comparisons

Lea, from the Imperial Cancer Research Fund, was the first to demonstrate a highly significant correlation between consumption of fats and oils and national mortality figures for breast cancer.[50] This was studied more extensively by Armstrong and Doll, who examined not only mortality but also incidence of breast cancer and food consumption in 37 countries.[51] Of all the dietary components, fat gave the highest correlation ($r = 0.79$) with breast-cancer incidence. However, an even more significant correlation was found between breast-cancer incidence and gross national product ($r = 0.83$). Dietary fat is closely correlated with gross national product. Breast-cancer development may arise from wealth-associated factors, which may not necessarily result from excess fat consumption.

Such comparisons, although interesting, give an unclear view of the situation. National food consumption is based not on what is eaten, but what is sold. Detailed studies of individuals rather than populations have led to conflicting results but certainly lend little support to any direct linkage between animal fat consumption and breast cancer.

Individual studies

The literature has recently been critically reviewed by Goodwin and Boyd.[52] They used the principles enunciated by Bradford Hill to infer causality, namely consistency of evidence, strength of association and a temporal relationship between putative cause and effect. No convincing evidence was found.

Of the four cohort studies examined, only one Japanese study reported a positive association with a relative risk of 3.8 for those who consumed meat daily compared with those eating meat less than once weekly.[53–6] Similar increases in relative risk were seen for egg eaters (2.9) and butter/cheese consumption (2.1). Another Japanese study showed no increase in relative risk, and a large study of US nurses found no difference in risk for those in the upper and lower quintiles of animal fat consumption.

Goodwin and Boyd[52] found 14 case-control studies of which eight studied fat intake and breast-cancer risk.[57–70] Only one study with a hospital-derived control group found any significant association. Six case-control studies examined fat content of foods and in none was there a significant association between all types of fat and breast cancer risk.[57–62] Miller found a significant association between saturated fat intake and risk

which was greatest among the postmeno-pausal.[59] Two studies reported that total calorie intake was associated with risk but did not analyse separately fat content and calories.

Goodwin and Boyd suggested that the discrepant data of international correlation and case-control studies result from the relatively narrow variations in national fat consumption.[52] To a large extent this can be overcome by using vegetarians and meat-eaters from the same populations where vegetarianism has been chosen either on religious or personal grounds. Follow-up of long-term vegetarians has shown no protective effect among those who were vegetarian from before puberty.

Another problem relates to the actual measurement of dietary content. Questionnaires give insufficiently accurate information, particularly when seeking secular changes in diet, up to 15 years before diagnosis of breast cancer.

The specificity of the relationship between dietary fat and breast cancer should hold after adjustment for known risk indicators. Gray et al examined international correlations, and corrected for height, weight and age at menarche.[71] A statistically significant association between dietary fat and breast carcinoma remained. Since height, weight and age at menarche are all indirect indicators of dietary intake, by which animal fats influence endocrine function, the residual significant association does suggest either an additional promotional effect or, alternatively, a possible role in the induction of breast cancers.

Migrant studies

Migrant populations provide a special opportunity to disentangle the respective contributions of nature and nurture in the aetiology of

Table 1.4 Comparative incidence of breast cancer among Japanese, American and Japanese-American women.[72]

Age	Japanese (%)	Issei* (%)	Nisei† (%)	US (%)
35–64	18	52	65	100
65–74	7	56	–	100

*Women born in Japan but moved to the USA.
†Japanese women born in the USA.

disease. Japanese women who have emigrated to the USA form a group of particular interest in the study of breast cancer since they derive from a population which has an incidence rate less than one-fifth of that in the USA. Buell reported incidence data from San Francisco/Oakland.[72] Of an entire population of 3 million women, there were 32 463 of Japanese origin. Comparative data were obtained for native white Americans and also from the Cancer Registry of Okayama, Japan. The results are summarized in Table 1.4.

Women aged 35–64, born in Japan, but who moved to the USA (Issei) developed a three-fold increase in the incidence rate which then became approximately half that of native-born American women. In the same age range, Japanese women born in the USA (Nisei) had a four-fold increase in incidence rate. There were insufficient Nisei aged over 65 years for any analysis to be conducted. Among the Issei aged 64–74 the incidence was 56 per cent of that of American women.

This suggests a fairly rapid assumption of American risk which is not dependent upon being exposed to an American lifestyle during puberty. Among Poles who migrated to the USA and Britain there is a rapid increase in breast-cancer incidence which has been attributed to rapid acculturation.[73,74]

These data do provide compelling evidence that the environment rather than the genetic make-up of individuals plays a major role in the aetiology of breast cancer. Of the aspects of lifestyle which are likely to be responsible for this change, diet is the prime suspect. However, atmospheric contamination, differential exposure to cosmic rays and different water supplies could also be responsible. As a long shot, the different flora and fauna and their associated viruses might also have an indirect role, although evidence for a viral aetiology of human breast cancer is very scant.

Diet and endocrine function

If dietary fat acts as a promoter of human mammary carcinogenesis, the mechanism might be endocrine. Because of the relatively narrow range of dietary fat consumption within nations, studies of diet and endocrine function have focused on comparisons of women from countries with high and low incidences of breast cancer. An alternative approach has been to examine vegetarians and vegans and compare their hormonal status with that of omnivorous controls.

Hill compared premenopausal white American women with South African black women, the former being deemed to be at higher risk of breast cancer.[75] The white American women had higher levels of prolactin and androgen in the plasma, but lower levels of oestradiol in both follicular and luteal phases. When the black South Africans were switched to a Western-style diet, their prolactin levels became elevated, but this may have been a stress response rather than a direct result of the high-fat low-fibre diet.

Teenage girls from Japan, USA, Chile and Papua New Guinea were studied by Gray, who found that despite major differences in diet, there were no significant differences in plasma prolactin and oestrogen, or in urinary oestrogens.[76] Gray also investigated teenage Californians, 23 vegetarians and 26 non-vegetarians.[77] Their endocrine profiles were similar, and analysis of the disparate diets showed a similar proportion of calories derived from fat, carbohydrate and protein.

Armstrong compared 50 postmenopausal vegetarians (Seventh Day Adventists) with 50 age-matched, non-vegetarian controls.[78] Plasma prolactin levels were slightly, but significantly, elevated in non-vegetarians. Furthermore, urinary oestriol and total oestrogens were significantly increased in non-vegetarians. Since MacMahon had shown that those at increased risk of breast cancer excreted less urinary oestriol, this suggested that the vegetarians might have an elevated risk of breast cancer.[79] Armstrong reported higher levels of SHBG in vegetarians (consistent with less free oestradiol) and higher levels of high-density lipoproteins (which may themselves stimulate the growth of human mammary cancer cells).

Goldin measured faecal, urinary and plasma levels of oestrogen in 10 vegetarian and 10 non-vegetarian premenopausal women.[80] Vegetarians excreted more faecal and less urinary oestrogen. This consistent finding suggested a possible increase in the risk of breast cancer.

Schultz and Leklem found lower plasma levels of oestrone and oestradiol in premenopausal vegetarian Seventh Day Adventists when compared with non-vegetarians of the same faith.[81] Levels of prolactin and androgens were similar in both groups.

A study was conducted at Guy's Hospital, London, to examine diurnal variations of endocrine function in normal premenopausal vegetarian and omnivorous women. Serial blood samples were taken every 2 hours for a 24-hour period from 25 vegetarians and 21 controls. No differences were found between prolactin secretion in the two groups, but the vegetarians displayed a singificant elevation of growth hormone.[82] Both groups had similar levels of SHBG and free oestradiol.[83] However, the proportion of oestradiol bound to SHBG was significantly lower among vegetarians and this could result in increased availability of oestrogens. Such an effect is suggested by the study of Mills who reported a lower risk of breast cancer in women who became vegetarians later in life, compared with those who were life-long vegetarians.[84]

Thus a vegetarian or low-fat diet may protect against heart disease and cancer of the colon. These are major benefits. However, for a woman deemed at extra risk of developing breast cancer, a change to a low-fat diet may not necessarily be in her best interests.

Caffeine

Attention was directed towards consumption of tea and coffee as a risk factor for breast cancer largely as a result of the work of Minton.[85] It was known that caffeine can act as a mutagen and also, in concert with unsaturated fats, as a promoter of the growth of dimethyl-benzanthracene (DMBA) induced cancers in the rat.[86,87] Minton reported elevated levels of cyclic adenosine monophosphate (cAMP) in human breast cancers. Subsequently, raised levels of cAMP were found in tissue from women with fibrocystic disease.[88] However, this was based on wet weight rather than DNA content, and the cellularity of the two types of tissue is very different.

The inference was made that, because

some women with fibrocystic disease were at increased risk of breast cancer, elevation of cAMP, induced by caffeine, might predispose to malignancy. This is not so. A series of case-control studies has shown either no association or a very weak one, and no relationship between either duration or dosage of caffeine ingested.[89–92] Studies of established human breast-cancer cell lines have shown that elevation of cAMP is associated with an inhibition of the growth of these cells.[93]

Alcohol

The putative relationship between alcohol and breast cancer which has emerged from several research studies may yet be recognized as the nadir of epidemiological achievement in the study of this disease. Alcohol has become inextricably woven into the fabric of Western society, resulting in subtle alterations in the behaviour of apparently normal individuals. Both case-control and cohort studies, which are assumed to be water-tight epidemiological vehicles, may develop stress fractures when used to investigate alcohol consumption.

One major problem is the selection bias within control groups. Those case-control studies which have shown a positive association between alcohol intake and risk of breast cancer have used hospital controls.[94–96] In order to be eligible for the control group, patients had to be hospitalized for diseases unrelated to alcohol consumption. No such exclusion applied to the cancer cases. Thus the very design of these studies predisposed to an under-representation of alcohol consumption within the control group and therefore led to an apparent over-representation among the cases. Among those case-control studies that used population controls, almost all did not show any

increase in relative risk among women who drank alcohol.[97–102]

The only exception was the study conducted by Harvey.[103] This compared 1524 cases with 1896 controls who took part in the Breast Cancer Detection Demonstration Project (BCDDP). Although there was no increase in relative risk for drinkers compared with non-drinkers, there was an apparent increase in relative risk with increase in alcohol consumption. Risk appeared to be increased in those who drank only one glass of wine per day and was exacerbated by drinking before age 30. When type of drink was considered, increased risk was borne only by those who consumed beer and spirits and not by wine drinkers, a biologically unlikely phenomenon.

Cohort studies would appear to be a less biased technique for approaching this problem. Theoretically, the alcohol consumption of a cohort would be ascertained and then related to subsequent development of breast cancer. This presupposes complete follow-up of the cohort. In two of the major studies, both of which have shown significant associations, there were considerable losses from the original cohort.

Willet enrolled 121 700 female registered nurses and then received replies to subsequent mailed questionnaires from 98 462 (81 per cent).[104] The loss of one in five would be of little importance if studying a factor unrelated to behaviour, such as family history. However, when examining alcohol consumption, bias may be introduced since it is likely that there will be an over-representation of alcohol abusers among the non-responders. This may lead to a spurious over-representation of alcohol abusers in the women with cancer who cannot escape because of their nominal entrapment within cancer registries.

The First National Health and Nutrition Examination Survey (NHANES) also reported an increase in risk of breast cancer with increase in alcohol consumption.[105]

The original cohort contained over-representation of individuals at risk of malnutrition, such as the elderly and the poor. Thus the conclusions may not be applicable to normal populations. The NHANES study suggested a 50–100 per cent increase in risk after consumption of 5 g alcohol per day (approximately three drinks per week), a very low threshold, which should give rise to a much higher increase in relative risk than shown by other studies.

Hiatt recruited a cohort of 69 000 women from the Northern California Kaiser Permanent Health Program, between 1979 and 1984, and compared the alcohol consumption of the 303 women who had developed breast cancer by the end of 1984 with 10 per cent of the entire group.[106] Consumption was measured as number of drinks per day. The relative risk was 1.3 for those drinking less than one drink per day (compared with unity for non-drinkers) and rose to 3.6 for those drinking more than six drinks per day.

The natural development of breast cancer probably takes place over a time-scale of 10–15 years, but the alcohol data were derived from only the latter 1–4 years of that time. It is tempting to conclude that alcohol consumption is an epiphenomenon such as a stress indicator. Threatening life events may be associated with excess alcohol consumption and may also act to promote the growth of cancer cells, possibly via elevation of prolactin. This might be amplified by the hyperprolactinaemia induced by alcohol.

Although carcinogenic properties have been ascribed to ethyl alcohol, the very weak association of alcohol and risk is more likely to be due to promotion rather than induction.

It is sensible for women to keep their alcohol intake below 25 g per week in order to avoid both hepatic and cardiovascular disease. A reduction of intake to below 5 g per week, suggested by some of the studies, would lead to an increase in unhappiness and little, if any, effect on the incidence of breast cancer.

Smoking

More deaths from cancer are known to be due to smoking than to any other cause. Predominantly this has manifested in an ever-increasing epidemic of lung cancer. As if to search for a silver lining within this blue cloud, it has been suggested that smoking might protect against breast cancer.[107] There is evidence suggesting that smoking may exert an anti-oestrogenic effect. MacMahon reported that premenopausal smokers excreted one-third less E_1, E_2 and E_3 than non-smokers during the luteal phase of the menstrual cycle.[108] In postmenopausal smokers, Khaw found that plasma androgens (dehydroepiandrosterone sulphate and androstenedione) were significantly elevated, compared with non-smoking controls.[109] An additional protective effect would be predicted from the earlier menopause which has been consistently reported among smokers, of the order of 1.5 years earlier than that of non-smokers.[110,111]

Supporting the anti-oestrogenic role of smoking are the findings of increased risk of osteoporosis and decreased risk of endometrial cancer in smokers.[112,113] Thus the endocrinology of smoking would argue in favour of a protective effect. Fortunately, the epidemiology tends to prove otherwise.

Those case-control studies that have used hospital-derived controls are summarized in Table 1.5.[27,43,114–21] Of these, half reported a relative risk of less than one. All controls were in hospital for diseases unrelated to cigarette smoking which would immediately reduce the cigarette intake of that group. Despite this, five studies showed no change in relative risk for smokers versus non-smokers.

This bias can be overcome using population-derived controls, and as is shown in Table 1.6, almost all of these studies have found no reduction in risk for smokers.[120,122–7] The exception was the study of O'Connell, which reported a relative risk of 0.75 for smokers.[99]

Table 1.5 Case-control studies of smoking and breast cancer using hospital controls.

No. of cases	No. of controls	Relative risk	Reference
340	340	1.0	27
799	2470	1.1	43
213	648	0.9	114
536	1550	1.0	115
1167	2380	0.9	116
1432	2650	0.8	117
332	1353	0.8	118
1176	1176	0.8	119
188	186	1.0	120
2160	717	1.0	121

Table 1.6 Case-control studies of smoking and breast cancer using community controls.

No. of cases	No. of controls	Relative risk	Reference
278	520	1.2	122
1473	1839	0.99	123
173	246	1.0	120
123	369	1.4	124
1547	1930	1.1	125
276	1519	0.75	99
456	1693	1.4	126
451	451	1.3	127

The controls were significantly older than the cases, and a positive interaction was reported between menopausal status and smoking. Nevertheless, the relative risk appeared to be unaffected by these confounding variables.

The two most recent studies not only showed no protection, but also suggested an increased relative risk for premenopausal women who smoked.[126,127]

Hiatt and Fireman studied the relationship between smoking and breast cancer in a cohort of women in a prepaid health plan.[128] There was an earlier menopause among smokers, but the relative risk of breast cancer was 1.1. After adjusting for age at menopause the relative risk was 1.08. Thus this study supports the multitude of others which have found no protective effect of smoking.

No woman should be advised or encouraged to smoke in order to reduce the breast cancer risk. A woman with a high risk of familial breast cancer will only delude herself that she will be able to prevent this disease by smoking. The only likelihood is that one potentially curable cancer will be replaced by an incurable, small-cell lung cancer.

Radiation

As a consequence of both medical and military irradiation of women, substantial data are available to confirm that this induces breast cancers. Unlike the majority of epidemiological studies which have examined promotional (endocrine) factors, this work has yielded important information concerning early stages of mammary carcinogenesis.

Shore studied 606 women who had breast irradiation for acute postpartum mastitis between 1940 and 1955.[129] These were compared with non-irradiated controls, and the dosage to the breast was 0.5–10.6 Gy. The relative risk for breast cancer was 2.2 for the irradiated women. There was a linear increase in relative risk with increase in dosage up to 4 Gy and then an apparent fall. Risk was equal for those irradiated before or after age 30 and the mean interval between irradiation and diagnosis of breast cancer was 15 years. Prince and Hildreth re-examined these data and adjusted for possible confounding variables such as selection bias and differential detection/verification of breast malignancy in cases and controls.[130] After adjustment the relative risk was 2.0, which remained statistically significant.

Boice and Monson followed 1764 women with pulmonary tuberculosis of whom 1047 (59 per cent) had repeated fluoroscopic monitoring for pneumothorax therapy.[131] There were 41 breast cancers in the fluoroscoped group but only 23 would have been expected (relative risk = 1.8). This work has been recently updated, and as more breast cancers have developed so it has become apparent that the risk persists and is inversely related to age at exposure.[132] Thus early reproductive life was the most sensitive time for X-ray-induced carcinogenesis which was unaffected by whether the total dose was given as a single exposure or in fractionated amounts. The mean interval from exposure to diagnosis of breast cancer was 15 years.

Similar increases in risk and comparable latent intervals have been reported in patients with childhood cancers treated by irradiation.[133–5] Such cases received radiotherapy to the breasts in dosages in the range 3–15 Gy. Information was lacking as to the risks of lower radiation doses, but important data have been provided recently by Modan who carried out a follow-up study of 10 834 children who received scalp irradiation for ringworm.[136] These were treated between 1949 and 1959, in Israel, and were compared with a similar number of population controls and 5392 sibling controls. Retrospective calculation of dosimetry was performed using phantoms. The scalp dosage was 3.5 Gy and the dose to the breast was calculated as 16 mGy. Until 1981, among the irradiated group the relative risk for breast cancer was 0.97. Between 1982 and 1986 this rose to 2.1. The relative risks for different ages at the time of scalp irradiation

Table 1.7 Relative risk of breast cancer after low-dose irradiation.[136]

Age at irradiation	Relative risk
< 5 years	0.59
5–9	12.0
10–15	0.58

are given in Table 1.7. This shows that the increased risk was carried entirely by those aged 5–9 at the time of irradiation. Such an observation could have profound implications. If very low dosages of radiation affect the breast through a particular window at age 5–9, background irradiation might play an important role in the induction of breast cancers, particularly in young women.

Supportive data can be derived from follow-up of atomic bomb survivors from Hiroshima and Nagasaki. The Radiation Effect Research Foundation (RERF) has conducted an extended lifespan study of a sample of 63 300 women who were unlucky enough to be within 2.5 km of the hypocentres.[137] Of this group, 564 have developed breast cancer and 395 cases have been confirmed by a panel of pathologists. The relative risks of breast cancer in relation to age at the time of the bombing and calculated dosage of radiation are shown in Table 1.8. This shows a clear rise in risk with increasing dosage for the younger age group, 0–9 years. Similarly, significant increases were found among those aged up to 39 years. Dosages in the range 50–199 Gy may have been protective in women aged 40–50, as a result of ovarian suppression.

Table 1.8 Relative risks of breast cancer in atomic-bomb survivors in relation to age and radiation dose.[137]

Age at time of bomb	Exposure in Gy					
	0	1–9	10–49	50–99	100–199	200+
0–9	1.0	2.0	3.1	13.0	9.0	4.8
10–19	1.0	0.9	1.7	2.3	3.4	7.2
20–29	1.0	0.9	1.4	1.6	2.6	4.1
30–39	1.0	1.1	0.7	0.9	3.0	4.9
40–49	1.0	0.8	1.4	0.2	0.8	1.6
50+	1.0	1.0	1.1	0.5	3.5	1.5
All ages	1.0	1.0	1.3	1.4	2.7	4.5

When the histopathology of the cancer in the exposed group was compared with that of tumours from non-irradiated controls, no differences were found. Thus radiation-induced tumours are not a special subgroup. Is this because radiation is responsible in part for the induction of the majority of breast cancers? Radiation-induced mammary tumours may be more than a model for breast cancer; they may hold the key to the DNA damage responsible for the disease.

Genetics

In 1926, Lane-Claypon conducted a case-control study and demonstrated that sisters and daughters of women with breast cancer had a three-fold increase in risk of dying from the disease.[138] Familial aggregation is well recognized, but this is not necessarily the same as an inherited predisposition for breast cancer. Since the disease behaves in a heterogeneous manner it is unlikely that the same genetic abnormality would be found in every case.

Anderson analysed family history of breast cancer and found an overall 2–3-fold increase in risk for first-degree relatives of cases.[139] This was present only in those with relatives who developed the disease whilst premenopausal. If the disease was bilateral, the relative risk was 5, and this rose to 9 if the breast cancer was not only bilateral but also developed premenopausally.

The risk of breast cancer in relatives of young women with the disease was examined in relatives of a series of 1137 patients, and 1001 population-derived controls.[140] For individuals whose sister had breast cancer the relative risk was 2.2, rising to 3.2 for mothers of cases. Women with both mothers and sisters with breast cancer had a ten-fold increase leading to a 50 per cent risk of development of the disease by age 65.

It has been suggested that at least three categories of familial breast cancer can be identified.[141] The first type comprises women with premenopausal disease, sometimes associated with ovarian cancer. The second group have a higher lifetime risk, unrelated to the menopause, and the third category have other associated malignancies such as brain tumours and sarcomas.

Based on work with the rare childhood tumour retinoblastoma, in which just under half have a germline mutation, Knudson proposed a two-stage developmental theory.[142] In hereditary cases because of a pre-existing mutation, only one event was necessary for malignant expression, but in non-hereditary cases, two events were necessary. Supportive evidence for this theory has been provided by Bodmer, who localized the gene for familial polyposis (which carries a high risk of development of cancer) to chromosome 5, and also reported the loss of this allele in sporadic cases of colonic carcinoma.[143,144]

Such a specific allele loss has not been found in patients with breast cancer. Ali extracted tumour DNA from 56 patients and found deletions from chromosome 11 sequences in 11 patients.[145] Lundberg studied both normal lymphocytes and tumour tissue and found loss of alleles on chromosome 13 in four patients.[146] Mackay reported that the highest rate of allele loss was on chromosome 22.[147] These findings would argue against a single breast-cancer susceptibility gene being responsible for all types of mammary malignancy.

Benign breast disease

The term 'benign breast disease' has been partly responsible for the protracted arguments which have shed little light on the relationship between fibrocystic change and breast cancer. As a result of haphazard clinical and pathological classifications, assertions were abundant but useful evidence was scarce. Unfortunately, matters were compounded by a lack of communication between diagnosticians (both radiologists and pathologists) and clinicians (almost invariably surgeons). This chaos has now been resolved, largely as a result of histologically controlled long-term follow-up studies.

Webber and Boyd critically analysed 36 cohort studied published before 1984, which had examined benign breast disease and subsequent risk of breast cancer.[148] They set standards for classification, follow-up and analysis of data. As intrinsic to classification, they required histological verification, definition of terms, observer variation and avoidance of bias. Follow-up criteria included duration, loss of cases and histological confirmation of malignancy. For analysis, requirements included numbers of observed and expected cases, calculation of relative risk, statistical methods, histological subtyping and consideration of other risk factors.

There were 22 studies which showed an increase in risk, 3 equivocal results and 11 which found no increase in risk. All the latter group were found to be lacking in terms of classification, follow-up and analysis. More criteria were met by the studies showing a risk and it was concluded that the positive association between benign breast disease and malignancy was real.

Much of the information concerning histological subtypes of benign breast disease and cancer risk has been provided by Page, who has extensively reviewed histological specimens from patients for whom long-term follow-up was available.[149] Page used the following histological categories of benign breast disease:

● Cyst

● Duct ectasia

- Sclerosing adenosis
- Fibroadenoma
- Apocrine change
- Papillary apocrine change
- Ductal hyperplasia
- Papillary epithelial hyperplasia
- Apocrine-like ductal hyperplasia
- Ductal hyperplasia with atypia
- Atypical ductal hyperplasia

Benign biopsies were reviewed from 1600 women, 94 per cent of whom had been followed for a minimum of 15 years. During this time 31 had developed breast cancer. Analysis showed that risk was carried only by those in whom the original biopsy showed evidence of proliferation. The relative risks are shown in Table 1.9. The highest relative risk was among women aged less than 45 years with atypical ductal hyperplasia.

However, this appeared to be the only histological risk factor in this age group.

Subsequent work by Page suggested that atypical ductal hyperplasia carried a 4–5-fold increase in risk of malignancy.[150] A doubling of breast cancer risk was seen in those who had a hyperplastic lesion and a first-degree family history of breast cancer. Confirmation of the risk of both hyperplasia and atypia has also been provided by the work of Kodlin[151] and Hutchinson.[152]

These studies have shown that there is a real risk of subsequent breast cancer in women who have had a benign breast biopsy but that the few at risk can be identified because of the presence of hyperplasia and atypia. Women who do not display these histological changes can be fully reassured and require no closer follow up than their non-biopsied neighbours. Those at risk because of histological changes, with or without a first-degree family history, may be suitable candidates for trials of systemic agents for the possible prevention of breast cancer.

Table 1.9 Relative risk of breast cancer in subtypes of benign breast disease

Subtype	Relative risk 31–45 years	>45 years
Atypical lobular hyperplasia	6.1	3.2
Ductal hyperplasia	1.1	2.7
Papillary apocrine change	1.0	2.7
Apocrine-like ductal hyperplasia	0.9	2.1

Cell biology

In order to compare the growth characteristics of normal mammary epithelium and malignant cells, cell culture would appear to be the ideal technique. In reality this aim has not yet been achieved and one of the major stumbling blocks has been the lack of methods for the characterization of cells in vitro. Ostensibly normal breast epithelial cells can be obtained from milk, reduction mammoplasty specimens and from biopsies from patients with fibroadenomas or fibrocystic disease. In the case of reduction mammoplasty material, organoids—that is, terminal ductolobular units—may be derived by collagenase digestion and culture on plastic dishes of floating collagen gels. Epithelium can be directly cultured from milk, once foam cells have been removed by allowing them to adhere to glass. Epithelium can be extruded from biopsy material by scraping (spillage technique).

None of these methods yields a homogeneous cell population and there may be contamination with fibroblasts, foam cells and myoepithelium. The latter may grow well in culture and, since they have epithelial morphology, can be mistaken for luminal epithelial cells which are the precursors of malignant cells. Comparison of growth characteristics of myoepithelial and malignant cells may lead to the observation of spurious differences that will not prove to have clinical usefulness. The detection of different cell lineages among morphologically indistinguishable cells has been enhanced greatly by the development of monoclonal antibody markers.[153,154]

The difficulties of culturing normal human mammary epithelium are as nothing compared with the problems of growing malignant cells. The growth and metastasis of breast-cancer cells can be unstoppable in vivo and yet these same cells are refractory to almost all attempts to culture them in vitro. Most laboratories that set out to culture human breast-cancer cells have found the task insurmountable and in order to maintain scientific output have reverted to the study of established cell lines or, worse still, rodent model systems.

Established human breast-cancer cell lines, of which MCF-7 is the best known, do provide an opportunity to work with large numbers of cells that were originally derived from a metastatic breast cancer.[155] However, it has to be appreciated that almost all the established lines were derived from malignant pleural effusions, which selects for particular variants able to grow in vivo in suspension culture. Long-term culture in vitro may also lead to selection of a phenotype which may be unrepresentative of cells in the primary tumour, even if oestrogen sensitivity is maintained. Long-term culture may

also lead to contamination with mycoplasma or cross-contamination from other cell lines, such as happened when what were thought to be human breast-cancer cells proved to be HeLa.[156]

For all these reasons, the results derived from cell culture of both benign and malignant breast epithelium have to be viewed with some caution. Nevertheless, certain tentative conclusions can be drawn. Experiments have shown the dependence of normal epithelium on stromal influences. Thus the growth of human mammary epithelium (HumE) can be stimulated by the presence of fibroblast feeder cells, or cell-free conditioned medium from a variety of sources.[157]

Although the primary alteration in malignancy is probably nuclear, the manifestations of cancer arise largely from cell-surface changes. One aspect of this is junctional intercellular communication. It was found that there was selectivity in communication among breast cells. Thus although both HumE and human mammary fibroblasts (HumF) were competent in communication, the cells did not communicate with one another as measured by ^{3}H-uridine transfer.[158] However, malignant mammary cells from both primary cultures and established lines showed loss of selectivity, either becoming unable to communicate directly or alternatively communicating promiscuously.[159]

The majority of studies of the growth of breast-cancer cells have used a combination of a synthetic medium with additional serum, either bovine or human. This can lead to problems because of the uncharacterized nature of factors in serum. Thus studies need to be carried out using defined medium, without serum. As an example, it has been shown that agents which elevate intracellular levels of cAMP lead to growth stimulation of normal HumE.[160] Studies using established lines cultured with serum suggested a similar effect with malignant cells.[161] However, when a series of established lines,

MCF-7, T47D and Cama-1, were grown in defined medium, there was consistent growth inhibition with several agents including cholera toxin, monobutyryl cAMP and prostaglandin E_2, all of which elevate intracellular cAMP.[93]

Lippman has conducted extensive studies of endocrine, autocrine and paracrine factors which influence the growth and function of human breast-cancer cells in culture, using a variety of established lines. In this model system, with cells in defined medium, physiological levels of oestradiol have been found to induce DNA synthesis and a plethora of enzyme activities associated with nucleic acid assembly in oestrogen-dependent lines such as MCF-7, T47D, CAMA-1 and ZR-75-1.[162] In addition, there was stimulation of differentiated functions including synthesis of progesterone-receptor protein and release of plasminogen activator.[163,164]

Cell lines possess a battery of receptors for growth factors such as insulin-like growth factor 1 (IGF-1), epidermal growth factor (EGF) and transforming growth factor alpha (TGFα), the latter two having a common receptor. Specific binding sites have also been found for the growth-inhibitory transforming growth factor beta (TGFβ). In culture, breast-cancer cells release these factors into the medium and this is stimulated in oestrogen-sensitive lines by the addition of E_2. Oestrogen-independent lines secrete more growth factors than their oestrogen-sensitive counterparts.

The administration of either tamoxifen or glucocorticoid leads to an inhibition of EGF and IGF-1 and an enhanced release of TGFβ. This would imply a range of anti-tumour activities for both tamoxifen and steroids, extending beyond effects mediated via oestrogen receptors. Thus this provides experimental backing for the observed benefit of tamoxifen in patients with oestrogen-receptor-negative tumours.

Ervin has recently reported the isolation of a growth-inhibitory polypeptide from conditioned medium derived from normal human mammary epithelial cells.[165] The inhibitor, dubbed mammastatin, differed from TGFβ and was present in normal cells, but in decreased amounts in cell lines, as measured by immunoperoxidase staining. Mammastatin appeared to be tissue-specific and did not affect the growth of non-mammary malignant cell lines.

Oncogenes

The term 'oncogene' was originally used to describe the sequence of retroviral DNA which was required to induce transformation of animal host cells.[166] Transformation was a state in which cells lost anchorage dependence, were enabled to grow in suspension culture and produced tumours in immune-suppressed rodents. This was deemed by many virologists to be synonymous with malignancy. Oncogene sequences were found to be a chimera of viral DNA and hijacked DNA from a prior host.[167]

Another property ascribed to oncogenes was that when transfected into mouse fibroblasts (3T3 cells), a transformed state was observed. This was of biological interest only until it was found the DNA extracted from human tumours could similarly transfect fibroblasts.[168]

When DNA from a human bladder cancer cell line was compared with that extracted from normal bladder epithelium it was found that the oncogene differed from a normal gene by substitution of one base-pair in the triplet code, a point mutation.[169] The homologous genes in normal cells were dubbed proto-oncogenes. It seemed as if the basis of DNA change in malignancy would be by point mutation. This proved to be an oversimplistic view.

Interest in oncogenes increased exponentially when it was shown that the protein encoded by the simian sarcoma virus oncogene (*v-sis*) bore a striking similarity to platelet-derived growth factor.[170] This factor is probably unrelated to human carcinomas, since epithelial cells have no PDGF receptor, although it could play a role in epithelial/stromal interaction. The subsequent demonstration that the protein product of *v-erbB* oncogene was closely homologous with epidermal growth factor receptor aroused great clinical excitement.[171] Human mammary epithelial cells growth is stimulated by EGF and the amount of the receptor in tumours had been shown to be positively associated with a poor prognosis.[172,173]

There are several different types of oncogene products, including nucleoproteins (*myc, fos*), nucleotide-binding proteins (ras), growth factors (*sis, int-2*) and protein kinases (*src, erbB1, erbB2*). In the latter group, the proteins encoded by the cellular oncogenes bind to peptide growth factors and activate protein kinases, whereas the products of the activated genes constitutively express the kinase.[174] This activation of oncogenes results either from overexpression or mutation.[175,176]

For the full expression of malignancy a concert of oncogenes is required in vitro. When transfected into normal cells, *myc* induces a state of immortality in culture, but the transformed cells do not display other features of malignancy unless *ras* gene is also inserted.[177]

More recent work has suggested that, rather than representing the primary alteration responsible for the malignant phenotype, the amplification of oncogene expression may be a reflection of the genetic instability of malignant cells.

Amplification of oncogene expression in human breast cancers has been examined by several groups using immunohistochemistry and the results are shown in Table 1.10.[178-82] A battery of oncogenes and proto-oncogenes has been studied and amplification of various oncogenes has been seen in 0–20 per cent of primary tumours. No consistent pattern of gene amplification was found although *c-erbB-2*, also known as *neu*, was the most

Table 1.10 Amplification of proto-oncogene/oncogene expression in breast carcinomas.

Reference	*myc*	*erbB-2*	*erbB-1*	*rasKi*	*RasHa*	*myb*	*Nmyc*	*sis*
178	8/57	9/60	0/35	1/50	0/65	1/59	0/31	0/34
179		4/20		6/20	13/20	5/20	4/20	
180		14/103						
181		17/195						
182		101/345						
TOTALS	8/57	145/723	0	7/70	13/85	6/79	4/51	0
%	14	20	10	15	8	8		

frequently overexpressed. No relationship was found between expression of *neu* and axillary-nodal status or steroid-receptor content.[181]

Hall studied 87 individuals with breast cancer in 12 extended families.[183] Leucocytes were isolated, transformed and cultured so the DNA could be extracted. After restriction enzyme digestion, DNA was hybridized with probes for *Hras, Kras2, Nras, myc, myh, erbA2, int2* and raf_1. None of the polymorphisms seen was found to be linked with breast cancer. It was concluded that these oncogenes were unrelated to susceptibility to breast cancer, but that the expression of the sequences might be linked to progression of metastasis. Thus it is likely that oncogene expression will prove to be a consequence of cancer rather than the primary abnormality responsible for the malignant genotype.

References

1 Moolgavkar SH, Stevens RG, Lee JAH, Effect of age on incidence of breast cancer, *J Natl Cancer Inst* (1979) **62**:493–501.

2 Doll R, An epidemiological perspective of the biology of cancer, *Cancer Res* (1978) **38**:3573–83.

3 Cairns, J, Mutation selection and the natural history of cancer, *Nature* (1975) **255**:197–200.

4 Armitage P, Doll R, The age distribution of cancer and a multi-stage theory of carcinogenesis, *Br J Cancer* (1954) **8**:1–2.

5 Moolgavkar SH, Day NE, Stevens RG, Two-stage model for carcinogenesis: epidemiology of breast cancer in females, *J Natl Cancer Inst* (1980) **65**:559–69.

6 Pike MC, Krailo MD, Henderson BE et al, Hormonal risk factors, breast tissue age and the age incidence of breast cancer, *Nature* (1983) **303**:767–70.

7 Ferguson DJP, Anderson TJ, Morphological evaluation of cell turnover in relation to the menstrual cycle in the resting human breast, *Br J Cancer* (1981) **44**:177–81.

8 Staszewski J, Age at menarche and breast cancer, *J Natl Cancer Inst* (1971) **47**:935–40.

9 Trichopoulos D, MacMahon B, Cole P, The menopause and breast cancer risk, *J Natl Cancer Inst* (1972) **48**:605–13.

10 MacMahon B, Feinleib M, Breast cancer in relation to nursing and menopausal history, *J Natl Cancer Inst* (1960) **24**:733–53.

11 Feinleib M, Breast cancer and artificial menopause: a cohort study, *J Natl Cancer Inst* (1968) **41**:315–29.

12 Longcope C, Pratt JH, Blood production rates of oestrogens in women with differing ratios of urinary oestrogen conjugates, *Steroids* (1977) **29**:483–92.

13 Bulbrook RD, Hayward JL, Spicer CC, Relation between urinary androgen and corticosteroid excretion and subsequent breast cancer, *Lancet* (1971) **ii**:395–7.

14 Adami HO et al, Serum concentrations of estrone, androstenedione, testosterone and sex-hormone binding globulin in postmenopausal women, *Ups J Med Sci* (1979) **84**:259–74.

15 Reed MJ, Cheng RW, Noel CT et al, Plasma levels of estrone, estrone sulphate and estradiol and the percentage of unbound estradiol in postmenopausal women with and without breast cancer, *Cancer Res* (1983) **43**:3940–3.

16 Henderson BE, Gerkin V, Rosario I et al, Elevated serum levels of estrogen and prolactin in daughters of patients with breast cancer, *N Engl J Med* (1975) **293**:790–5.

17 Boffard K, Clark GMG, Irvine JBD et al, Serum prolactin, androgens, oestradiol and progesterone in adolescent girls with or without a family history of breast cancer, *Eur J Cancer Clin Oncol* (1981) **17**:1071–7.

18 Moore JW, Hoare SA, Quinlan MK et al, Centrifugal ultrafiltration dialysis for non-protein-bound oestradiol in blood: import-

ance of the support, *J Steroid Biochem* (1987) **28**:677–8.

19 Siiteri PK, Hammond GL, Nisker JA, Increased availability of serum estrogens in breast cancer: a new hypothesis. In: Pike MC, Siiteri PK, Welsch CW, eds. *Hormones and Breast Cancer.* (Banbury Report 8, Cold Spring Harbor Laboratory: New York 1981) 87–101.

20 Moore JW, Clark GMG, Bulbrook RD et al, Serum concentrations of total and non-protein bound oestradiol in patients with breast cancer and normal controls, *Int J Cancer* (1982) **29**:17–21.

21 Langley MS, Hammond GL, Bardsley A et al, Serum steroid binding proteins and the bioavailability of estradiol in relation to breast diseases, *J Natl Cancer Inst* (1985) **75**:823–9.

22 Bruning PF, Hart AAM, Non-protein bound estradiol, sex hormone binding globulin, breast cancer and breast cancer risk. *Br J Cancer* (1985) **51**:479–81.

23 Moore JW, Hoare SA, Millis RR et al, Binding of oestradiol to blood proteins and the aetiology of breast cancer, *Int J Cancer* (1986) **38**:625–30.

24 Siiteri PK, Simberg N, Murai J, Estrogens and breast cancer, *Ann NY Acad Sci* (1984) **464**:100–5.

25 Pike MC, Henderson BE, Casagrande JT et al, Oral contraceptive use and early abortion risk factors for breast cancer in young women, *Br J Cancer* (1981) **43**:72–9.

26 Henderson BE, Powell D, Rosano I, An epidemiologic study of breast cancer, *J Natl Cancer Inst* (1974) **53**:609–14.

27 MacMahon B, Cole P, Lin TM et al, Age at first birth and breast cancer risk, *Bull WHO* (1970) **43**:209–21.

28 Trichopoulos D, Hsieh CC, McMahon B et al, Age at any birth and breast cancer risk, *Int J Cancer* (1983) **31**:701–4.

29 Hunt SC, Williams RR, Skolnick MH et al, Breast cancer and reproductive history from

geneological data, *J Natl Cancer Inst* (1980) **64**:1047–53.

30 Shiu RPC, Friesen HG, Mechanism of action of prolactin in the control of mammary gland function, *Ann Rev Physiol* (1980) **42**:83–96.

31 Holdaway IM, Friesen HG, Hormone binding by human mammary carcinoma, *Cancer Res* (1977) **37**:1946–9.

32 Boston Collaborative Drug Surveillance Program, Reserpine and breast cancer, *Lancet* (1974) **ii**:669–71.

33 Armstrong B, Skegg D, White G et al, Rauwolfia derivatives and breast cancer in hypertensive women, *Lancet* (1976) **ii**:8–12.

34 Ross RK, Paganini-Hill A, Krailo M et al, Effects of reserpine on prolactin levels and incidence of breast cancer in postmenopausal women, *Cancer Res* (1984) **44**:3106–8.

35 Stanford JL, Martin EJ, Brinton LA et al, Rauwolfia use and breast cancer: a case-control study, *J Natl Cancer Inst* (1986) **76**:817–22.

36 Malarkey WB, Schroeder LL, Stevens VL et al, Disordered nocturnal prolactin regulation in women with breast cancer, *Cancer Res* (1977) **37**:4650–4.

37 Wang DY, de Stavola BL, Bulbrook RD et al, The relationship between blood prolactin levels and risk of breast cancer in premenopausal women, *Eur J Cancer Clin Oncol* (1987) **23**:1541–4.

38 Wang DY, de Stavola BL, Bulbrook RD et al, The permanent effect of reproductive events on blood prolactin levels and its relation to breast cancer risk: a population study of postmenopausal women, *Eur J Cancer Clin Oncol* (1988) **24**:1225–31.

39 Bulbrook RD, Wang DY, Hayward JL, Plasma prolactin levels and age in a female population relating to breast cancer, *Int J Cancer* (1981) **28**:43–5.

40 Byers T, Graham S, Rzepka T et al, Lactation and breast cancer: evidence for a negative association in premenopausal women, *Am J Epidemiol* (1985) **121**:664–74.

41 Anderson JD, Breast feeding and breast cancer, *S Afr Med J* (1975) **49**:479–82.

42 Lubin JH, Buras PE, Blot WJ et al, Risk factors for breast cancer in women in northern Alberta, Canada, as related to age at diagnosis, *J Natl Cancer Inst* (1982) **68**:211–17.

43 Valoaras VG, MacMahon B, Trichopoulos P et al, Lactation and reproductive histories of breast cancer patients in greater Athens, *Int J Cancer* (1969) **4**:350–63.

44 Ravnihar B, MacMahon B, Lindtner J, Epidemiologic features of breast cancer in Slovenia 1965–1967, *Eur J Cancer* (1971) **7**:295–306.

45 McTiernan A, Thomas DB, Evidence for a protective effect of lactation on risk of breast cancer in young women, *Am J Epidemiol* (1986) **124**:353–8.

46 De Waard F, Breast cancer incidence and nutritional status with particular reference to body weight and height, *Cancer Res* (1975) **35**:3351–6.

47 Lew EA, Garfinkel L, Variations in mortality by weight among 750,000 men and women, *J Chron Dis* (1979) **32**:563–76.

48 Tornberg SA, Holm LE, Carstensen JM, Breast cancer risk in relation to serum cholesterol serum beta-lipoprotein, height, weight and blood pressure, *Acta Oncologica* (1988) **27**:31–7.

49 Rudling MJ, Stahle L, Peterson CO et al, Content of low density lipoprotein receptors in breast cancer tissue related to survival of patients, *Br Med J* (1986) **292**:580–3.

50 Lea AJ, Dietary factors associated with death rates from certain neoplasms in man, *Lancet* (1966) **ii**:332–3.

51 Armstrong B, Doll R, Environmental factors and cancer incidence and mortality in different countries with particular reference to dietary practices, *Int J Cancer* (1975) **15**:617–31.

52 Goodwin PJ, Boyd NF, Critical appraisal of the evidence that dietary fat intake is related to breast cancer risk in humans, *J Natl Cancer Inst* (1987) **79**:473–85.

53 Willett WC, Stampfer MJ, Colditz GA et al, Dietary fat and breast cancer, *N Engl J Med* (1987) **316**:22–6.

54 Hirayama T, Epidemiology of breast cancer with special reference to diet, *Prev Med* (1978) **7**:173–95.

55 Hirayama T, Diet and cancer, *Nutr Cancer* (1979) **1**:67–81.

56 Phillips RL, Snowdon DA, Association of meat and coffee use with cancers of the large bowel, breast and prostate among Seventh-Day Adventists: preliminary results, *Cancer Res* (1983) **43**:2403–8.

57 Phillips RL, Role of life style and dietary habits in risk of cancer among Seventh-Day Adventists, *Cancer Res* (1975) **35**:3513–27.

58 Nomura A, Henderson BE, Lee J, Breast cancer and diet among the Japanese in Hawaii, *Am J Clin Nutr* (1978) **31**:2020–5.

59 Miller AB, Kelly A, Choi NW et al, A study of diet and breast cancer, *Am J Epidemiol* (1978) **107**:499–509.

60 Lubin JH, Burns PE, Blot WJ et al, Dietary factors and breast cancer risk, *Int J Cancer* (1981) **28**:685–9.

61 Graham S, Marshall J, Mettlin C et al, Diet in the epidemiology of breast cancer, *Am J Epidemiol* (1982) **116**:68–75.

62 Sarin R, Tandon RK, Paul S et al, Diet, body fat and plasma lipids in breast cancer, *Indian J Med Res* (1985) **81**:493–8.

63 Hislop TG, Coldman AJ, Elwood JM et al, Childhood and recent eating patterns and risk of breast cancer, *Cancer Detect Prev* (1986) **9**:47–58.

64 Katsouyanni K, Trichopoulos D, Boyle P et al, Diet and breast cancer: a case control study in Greece, *Int J Cancer* (1986) **38**:815–20.

65 Kolonel LN, Nomura AM, Hinds MW et al, Role of diet in cancer incidence in Hawaii, *Cancer Res* (1983) **43**:2397–402.

66 Talamani R, La Vecchia C, De Carli A et al, Social factors, diet and breast cancer in a

northern Italian population, *Br J Cancer* (1984) **49**:723–9.

67 Zelma B, The role of skeletal dietary elements in breast cancer among native and migrant populations in Poland, *Nutr Cancer* (1984) **6**:187–95.

68 Nomura AM, Hirohata T, Kolonel LN et al, Breast cancer in caucasian and Japanese women in Hawaii, *Natl Cancer Inst Monogr* (1985) **69**:187–90.

69 Hirohata T, Shigematsu T, Nomura AM et al, Occurrence of breast cancer in relation to diet and reproductive history. A case control study from Fukuoka, Japan, *Natl Cancer Inst Monogr* (1985) **69**:187–90.

70 Lubin F, Wax Y, Modan, B, Role of fat, animal protein, and dietary fiber in breast cancer etiology: a case control study, *J Natl Cancer Inst* (1986) **77**:605–12.

71 Gray GE, Pike MC, Henderson BE, Breast cancer incidence and mortality rates in different countries in relation to known risk factors and dietary practices, *Br J Cancer* (1979) **39**:1–7.

72 Buell P, Changing incidence of breast cancer in Japanese-American women, *J Natl Cancer Inst* (1973) **51**:1479–83.

73 Staszewski J, Haenszel W, Cancer mortality among the Polish-born in the United States, *J Natl Cancer Inst* (1965) **35**:291–7.

74 Adelstein AM, Staszewski J, Muir CS, Cancer mortality in 1970–1972 among Polish-born migrants to England and Wales, *Br J Cancer* (1979) **40**:464–75.

75 Hill P, Garbaczewski L, Helman P et al, Diet lifestyle and menstrual activity, *Am J Clin Nutr* (1980) **33**:1192–8.

76 Gray GE, Pike MC, Hirayama T et al, Diet and hormone profiles in teenage girls in four countries at different risk of breast cancer, *Prev Med* (1982) **11**:108–13.

77 Gray GE, Williams P, Gerkins V et al, Diet and hormone levels in Seventh-Day Adventist teenage girls, *Prev Med* (1982) **11**:103–7.

78 Armstrong BK, Brown JB, Clark HT et al, Diet and reproductive hormones: a study of vegetarian and non-vegetarian women, *J Natl Cancer Inst* (1981) **67**:761–7.

79 McMahon B, Cole P, Brown JB et al, Oestrogen profiles of Asian and North American women, *Lancet* (1971) **ii**:900–2.

80 Goldin BR, Adlercreutz H, Gorbach SL et al, Estrogen excretion patterns and plasma levels in vegetarian and omnivorous women, *N Engl J Med* (1982) **30**:1542–7.

81 Schultz TD, Leklem JE, Nutrient intake and hormonal status of premenopausal vegetarian Seventh-Day Adventists and premenopausal non-vegetarians, *Nutr Cancer* (1982) **4**:247–59.

82 Fentiman IS, Caleffi M, Wang DY et al, Diurnal variations in prolactin and growth hormone levels in normal premenopausal vegetarians and omnivorous women, *Nutr Cancer* (1986) **8**:239–45.

83 Fentiman IS, Caleffi M, Wang DY et al, The binding of blood-borne oestrogens in normal vegetarian and omnivorous women and the risks of breast cancer, *Nutr Cancer* (1988) **11**:101–6.

84 Mills PK, Annegers JF, Phillips RC, Animal product consumption and subsequent fatal breast cancer risk among Seventh-Day Adventists, *Am J Epidemiol* (1988) **127**:440–53.

85 Minton JP, Wisenbaugh T, Matthews RH, Elevated cyclic AMP levels in human breast cancer tissue, *J Natl Cancer Inst* (1974) **53**:283–7.

86 Ritter EJ, Scott WJ, Wilson JG et al, Potentiative interactions between caffeine and various teratogenic agents, *Teratology* (1982) **25**:91–100.

87 Minton JP, Abou-Issa H, Foecking MK et al, Caffeine and unsaturated fat diet significantly promotes DMBA-induced breast cancer in rats, *Cancer* (1983) **51**:1249–53.

88 Minton JP, Foecking MK, Webster DJT et al, Caffeine, cyclic nucleotides and breast disease, *Surgery* (1979) **86**:105–9.

89 Lawson DH, Jick H, Rothman KJ, Coffee and tea consumption and breast disease, *Surgery* (1981) **90**:801–3.

90 Lubin F, Ron E, Wax Y et al, Coffee and methylxanthines and breast cancer: a case-control study, *J Natl Cancer Inst* (1985) **74**:569–73.

91 La Vecchia C, Talamini R, Decarli A et al, Coffee consumption and the risk of breast cancer, *Surgery* (1986) **100**:477–81.

92 Phelps H, Phelps CE, Caffeine ingestion and breast cancer. A negative correlation, *Cancer* (1988) **61**:1051–4.

93 Fentiman IS, Duhig T, Griffiths AB et al, Cyclic AMP inhibits the growth of human breast cancer cells in defined medium, *Mol Biol Med* (1984) **2**:81–8.

94 Rosenberg L, Slone D, Shapiro S et al, Breast cancer and alcoholic beverage consumption, *Lancet* (1982) **i**:267–71.

95 Le MG, Hill C, Kramar A et al, Alcoholic beverage consumption and breast cancer in a French case-control study, *Am J Epidemiol* (1984) **120**:350–7.

96 La Vecchia C, De Carli A, Franceschi S et al, Alcohol consumption and the risk of breast cancer in women, *J Natl Cancer Inst* (1985) **75**:61–5.

97 Paganini-Hill A, Ross RK, Breast cancer and alcohol consumption, *Lancet* (1983) **ii**:626–7.

98 Webster LA, Wingo PA, Lande PM et al, Alcohol consumption and risk of breast cancer, *Lancet* (1983) **ii**:724–6.

99 O'Connell DL, Hulka BS, Chambless LE et al, Cigarette smoking, alcohol consumption and breast cancer risk, *J Natl Cancer Inst* (1987) **78**:229–34.

100 Rohan TE, McMichael AJ, Alcohol consumption and risk of breast cancer, *Int J Cancer* (1988) **41**:695–9.

101 Adami H-O, Lund E, Bergstrom R et al, Cigarette smoking, alcohol consumption and risk of breast cancer in young women, *Br J Cancer* (1988) **58**:832–7.

102 Schatzkin A, Carter CL, Green SB et al, Is alcohol consumption related to breast cancer? Results from the Framingham Heart Study, *J Natl Cancer Inst* (1988) **81**:31–3.

103 Harvey EB, Schairer C, Brinton LA, Alcohol consumption and breast cancer, *J Natl Cancer Inst* (1987) **78**:657–61.

104 Willett WC, Stampfer MJ, Colditz GA et al, Moderate alcohol consumption and the risk of breast cancer, *N Engl J Med* (1987) **316**:1174–80.

105 Schatzkin A, Jones DY, Hoover RN et al, Alcohol consumption and breast cancer in the epidemiologic follow-up study of the First National Health and Nutrition Examination Survey, *N Engl J Med* (1987) **316**:1169–73.

106 Hiatt RA, Klatsky AL, Armstrong MA, Alcohol consumption and the risk of breast cancer in a prepaid health plan, *Cancer Res* (1988) **48**:2284–7.

107 Baron JA, Smoking and estrogen-related disease, *Am J Epidemiol* (1984) **119**:9–22.

108 MacMahon B, Trichopoulos D, Cole P et al, Cigarette smoking and urinary estrogens, *N Engl J Med* (1982) **307**:1062–5.

109 Khaw K-T, Tazuke S, Barrett-Connor E, Cigarette smoking and levels of adrenalandrogen in postmenopausal women, *N Engl J Med* (1988) **318**:1705–9.

110 Kaufman DW, Slone D, Rosenberg L et al, Cigarette smoking and age at natural menopause, *Am J Public Health* (1980) **70**:420–2.

111 Willett W, Stampfer MJ, Bain C et al, Cigarette smoking, relative weight and menopause, *Am J Epidemiol* (1983) **117**:651–8.

112 Daniell HW, Osteoporosis of the slender smoker, *Arch Intern Med* (1976) **136**:298–304.

113 Weiss NS, Farewell VT, Szekely DR et al, Oestrogens and endometrial cancer: effect of other risk factors on the association, *Maturitas* (1980) **2**:185–90.

114 Lin TM, Chen KP, MacMahon B, Epidemiologic characteristics of cancer of the breast in Taiwan, *Cancer* (1971) **27**:1497–504.

115 Mirra AP, Cole P, MacMahon B, Breast cancer in an area of high parity: Sao Paulo, Brazil, *Cancer Res* (1971) **31**:77–83.

116 Williams RR, Horm JW, Association of cancer sites with tobacco and alcohol consumption and socio-economic status of patients: interview study from the Third National Cancer Survey, *J Natl Cancer Inst* (1977) **58**:525–47.

117 Paffenbarger RS, Kampert JB, Chang H-G, Oral contraceptives and breast cancer risk, *INSERM* (1979) **83**:93–114.

118 Kelsey JL, Fischer DB, Holford DM et al, Breast cancer and oral contraceptive use: a case-control study, *J. Chronic Dis* (1983) **36**:639–46.

119 Vessey M, Baron J, Doll R et al, Oral contraceptives and breast cancer. Final report of an epidemiological study, *Br J Cancer* (1983) **47**:455–62.

120 Porter JB, Jick H, Breast cancer and cigarette smoking, *N Engl J Med* (1983) **309**:186.

121 Rosenberg L, Schwingl PJ, Kaufman DW et al, Breast cancer and cigarette smoking, *N Engl J Med* (1984) **310**:92–4.

122 Janerich DT, Polednak AP, Glebatis DM et al, Breast cancer and oral contraceptive use: a case-control study, *J Chronic Dis* (1983) **36**:639–46.

123 Centers for Disease Control, Long-term oral contraceptive use and the risk of breast cancer, *JAMA* (1983) **249**:1591–3.

124 Schecter MT, Miller AB, Howe GP, Cigarette smoking and breast cancer: a case-control study of screening program participants, *Am J Epidemiol* (1985) **121**:479–87.

125 Brinton LA, Schairer C, Stanford JL et al, Cigarette smoking and breast cancer, *Am J Epidemiol* (1986) **123**:614–22.

126 Brownson RC, Blackwell CW, Pearson DK et al, Risk of breast cancer in relation to cigarette smoking, *Arch Intern Med* (1988) **148**:140–4.

127 Rohan TE, Baron JA, Cigarette smoking and breast cancer, *Am J Epidemiol* (1989) **129**:36–47.

128 Hiatt RA, Fireman BH, Smoking, menopause and breast cancer, *J Natl Cancer Inst* (1986) **76**:833–8.

129 Shore RE, Hempelmann LH, Kowaluk E et al, Breast neoplasms in women treated with x-rays for acute post-partum mastitis, *J Natl Cancer Inst* (1977) **59**:813–22.

130 Prince MM, Hildreth NG, The influence of potential biases on the risk of breast tumors among women who received radiotherapy for acute post-partum mastitis, *J Chronic Dis* (1986) **39**:553–60.

131 Boice JD, Monson RR, Breast cancer in women after repeated fluoroscopic examinations of the chest, *J Natl Cancer Inst* (1977) **59**:823–32.

132 Hrubec Z, Boice JD, Monson RR et al, Breast cancer after multiple chest fluoroscopies: second follow-up of Massachusetts women with tuberculosis, *Cancer Res* (1989) **49**:229–34.

133 Li FP, Corkery J, Vawter G et al, Breast carcinoma after cancer therapy in childhood, *Cancer* (1983) **51**:521–3.

134 Meadows AT, Baum E, Fossati-Bellani F et al, Second malignant neoplasms in children: an update from the Late Effects Study Group, *J Clin Oncol* (1985) **3**:532–8.

135 Ivins JC, Taylor WF, Wold LE, Elective whole-lung irradiation in osteosarcoma treatment: appearance of bilateral breast cancer in the long-term survivors, *Skeletal Radiol* (1987) **16**:133–5.

136 Modan B, Chetrit A, Alfandary E et al, Increased risk of breast cancer after low-dose irradiation, *Lancet* (1989) **ii**:629–30.

137 Tokunaga M, Land CE, Yamamoto T et al, Breast cancer among atomic bomb survivors. In Boice JD, Fraumeni JF, eds. *Radiation carcinogenesis: epidemiology and biological significance.* (Raven Press: New York 1984) 45–56.

138 Lane-Claypon JE, A further report on cancer of the breasts, with special reference to its association antecedent conditions, *Reports of the Ministry of Health, London* (1926) No 32.

139 Anderson DE, A genetic study of human breast cancer, *J Natl Cancer Inst* (1972) **48**:1029–34.

140 Schwartz AG, King M-C, Belle SH et al, Risk of breast cancer to relatives of young breast cancer patients, *J Natl Cancer Inst* (1985) **75**:665–8.

141 Go RCP, King M-C, Bailey-Wilson J et al, Genetic epidemiology of breast cancer and associated cancers in high-risk families. 1. Segregation analysis, *J Natl Cancer Inst* (1983) **71**:455–61.

142 Knudson AG, Mutation and cancer: statistical study of retinoblastoma, *Proc Natl Acad Sci USA* (1971) **68**:820–3.

143 Bodmer WF, Bailey CJ, Bodmer J et al, Localisation of the gene for familial adenomatous polyposis on chromosome 5, *Nature* (1987) **328**:614–16.

144 Solomon E, Voss R, Hall V et al, Chromosome 5 allele loss in human colorectal carcinomas, *Nature* (1987) **328**:616–19.

145 Ali IV, Lidereau R, Theillet C et al, Reduction to homozygosity of genes on chromosome 11 in human breast neoplasia, *Science* (1987) **238**:185–8.

146 Lundberg C, Skoog L, Cavenee WK et al, Loss of heterozygosity in human ductal breast tumors indicates a recessive mutation on chromosome 13, *Proc Natl Scand Sci USA* (1987) **84**:2372–6.

147 Mackay J, Steel CM, Elder PA et al, Allele loss on short arm of chromosome 17 in breast cancers, *Lancet* (1988) **ii**:1384–5.

148 Webber W, Boyd N, A critique of the methodology of studies of benign breast disease and breast cancer risk, *J Natl Cancer Inst* (1986) **77**:397–404.

149 Page DL, Vander Zwaag R, Rogers LW, Relation between component parts of fibrocystic disease complex and breast cancer, *J Natl Cancer Inst* (1978) **61**:1055–63.

150 Page DL, Dupont WD, Rogers LW, Breast cancer risk of lobular-based hyperplasia: 'ductal' pattern lesions, *Cancer Detect Prev* (1986) **9**:441–8.

151 Kodlin D, Winger EE, Morgenstern NL et al, Chronic mastopathy and breast cancer. A follow up study, *Cancer* (1977) **39**:2603–7.

152 Hutchinson WB, Thomas DB, Hamlin WB et al, Risk of breast cancer in women with benign breast disease, *J Natl Cancer Inst* (1980) **65**:13–20.

153 Arklie J, Taylor-Papadimitriou J, Bodmer W et al, Differentiation antigens expressed by epithelial cells in the lactating breast are also detectable in breast cancers, *Int J Cancer* (1981) **28**:23–9.

154 Bartek J, Durban EM, Hallowes RC et al, A subclass of luminal epithelial cells in the human mammary gland, defined by antibodies to cytokeratins, *J Cell Sci* (1985) **75**:17–33.

155 Soule HD, Vasquez J, Long A et al, Human cell line from a breast carcinoma, *J Natl Cancer Inst* (1973) **51**:1409–15.

156 Nelson-Rees WA, Flander Meyer RR, Hawthorne PK, Distinctive banded chromosomes of human tumour cells lines, *Int J Cancer* (1975) **16**:74–82.

157 Taylor-Papadimitriou J, Shearer M, Stoker MGP, Growth requirements of human mammary epithelial cells in culture, *Int J Cancer* (1977) **20**:903–8.

158 Fentiman IS, Taylor-Papadimitriou J, Stoker M, Selective contact-dependent cell communication, *Nature* (1976) **264**:760–2.

159 Fentiman IS, Cell communication in breast cancer, *Ann R Coll Surg Engl* (1980) **62**:280–6.

160 Taylor-Papadimitriou J, Purkis P, Fentiman IS, Choleratoxin and analogues of cyclic AMP stimulations on the growth of cultured human mammary epithelial cells, *J Cell Physiol* (1980) **102**:317–21.

161 Sheffield LG, Welsch CW, Choleratoxin enhanced growth of human breast cancer cells in vitro and in vivo: interaction with estrogen, *Int J Cancer* (1985) **36**:479–83.

162 Lippman ME, Dickson RB, Bates S et al, Autocrine and paracrine growth regulation of human breast cancer, *Breast Cancer Res Treat* (1986) **7**:59–70.

163 Horwitz KB, Is a functional estrogen receptor always required for progesterone receptor induction in breast cancer? *J Steroid Biochem* (1981) **15**:209–17.

164 Huff KK, Lippman MF, Hormonal control of plasminogen activator secretion in 2R-75-1 human breast cancer cells in culture, *Endocrinology* (1984) **114**:1665–71.

165 Ervin PR, Kaminski MS, Cody RL et al, Production of mammastatin, a tissue-specific growth inhibitor, by normal human mammary cells, *Science* (1989) **244**:1585–7.

166 Bishop JM, Cellular oncogenes and retroviruses, *Ann Rev Biochem* (1983) **52**:301–54.

167 Stehelin D, Varmus HE, Bishop JM et al, DNA related to the transforming gene(s) of avian sarcoma viruses is present in normal avian DNA, *Nature* (1976) **260**:170–3.

168 Shih C, Padhy LC, Murray M et al, Transforming genes of carcinomas and neuroblastomas introduced into mouse fibroblasts, *Nature* (1981) **290**:261–4.

169 Reddy EP, Reynolds RK, Santos E, A point mutation is responsible for the acquisition of transforming properties by the T24 human bladder carcinoma oncogene, *Nature* (1982) **300**:149–52.

170 Waterfield MD, Scrace GJ, Whittle N et al, Platelet-derived growth factor is structurally related to the putative transforming protein p28[sis] of simian sarcoma virus, *Nature* (1983) **304**:35–9.

171 Downward J, Yarden Y, Mayes E et al, Close similarity of epidermal growth factor receptor and v-erbB oncogene protein sequences, *Nature* (1984) **307**:521–7.

172 Stoker MGP, Pigott D, Taylor-Papadimitriou J, Response to epidermal growth factors of cultured human mammary epithelial cells from benign tumours, *Nature* (1976) **264**:764–7.

173 Sainsbury JRC, Nicholson S, Angus B et al, Epidermal growth factor receptor status of histological sub-types of breast cancer, *Br J Cancer* (1988) **58**:458–60.

174 King CR, Giese NA, Robbins KC et al, In vitro mutation of the v-sis transforming gene defines functional domains of its growth factor-related product, *Proc Natl Acad Sci USA* (1987) **84**:2980–4.

175 Nowell PC, Final J, Dalla-Favera R et al, Association of amplified oncogene c-myc with an abnormally banded chromosome 8 in a human leukaemia cell line, *Nature* (1983) **300**:143–9.

176 Blair DG, Oskarsson M, Wood TG et al, Activation of the transforming potential of a normal cellular sequence: a molecular model for carcinogenesis, *Science* (1981) **212**:941–3.

177 Land H, Parada LF, Weinberg RA et al, Tumorigenic conversion of primary embryo fibroblasts requires at least two cooperating oncogenes, *Nature* (1983) **304**:596–602.

178 Masuda H, Battifora H, Yokota J et al, Specificity of proto-oncogene amplification in human malignant diseases, *Mol Biol Med* (1987) **4**:213–27.

179 Biunno I, Pozzi MR, Pierotti MA et al, Structure and expression of oncogenes in surgical specimens of human breast carcinomas, *Br J Cancer* (1988) **57**:464–8.

180 Gusterson BA, Machin LG, Gullick WJ et al, c-erbB-2 expression in benign and malignant breast disease, *Br J Cancer* (1988) **58**:453–7.

181 Barnes DM, Lammie GA, Millis RR et al, An immunohistochemical evaluation of c-erbB-2 expression in human breast carcinoma, *Br J Cancer* (1988) **58**:448–52.

182 Slamon DJ, Godolphin W, Jones LA et al, Studies of the Her-2/neu proto-oncogene in human breast and ovarian cancer, *Science* (1989) **244**:707–12.

183 Hall JM, Zuppan PJ, Anderson LA et al, Oncogenes and human breast cancer, *Am J Hum Genet* (1989) **44**:577–84.

CHAPTER 2

PRESENTING FEATURES OF BREAST CANCER

Between the idea
And the reality
Between the motion
And the act
Falls the Shadow.

TS Eliot

Nobody should be surprised that the disparate diseases which parade under the banner of breast cancer present in protean clinical disguises. However, most doctors still expect that patients with breast cancer will complain of a painless lump. The archetypal 53-year-old woman giving a 6-week history of a non-tender lump who is found to have a 2.5 cm mass may soon become an historical curiosity as screening becomes more widely available.

These straightforward cases are not difficult to diagnose. No great clinical skills or radiological expertise are required. The much more demanding problem is to sort out the few patients with early malignancy from the majority of women with breast symptoms. Towards the end of a long clinic spent reassuring worried women that their symptoms of tender lumpiness are not due to malignancy, it can be easy to miss subtle signs of early breast cancer.

The Yorkshire Breast Group reported the symptoms and signs in 1205 women presenting with early breast cancer between 1976 and 1981.[1] The features are summarized in Table 2.1. The commonest problem was a lump. On close questioning, one-third of patients stated that this was tender, either spontaneously or on palpation.

Table 2.1 Presentation of 1205 patients with operable breast cancer.[1]

Symptom	Percentage of patients
Lump	76
Swelling	8
Pain	5
Paget's disease	3
Nipple retraction	4
Nipple discharge	2
Skin puckering	1
Axillary lump	1

Clinical history

It is valuable to elicit a full history, not only as a step towards diagnosis, but also to begin to establish a relationship with the patient and assess the burden of anxiety that she may be carrying, possibly as the result of the death of a relative from cancer. In addition, the response of the patient to questioning can yield important clues as to her cognition as well as her capacity for denial. This helps with the assessment of likely duration of symptoms and provides an indication of how much the individual is likely to wish to know about her condition.

The commonest breast symptom in women consulting general practitioners is breast pain.[2] The majority of these patients are never referred to surgeons so that the most frequent symptom in patients attending breast clinics is a breast lump or lumpiness, the two not being mutually exclusive. Often the association of the lump with tenderness, changing cyclically in the premenopausal woman, will give clues as to its likely benign nature.

Details of any change in breast shape, nipple retraction or discharge will also be sought together with information about prior breast problems, general health, current medication and family history. It is customary in many clinics to ask a battery of epidemiological questions such as age at menarche, first baby, lactational history and length of pill usage, but these are of little immediate benefit to either clinician or patient. The present information recorded at Guy's Hospital Breast Unit from patients at their first attendance is shown in Figure 2.1.

The patient's menstrual history is of importance, together with knowledge of recent pregnancies. With increasing frequency, patients will be referred who will be taking or have taken hormone replacement therapy. This change in endocrine milieu is likely to lead to a rewriting of the natural history of both benign and malignant breast disease in middle-aged women. Thus cysts may become more common in women in their late fifties, more of whom may also develop breast cancer.

Clinical examination

After being asked to undress down to the waist, the patient is examined on a hinged couch with the head-end raised to 45 degrees. This is kinder to the patient who does not have the examiner towering over her and it provides a good position for breast examination. The couch can be laid flat if necessary for abdominal palpation. One of the most important requirements, apart from an atmosphere of apparent unhurried calm, is a good light. Tell-tale signs of malignancy may be missed in the semi-gloom which pervades many outpatient departments. Because of this it can happen that the pre-existing peau d'orange will become apparent only when the patient is re-examined under the lights of the operating theatre, at the time of surgery. This may lead to a change in treatment plan, possibly from breast conservation to mastectomy, or alternatively the decision that a mastectomy will not be technically possible so that radiotherapy becomes first-line treatment.

The patient is asked to identify the site of the symptom(s) and then the arms are lifted above the head, with the elbows flexed, to demonstrate whether skin tethering is present. For a few younger patients this will be linear tethering due to phlebitis in lateral

Figure 2.1   Baseline data sheet used for patients attending Breast Clinic at Guy's Hospital.

NAME: _____ Age: _____ DOB: _____

SYMPTOMS ON FIRST PRESENTATION

Date of onset: _____
Swelling: _____
Pain: _____
Nipple discharge: _____
Nipple inversion: _____
Other: _____
No symptoms: _____

PAST HISTORY

Breast disease and treatment: YES/NO (if yes, dictate notes to secretary)
Any other disease and treatment: YES/NO (if yes, dictate notes to secretary)

FAMILY HISTORY OF BREAST CANCER

Mother: YES/NO   If yes, age at diagnosis _____
Sister: YES/NO   If yes, age at diagnosis: _____
Daughter: YES/NO   If yes, age at diagnosis: _____
Maternal grandmother: YES/NO
Paternal grandmother: YES/NO

PREGNANCIES

Number of births/stillbirths: _____
Age of children: _____
Number of children breast fed for 2 weeks or more: _____
Number of miscarriages or terminations: _____
Reason for no children: CHOICE/INFERTILITY

MENSTRUAL HISTORY

Menarche age: _____
Date LMP: ___/___/___ (year only in case of postmenopausals)
Hysterectomy before menopause: YES/NO
Oöphorectomy before menopause: YES/NO
Contraceptive pill: Ever on   YES/NO   On now   YES/NO
                         On more or less than 6 months in all   MORE/LESS
Postmeno hormone replacement therapy: Ever on   YES/NO   On now   YES/NO
                                           Brand: _____
                                           Age therapy started: _____
                                           Age therapy stopped: _____

CONDITION ON FIRST ATTENDANCE

On examination: (dictate notes to secretary)
Clinical diagnosis (provisional):   _____

Primary treatment advised: Mammography and discharge
                           Mammography and follow-up
                           Follow-up
                           Trucut/Biopty-cut® and follow-up
                           TCA for minor op under LA
                           TCI Hedley Atkins Unit

Occupation: _____
Husband's Occupation: _____
Ethnic Origin: _____

thoracic veins (Mondor's syndrome)[3] which is of no consequence other than as a source of unnecessary worry. The skin is inspected for evidence of puckering, peau d'orange, erythema and ulceration after which the breasts are palpated, starting with the non-symptomatic side. After this the axillae are examined and the patient is then instructed to turn half on her side away from the examiner, with the arm rested above the head. In this way the lateral aspect of the breast can be more thoroughly checked, together with the axilla. The patient is then asked to turn half on her side towards the examiner so that the outer part of the other breast and axilla can be examined.

By this time the examiner will have a suspicion or certainty of the diagnosis and if this is probably malignant, will proceed to a more general examination including the neck, chest and abdomen. If the patient has mastalgia particular attention will be paid to the localization or otherwise of the pain, the presence of trigger points, bone tenderness or musculoskeletal conditions which may produce pain apparently arising from the breast. After this the examiner will usually have allotted the patient to one of four categories:

● Benign, lump-free
● Benign lump
● Malignant lump
● Possibly malignant

majority will require no treatment other than reassurance. A few will have severe pain, present for more than 6 months, which has had a damaging effect on their working, social and sexual lives. These women may ask for specific treatment for their mastalgia. It is customary to arrange bilateral mammography for those aged 35 or older to exclude non-palpable cancers. The patients should be asked to complete pain analogue cards for a 6-week run-in period, before starting treatment. At Guy's it has been the policy to review these cases at a special mastalgia clinic, set up to carry out trials of therapy. Despite the stringency of criteria for severity and chronicity of pain, only 60 per cent of those originally thought to need treatment will actually require therapy when returning 6 weeks later.[4] Such is the power of reassurance.

For women who are deemed to be benign, without a lump or severe mastalgia, it has been the policy to arrange X-ray mammography for those over 35, even though the diagnostic yield of subclinical cancer in those aged 35–40 is very low. It was the policy at Guy's to review all patients 6 weeks later, so that the premenopausal could be checked during a different phase of the menstrual cycle. This involved an unnecessary extra visit for most so that in the absence of any worrying features, and provided that the patient's anxiety has been assuaged, the majority can be reassured and told that they need return only if they have any new problems.

Benign, lump-free

These will form the majority of symptomatic cases. Many have lumpiness, that is a change of texture in one or several parts of the breasts, particularly the upper outer quadrants, but without any discrete lump or any other abnormal physical signs. Some of these patients will have cyclical mastalgia and the

Benign lump

For women under the age of 30 who are not lactating but have a discrete mobile mass, without evidence of inflammation, this is likely to be a fibroadenoma. Whenever possible this diagnosis should be confirmed cytologically. Provided that the lump is small (less than 2 cm) and not producing pain, it is not necessary to excise a fibroadenoma in a woman aged under 30 years. Patients can be reassured and told that it will be necessary to remove the lump if it enlarges or becomes symptomatic. Larger lumps or suddenly expanding lesions will require excision biopsy, irrespective of age. Despite efforts by surgeons to avoid operating on young women with proven fibroadenoma, approximately 50 per cent of patients will ask for removal of their breast lump.[4] One possible source of confusion which can have tragic consequences is unilateral breast enlargement in a pubertal girl. Asynchronous development is common and it is important that the breast bud is not mistaken for a fibroadenoma and excised, producing unilateral amazia. Patient observation should be the almost invariable rule for adolescent breast lumps.

Smaller, fibroadenotic nodules can give more problems. It is difficult to sample these by fine-needle aspiration and both ultrasound and X-ray mammography will be unhelpful. Although the majority of these lesions are usually observed, in women over the age of 35 consideration should be given to biopsy under local anaesthesia, since a few will prove to be small carcinomas.

Malignant lump

Signs of skin tethering, infiltration, peau d'orange or ulceration will strongly suggest the diagnosis, although all can be mimicked by non-malignant conditions. Hardness or irregularity of a lump, although likely to be due to cancer, can be signs of a cyst in the 40–50 age group, where diagnostic uncertainty can be at its greatest. When the diagnosis is borderline, needle aspiration is worthwhile since a cyst may feel like a cancer. If this is negative, it should be followed by fine-needle aspiration for cytology where this is available, or alternatively by either needle biopsy or arrangement for surgical excision.

It is at the time that the examiner becomes convinced that the lump is malignant that these thoughts should be shared with the patient. A direct approach, including the word 'cancer' will establish for the patient that she is being treated by someone who keeps her informed, and who is not fearful of the consequences of an unnamed disease. At this stage it is important to keep matters as simple as possible. Thus the patient should be told that it is likely that the lump is a cancer, many treatments are available to deal with this, and that the diagnosis of breast cancer is not a sentence of death. It may also be possible to speak in terms of whether breast conservation would be an appropriate option but it is important not to confuse the patient with too much detail. Extremely anxious patients remember only the headlines, not the small print. Later, when the patient has come to terms with the diagnosis and if possible when she is accompanied by her partner, it will be the right time to discuss detail and prognosis.

Possibly malignant

There will be some patients who have fibroadenosis but in whom the nodularity is very localized, and there may be genuine doubt as to the nature of this. If an ultrasound scanner is available in the clinic this may help to show the texture of the tissue to be similar to that of the rest of the breast. Additional confirmation may be obtained by normal cytology. A needle biopsy is of no value in the provenance of benignity. Thus a few of these women despite normal investigation, and possibly because of a family history, will undergo excision biopsy.

Nipple inversion without the presence of a mass in a 60-year-old woman is probably due to duct ectasia. This may be suggested radiographically but the duct thickening may lead to a rather indurated mass with some distortion of the surrounding breast, so that sometimes surgical confirmation will be required.

Nipple discharge

This may be of particular worry to patients, particularly when the discharge is blood-stained, although it is rare for nipple discharge in the absence of an associated lump to be due to serious underlying pathology. For diagnostic purposes, nipple discharge may be subdivided into bilateral/unilateral, single-duct/multiple-duct and blood-containing—Hb positive/Hb negative. An outline of likely causes is given in Table 2.2.

Bilateral milky discharge in non-lactating women (galactorrhoea) is usually an aberration of normal involution, or very rarely the result of hyperprolactinaemia from a pituitary adenoma or microadenoma. It is customary to check serum prolactin but rarely does this prove to be abnormal, particularly in women with normal menstrual cycles.

Duct ectasia may give rise to discharge which can be a variety of colours from pale straw through to blue/brown. Often this involves more than one duct and it is unusual for the discharge to contain haemoglobin on testing. It is the single-duct discharges which can pose a problem. Irrespective of the colour, if haemoglobin is present it has been the practice at Guy's to advise a microdochectomy. In the absence of any mammographic abnormality and without frank blood staining others have advised a policy of observation.[5]

Since microdochectomy not only confirms the histological nature of the underlying cause but also rids the patient of unpleasant symptoms this remains the management at Guy's.[6] A review of 270 women managed in this way who had a total of 292 microdochectomies revealed that 132 (45 per cent) had

Table 2.2 Causes of nipple discharge.

Bilateral	Unilateral		
	Multiple-duct	Single-duct	
Lactation			
Galactorrhoea			
Duct ectasia	Duct ectasia	Hb+	Hb−
		Duct ectasia	Duct ectasia
		Cystic disease	
		Intraduct papilloma	
		Carcinoma (intraduct)	
		Carcinoma (infiltrating)	

Table 2.3 Histopathology of 292 microdochectomy specimens.

Lesion	No of patients	%	Hb+	Hb−	Hb ?
Intraduct papilloma	132	45	107	19	6
Duct ectasia	94	32	67	25	2
Cystic disease	28	10	13	15	0
Carcinoma	16	5	16	0	0
No abnormality	22	8	12	10	0

intraduct papilloma, 94 (32 per cent) had duct ectasia change and 8 per cent had no specific changes, as shown in Table 2.3. Only 5 per cent of those patients had an underlying carcinoma. Of the 16 carcinomas, half were DCIS and the other half had infiltrating carcinoma with a DCIS component. All had haemoglobin-positive nipple discharges.

Mimicry by malignancy

Any breast symptom or sign can be mimicked by cancer. Care needs to be taken so that as few patients as possible fall through the diagnostic net and return some months later with an obvious and sometimes inoperable cancer which might have been treated curatively at the time of first presentation.

Pain mimicry

Cancer does not give rise to symptoms of cyclical mastalgia but a few patients, particularly those who are approaching the menopause, will have an impalpable infiltrating or non-infiltrating carcinoma which may be detectable radiographically. Malignancy can give rise to a very localized pain which the patient can pinpoint within the breast and which is not related to underlying bone, muscle or nerve. Even in the presence of normal mammograms these individuals do require close follow-up.

Lump mimicry

In younger women there is a natural tendency for clinicians to diagnose a fibroadenoma when the patient has a smooth mobile mass. However, a few of these will be small cancers so that unless there is unequivocal cytological proof of the lump being a fibroadenoma it should be excised, particularly in women aged over 30.

Discharge mimicry

If it is a rule to carry out microdochectomy when a discharge containing haemoglobin is found coming from a single duct, very few cancers will be missed. However, there will be a very small number of women with an intraduct carcinoma producing a haemoglobin-negative discharge. If the discharge is persistent and localized, ductography should be carried out and, if equivocal, a microdochectomy should be performed.

Cyst mimicry

Approximately 1 per cent of patients who present with a breast cyst prove to have an underlying carcinoma. Routine cytological examination of cyst fluid is a redundant pastime. Cancers will not be missed, provided that three conditions are met:

● The cyst fluid is not blood-stained
● After aspiration the cyst disappears
● At follow-up the cyst has not recurred

If any of these three conditions are not fulfilled the mass requires excision. These criteria were laid down before mammography became a routine examination and thus it could be questioned whether it is necessary to review all patients with cysts, provided the first two conditions are fulfilled and when mammography shows no evidence of malignancy.

A review was conducted of 400 patients seen at Guy's Hospital Breast Unit between

1978 and 1980.[7] At the first visit there was a residual mass after aspiration in five patients and one had a blood-stained discharge. Only two of these proved to have a carcinoma when biopsy was carried out. At the return visit, usually 6 weeks later, there was a mass at the site of the cyst aspiration in 64 cases (16 per cent). A new cyst in either another quadrant or the opposite breast was present in 22 (5 per cent). Of the recurrent lumps, complete aspiration was possible in 44 (11 per cent), but in 20 a residual mass was present after aspiration. All 20 had an excision biopsy and two proved to have infiltrating carcinomas. No cases of subclinical carcinoma were diagnosed mammographically.

Thus, although a few cases of carcinoma will be picked up as a result of follow-up of women with apparently completely aspirated cysts, the yield is low. Nevertheless, since 16 per cent will have a recurrent lump it is worthwhile reviewing these women in order to settle their anxiety.

References

1 The Yorkshire Breast Cancer Group, Symptoms and signs of operable breast cancer, *Br J Surg* (1983) **70**:350–3.

2 Nichols S, Waters WE, Wheeler MJ, Management of female breast disease by Southampton General Practitioners, *Br Med J* (1980) **281**:1450–3.

3 Mondor H, Tronculite sous-cutanee subaigue de la paroi thoracique antero-lateral, *Mem Acad Chir* (1939) **65**:1271.

4 Fentiman IS, Caleffi M, Brame K et al, Tamoxifen therapy for mastalgia: a double-blind controlled trial, *Lancet* (1986) **i**:287–8.

5 Locker AP, Galea MH, Ellis IO et al, Microdochectomy for single duct discharge from the nipple, *Br J Surg* (1988) **75**:700–701.

6 Chaudary MA, Millis RR, Davies GC et al, Nipple discharge. The diagnostic value of testing for occult blood, *Ann Surg* (1982) **196**:651–5.

7 Hamed H, Cody A, Chaudary MA et al, Follow-up of patients with aspirated breast cysts. Is it necessary? *Arch Surg* (1989) **124**:253–5.

CHAPTER 3

MAKING THE DIAGNOSIS

What hand and brain went ever paired,
What heart alike conceived and dared,
What act proved all its thought had been,
What will but felt the fleshly screen?

Robert Browning

A multitude of factors determine whether a woman who is being examined by a surgeon will have a biopsy performed. In part this will depend upon physical signs, such as a dominant lump or a blood-stained nipple discharge, but also upon the extent to which the patient's anxiety can be assuaged by non-invasive investigation and reassurance. The biopsy threshold of both patient and surgeon will probably be lowered if she has a first-degree relative with premenopausal breast cancer.

Clinical examination alone may be sufficient to convince the examiner that there is a problem which requires further investigation. Much more commonly, clinical examination may be either normal or indicate signs of nodularity that are consistent with fibroadenosis but also compatible (more rarely) with early breast cancer. Where no abnormality is present it is customary to carry out mammography in those women aged over 35. When signs are fairly localized, but non-specific in the form of nodularity or tenderness, it is likely that this will be augmented with cytology and ultrasound scanning, when available. The combination of clinical examination, fine-needle aspiration cytology and X-ray mammography has been dubbed triple assessment. It is probably the best presently available combination for the exclusion of malignancy in symptomatic women. Triple assessment alone may be of less value in the evaluation of patients with breast cancer.

Evaluation of diagnostic tests

In order to quantify the usefulness of diagnostic tests, a variety of standard measurements have been adopted and their definitions are as follows:

$$\text{Sensitivity} = \frac{TP}{TP + FN} \times 100$$

$$\text{Specificity} = \frac{TN}{TN + FP} \times 100$$

$$\text{Positive predictive value} = \frac{TP}{TP + FP} \times 100$$

$$\text{Negative predictive value} = \frac{TN}{TN + FN} \times 100$$

$$\text{Accuracy} = \frac{TP + TN}{TP + TN + FP + FN} \times 100$$

where TP = true positive, FP = false positive, TN = true negative and FN = false negative.

X-ray mammography

The technique of using X-rays to obtain images of the breast was first reported by Warren in 1930, after he had examined 100 women using sagittal views.[1] The radiological characteristics which he described were scarring and irregularity of surrounding tissue. Some of the cases were so advanced that direct pleural infiltration could be seen. With this simple technique a sensitivity of 75 per cent and a specificity of 100 per cent was obtained, although all tumours were clinically apparent.

In 1953 Raul Leborgne, in a monograph entitled *The Breast in Roentgen Diagnosis*, described the typical spiculated density of scirrhous (infiltrating ductal) carcinoma.[2] An example is shown in Figure 3.1. In addition he stressed the diagnostic value of calcifications on X-ray scans: 'Calcifications in carcinoma are generally tiny, dot-like or somewhat elongated, innumerable and irregularly grouped very close together in an area of the breast, resembling a powdering of fine grains of salt'. Figure 3.2 shows such an example. Leborgne found this pattern of microcalcification to be present in 30 per cent of breast cancers.

It was Egan who carried out the major developmental work on mammography.[3] In a series of 1000 cases, albeit containing some advanced breast cancers, a sensitivity of 97 per cent was reported suggesting that this

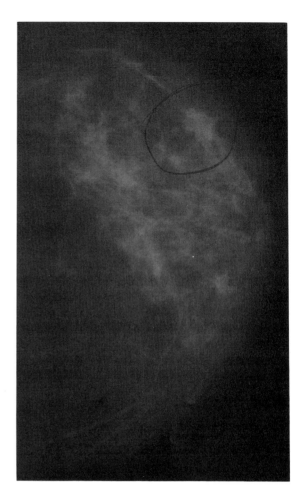

Figure 3.1 Cranio-caudal view of left breast showing spiculated density.

was a technique which was going to play a very important role in the evaluation of patients with breast lumps.

With only minor additions, these criteria of malignancy reported by the pioneers are

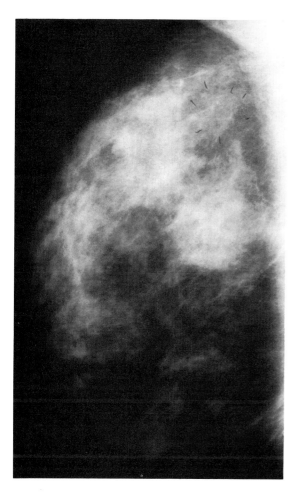

Table 3.1 Sensitivity of mammography in patients with palpable breast lumps.

No of patients	Sensitivity (%)	Reference
80	73	4
98	61	5
156	87	6
50*	42	7
520	79	8
154†	70	8
366‡	83	8
499	78	9
139†	56	9
360‡	87	9

* <45 years old.
† <50 years old.
‡ >51 years old.

Figure 3.2 Axillary view of right breast showing microcalcification.

those that the radiologists still seek. It should be noted that these changes arise from the infiltrative behaviour of ductal carcinoma together with the tendency of hypoxic intraductal carcinoma cells to undergo necrosis and subsequent calcification. These features may not be observed in patients with infiltrating lobular carcinoma where the indian-file pattern of diffuse invasion may not give rise to a clinically obvious lump, and may not manifest radiologically as either a spiculated mass or an area of microcalcification. It is because of such cases that the much less specific changes of asymmetry may have to be taken more seriously, in conjunction with an area of nodularity. Infiltrating lobular carcinoma can lead to palpable lesions being missed radiologically.

The sensitivity of mammography in patients with palpable lesions reported in major series is summarized in Table 3.2.[4-9] An average sensitivity of 70 per cent was obtained. For women under the age of 50 years the average sensitivity was 56 per cent but rose to 78 per cent for those aged over 51 years. Thus for patients in whom there is likely to be the greatest amount of clinical uncertainty the sensitivity of mammography is at its lowest for both exclusion and confirmation of malignancy. The inevitable sequel was the dictum that all women with palpable breast lumps should have them excised, irrespective of apparently benign or normal mammograms. This surgical reflex may have to be unlearned, as wider availability of cytopathological expertise enables more confident exclusion of malignancy using fine-needle aspiration.

Ultrasound

Real-time, hand-held ultrasonography is now used not only in radiology departments as an adjunct to X-ray mammography but also in the clinic to assist in the evaluation of breast lumps. It cannot be used as a replacement for mammography in attempted 'screening' of younger women as it does not detect the subtle changes of focal microcalcification or minor architectural distortion which can characterize early malignancy. Nevertheless, it is a good technique for distinguishing between solid and fluid-filled masses.

The criteria for the identification of breast abnormalities have been described by Kobayashi et al[10] and Jellins et al.[11] The ultrasonic characteristics of a cyst are the presence of smooth contour, a well-defined posterior wall and absent internal echoes other than anterior sound reverberations. This can enable a confident diagnosis to be made so that the cyst can be aspirated or observed. Fibroadenomas display a mass lesion with associated displacement of breast architecture, but well-defined internal echoes and borders. Unfortunately, carcinoma may display similar features or alternatively may not be imaged. This results in a reduction of specificity.

Table 3.2 Ultrasound in the diagnosis of palpable breast lumps.

No of patients	No of cancers	Sensitivity (%)	Specificity (%)	PPV (%)	NPV (%)	Reference
235	120	83	93	93	84	12
268	97	90	94	90	94	13
77	31	68	93	88	81	14
148	45	87	90	80	94	15
223	166	93	74	91	79	16
	—	—	—	—	—	
	AVERAGE	84	89	88	86	

PPV = Positive predictive value.
NPV = Negative predictive value.

A malignant lesion typically possesses an irregular border, mixed echogenic core and posterior attenuation. Representative reports of the use of ultrasound in evaluation of solid lumps are summarized in Table 3.2.[12–16] The overall sensitivity was 84 per cent. Thus approximately one in five cancers will not show characteristic ultrasonic features. The specificity was 89 per cent so that one in ten lesions which ultrasonically appear malignant will prove to be benign.

Not surprisingly, ultrasound is better at detecting larger tumours. Sickles et al studied 64 patients with histologically confirmed carcinoma and detected 37 (58 per cent) by ultrasound and 62 (97 per cent) on X-ray mammography.[17] Of the tumours measuring less than 1 cm in diameter, 92 per cent were detectable radiologically but only 8 per cent ultrasonically. Of the axillary node-negative cases only 48 per cent were identified by ultrasound compared with 95 per cent shown radiologically.

Fine-needle aspiration (FNA) cytology

The technique of taking specimens by FNA is deceptively simple. After the skin over the lump has been cleaned, a standard (20–23) gauge needle (0.6–0.9 mm), attached to a glass or plastic syringe, is pushed through the skin in a single firm movement. When the tip of the needle enters the suspect mass, a vacuum is created and the needle passed through the tumour eight to ten times. The vacuum is released, the needle withdrawn and firm pressure applied to the puncture site to minimize haematoma formation.

The needle is removed from the syringe into which air is drawn so that after replacement of the needle the cells within the syringe can be expelled onto a glass slide. The aspirate is gently smeared and the slide is either air-dried or fixed in alcohol. The cells are then stained by either the May-Grünwald-Giemsa method or the Papanicolaou technique.

It is customary for the cytopathologist to report the specimen as being in one of five categories: unsatisfactory (where an acellular aspirate has been obtained), benign, atypical, suspicious and definitely malignant. Optimal results depend upon three factors: the patient's tumour, the technique of the aspirator and the experience of the cytopathologist. Only the final two are susceptible to improvement by practice. Even when experienced clinicians work with trained cytologists, there will always be a hard core of cancers which will elude cytological diagnosis.

In a large series to evaluate FNA, unsatisfactory (acellular) smears were obtained from 9 per cent of cancers and 13 per cent of lumps which were significantly proven histologically to be benign.[18–25] Representative studies are summarized in Table 3.3 and indicate an overall sensitivity of 87 per cent.[18,19,21–8] False positive diagnoses occur but are rare so that the specificity is 99 per cent.

Thus a cytological report stating that malignant cells are present can be taken as almost certain confirmation that malignancy is present. However, this may not necessarily provide sufficient information upon which to plan treatment. In an elderly patient with a palpable lump, a spiculated mass on mammograms and positive cytology, it is very likely that the patient has an infiltrating carcinoma. However, a 50-year-old woman with an indefinite mass, microcalcification and positive cytology may have ductal carcinoma in situ (DCIS), the treatment of which will differ from that of a patient with an infiltrating carcinoma.

DCIS is a relatively rare condition so that, overall, progression to either a mastectomy or a breast-conserving treatment including axillary clearance will not represent overtreatment for too many patients. However,

Table 3.3 Evaluation of FNA cytology in diagnosis of breast lumps.

No of patients	No of cancers	Sensitivity (%)	Specificity (%)	PPV	NPV	Reference
1680	873	89	97	97	89	18
2772	1745	88	99	99	94	19
3545	368	90	98	85	99	26
1173	534	67	98	97	78	27
449	156	88	98	97	94	28
853	297	88	97	95	94	21
369	96	89	99	96	96	22
398	136	90	100	100	95	23
480	276	95	100	100	93	24
590	133	85	100	100	96	25
	AVERAGE	87	99	97	93	

PPV = Positive predictive value.
NPV = Negative predictive value.

for women under the age of 60 years the use of FNA diagnosis of malignancy will mean that up to 10 per cent of patients could have inappropriate treatment. This can be avoided by the use of needle biopsy rather than aspiration cytology.

Needle biopsy

The aim of needle biopsy is to achieve an outpatient histological diagnosis of breast cancer in a patient with a suspicious lump. It is not of value in confirmation of the benign nature of a breast lump or lumpiness since it cannot exclude small foci of malignancy. The technique is now in widespread use and most centres have shown consistent results for trucut biopsy, once the technique has been learnt and practised.

Trucut biopsy can be performed easily as an outpatient procedure and requires minimal special equipment. After the skin has been cleansed a small wheal is raised using 1 per cent lignocaine and then a small puncture is made with a size 15 scalpel blade. The closed needle is inserted through the puncture until the tip abuts against the tumour, and then the central trocar is advanced into the mass. This central trocar is then fixed and the outer cutting sheath is advanced, to take a core of tissue. With the trocar and sheath held in the closed position the two are withdrawn and gentle pressure is applied to the skin puncture.

Although the diagnosis will ultimately be made by the histopathologist, a rule of thumb as to the adequacy of the specimen is its behaviour when put into formol saline. Specimens that sink are likely to contain diagnostic material whereas those that float are fat and less likely to be positive histologically. Thus a floating specimen is an indication to carry out a second attempt at trucut biopsy.

A summary of series reporting results of trucut needle biopsy is given in Table 3.4[29-35] Overall, the sensitivity of the technique was found to be 82 per cent, which is slightly lower than that of FNA cytology (87 per cent). The specificity was 100 per cent. The only false-positive results are those reported by authors who combined trucut biopsy with frozen section of the resulting specimens. Gonzales et al reported eight suspicious needle biopsies, although none were actually labelled malignant by the pathologist.[32] Bradbeer had one false positive report.[33] Thus although the concept of trucut biopsy and frozen section is enticing because the patient may be given a histological diagnosis at the time that she is first seen in the clinic, it may cause a return to some of the problems implicit in the use of frozen sections.

Techniques which may appeal to the clinician may not necessarily be viewed in the same way by patients. For this reason, a postal questionnaire was sent to 58 patients diagnosed by trucut biopsy. Most of the patients (94 per cent) had no problem with the procedure and only 6 per cent found the biopsy to be very painful. Biopsy under local anaesthesia was preferred by 85 per cent. Almost all patients expressed a preference

Table 3.4 Studies evaluating trucut needle biopsy for confirmation of malignancy in breast lumps.

No of patients	No of cancers*	Sensitivity	Specificity	PPV	NPV	Reference
102	87 (85)	74	100	100	39	29
368	278 (76)	73	100	100	45	30
151	135 (89)	79	100	100	36	31
162	103 (64)	75	100	100	69	32
194	170 (88)	89	96	99	56	33
151	112 (74)	88	100	100	70	34
140	130 (93)	95	100	100	59	35
	AVERAGE	82	100	100	53	

*Percentage in parentheses.
PPV = Positive predictive value.
NPV = Negative predictive value.

for being at home rather than in hospital while waiting for a definite diagnosis.

One in five of these biopsies will be negative. Because of sampling problems it is essential that an excision biopsy be performed to exclude malignancy. Reasons for failure can be multiple, the first being inexperience of the operator. Smaller tumours are more difficult to biopsy and at Guy's approximately 50 per cent of those patients with tumours measuring less than 2 cm (clinically) were positive on trucut biopsy. The other major determinant of success is the texture of the tumour. Very soft lesions may give problems as may sclerotic lesions, into which the needle may not penetrate.

Antagonists of needle biopsy would argue that the delay between needle biopsy and definitive surgery might adversely affect survival as incision of the tumour and local release of tumour cells might expedite vascular invasion and metastasis. To examine this a study was performed to compare the outcome (as measured by freedom from relapse and overall survival) of 103 patients diagnosed by trucut and 189 by excision biopsy.[36] After 5 years of follow-up there was no significant difference for those whose original trucut biopsies were positive or false negative, compared with those who had excision biopsies. Thus trucut biopsy is a safe procedure. In addition, steroid-receptor measurements were not compromised in individuals whose tumours were originally sampled by trucut biopsy.

Comparison of trucut biopsy and fine-needle aspiration (FNA) cytology

Only one study has compared directly the results of trucut biopsy and FNA in a series of patients with breast lumps, all of which were excised so that definitive histology was available. This was carried out in Nottingham and 163 patients were studied, of whom 119 had cancers and 44 had benign lumps.[30] The sensitivity of trucut biopsy was 72 per cent and that of FNA 52 per cent. The specificity of trucut biopsy was 100 per cent but there were 5 false-positive diagnoses after FNA, leading to a specificity of 89 per cent.

In a smaller series, Shabot et al reported a specificity of 100 per cent for both techniques, but not all cases had trucut biopsy, FNA and excision biopsy.[37] The sensitivity was 92 per cent for FNA and 71 per cent for trucut biopsy, the former being higher than mean FNA sensitivity and the latter lower than trucut sensitivity reported in other series (Table 3.4).

Optimally, the two techniques should be used in a complementary manner, tailoring the test to the information that is being sought. Thus a young woman with a suspected fibroadenoma can have the diagnosis confirmed by FNA. A middle-aged woman with clinical fibroadenosis and mammographic asymmetry should have FNA cytology of the predominant area. A patient with a lump suspected to be malignant should have a trucut biopsy in order to obtain a tissue diagnosis and plan treatment. Confirmation of the presence of infiltration is necessary if the trucut biopsy shows the presence of DCIS, without infiltration. This is an indication for excision biopsy in order that the lump can be more thoroughly studied histologically.

Trucut biopsies, like ordinary surgical biopsies, may be used to obtain more than just histological information. Baildam et al studied 140 patients who had trucut biopsies to determine how many other data could be collected.[35] In 90 per cent of biopsies it was possible for the pathologist to type the tumour and carry out grading in 70 per cent. Steroid receptors were measured in 45 per

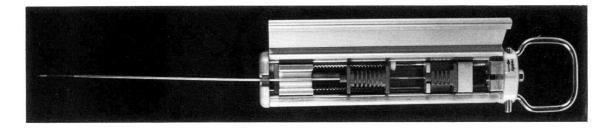

Figure 3.3   Bioptycut® needle biopsy system, open.

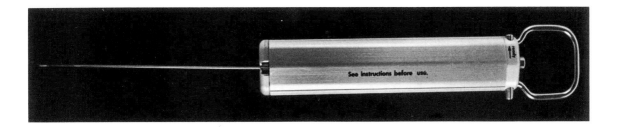

Figure 3.4   Bioptycut® needle biopsy system, closed.

cent and the distribution of positivity and negativity was similar to that in resected tumours. In a further 30 per cent it was possible to carry out DNA flow cytometry, the results of which were also similar to those in the ultimately resected cancers.

One of the major technical problems in needle biopsy is the need to fix the tumour and the central trocar whilst advancing the outer cutting sheath. Failure to do this results in either a very small specimen or one that has been so damaged that histological examination is difficult. Various techniques have been used to aid in needle biopsy.

One such device is the Bioptycut® system which has recently been used at Guy's. The spring-loaded, hand-held device is shown in Figures 3.3 and 3.4. So far, 120 biopsies have been performed with a sensitivity of 90 per cent and a specificity of 100 per cent. Because a fine needle is available, the technique can be performed without local anaesthetic which enables a tissue diagnosis to be made very simply, without interruption of clinic routine.

Excision biopsy

Despite the use of both FNA and trucut biopsy, there will still be some breast lumps whose nature is undetermined so that they are excised under either local or general anaesthesia.

Whenever possible, breast incisions should be based on Langer's lines or, for central small lesions, a circumareolar approach yields a cosmetically acceptable scar. However, the surgeon carrying out the biopsy must consider what the likely treatment will be for the patient if the lump proves to be a carcinoma. Thus if a patient has a 5 cm diameter mass in the upper outer quadrant, a circumferential incision may lead to major difficulties in planning skin flaps for a subsequent mastectomy. Thus an oblique excision, which can be incorporated into the resected specimen, is better.

Use of scissors rather than a knife to dissect out the lump leads to the removal of less surrounding normal tissue. If breast conservation is being considered, so should the use of a vacuum drain. Haematomas followed by radiotherapy can mar cosmetic outcome.

Frozen-section diagnosis

Use of frozen-section diagnosis followed by immediate mastectomy is a totally inappropriate method to diagnose and treat breast cancer. It had great appeal to those surgeons who were reluctant to use the word 'cancer' in their patients' hearing, and who did not possess the aptitude for discussion of options with their luckless patients.

Frozen-section diagnosis puts pressure upon the pathologist to make an almost instant diagnosis on a suboptimally prepared specimen. Mistakes are made. In a review of long-term survivors after mastectomy, re-evaluation of paraffin sections showed that three out of 230 (1 per cent) had benign lesions.[38] Worldwide, how many women have had unnecessary mastectomies because of misdiagnosis by frozen section?

Equally importantly, the 'smash and grab approach' to breast cancer surgery can be very harmful to the psyche of the patient. There is no evidence that a delay of up to one month between the time of biopsy and definitive treatment makes for any worsening of prognosis. It is important for the patient that she does have time to come to terms with the diagnosis of breast cancer and its implications and does not feel railroaded into making a decision which she subsequently regrets.

Proceeding immediately to definitive treatment, often mastectomy, will mean that a few patients with detectable metastases will have had inappropriately aggressive local therapy. Of course, there are a few who will not wish to discuss matters, are happy to leave the decision to the surgeon and are prepared to undergo full preoperative staging and then have a frozen-section diagnosis and immediate mastectomy. Such women are rare. Frozen-section diagnosis of breast cancer is best consigned to the dustbin of history, as a technique whose danger is now manifest.

Needle localization and excision of non-palpable breast lesions

With increasing frequency, surgeons are being sent women who are asymptomatic but who have had an abnormality detected on screening mammograms. Rapid, efficient and sensitive management of these worried women is required so that the majority can be reassured and the few with malignant lesions can have appropriate treatment.

The decision to localize and biopsy such lesions will depend upon close cooperation between surgeon, radiologist and pathologist. In recent series reporting results of localization the most common reason for biopsy was the presence of microcalcification (52 per cent).[39–43] The next most common indication was the presence of a mass (45 per cent), which was spiculated in 3 per cent and associated with microcalcification in 6 per cent. In 3 per cent of cases there was an increased density or distortion.

The distribution of microcalcification can be used to determine the likelihood of malignancy. Sigfusson et al divided mammograms with more than five focal microcalcifications into four risk groups, as shown in Table 3.5.[44] Those with round, cloudy or sedimented (tea-cup) calcifications were at very low risk. None was due to invasive cancer and only three cases of lobular carcinoma in situ (LCIS) were discovered, and these were incidental findings. The highest risk was borne by those with irregular microcalcification, distributed linearly and in branching patterns. Of these, 96 per cent had breast cancer. Those with slightly irregular microcalcification and a suggestion of linear orientation had an intermediate risk.

Abbes et al related the type of microcalcification on mammograms to the histological diagnosis in 112 cases.[45] Cancers were more commonly associated with more than 10

Table 3.5 Risk groups for malignancy based on type of microcalcification on mammograms.[44]

Risk	Calcification	Total*	Invasive carcinoma	Non-invasive carcinoma
None	Round, cloudy sedimented	65 (26)	–	3
Low	As above with some irregularity	95 (38)	7	11
Moderate	Irregular and linear	66 (26)	8	16
High	Irregular, linear, branching	26 (10)	15	10

*Percentage in parentheses.

Table 3.6 Histological outcome of biopsies for non-palpable, mammographically-detected lesions.

No of patients	Malignant	Infiltrating	DCIS	LCIS	Reference
203	70	30	30	10	44
557	175	116	45	14	39
162	50	21	22	7	46
653	147	59	65	23	41
179	41	32	9	–	40
112	56	29	27	–	45
678	78	53	20	5	43
2544	617	340 (55%)	218 (35%)	59 (10%)	

microcalcifications, resembling irregular salt grains and measuring between 0.1 and 0.5 mm. Heterogeneous microcalcification within ducts was also a frequent indicator of malignancy.

Once the decision has been made to excise a mammographic abnormality, approximately one-third of such cases will prove to have carcinoma. Table 3.6 gives the histological outcome after excision of non-palpable lesions detected mammographically.[39–41,43–6] Of the cancers, 55 per cent were infiltrating, DCIS was present in 35 per cent and LCIS in 10 per cent.

For the surgeon to excise the abnormality accurately, a localization technique is required. The particular methodology employed may be less important than the spirit with which the clinicians and diagnosticians

cooperate. Although a few surgeons use external skin markers or a system of segmentalization of the breast with removal of the suspected segment, most techniques involve needle localization. One approach has been for radiologists to inject 0.5 ml dye into the region of the lesion.

At present, most assessment teams use needle localization, with the insertion of a hooked needle into the site of the abnormality. The problem with these needles is that they can migrate—sometimes a great distance. Thus a marker which does not move from its site of placement is a great advantage. Dr John Reidy, Consultant Radiologist at Guy's Hospital, has designed a new needle which has proved to be very satisfactory in localization of mammographic lesions (Figure 3.5). It is thicker than most needles in

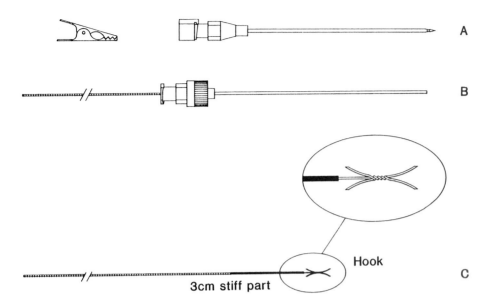

A

B

Hook

3cm stiff part

C

Figure 3.5 Diagram of Reidy needle.

use and has an x-shaped barb at the end. This not only fixes the tip but also makes palpation easier for the surgeon.

Radiological technique of marker placement

This is performed just prior to surgery, in the X-ray department. The breast is compressed with a transparent grid. When the lesion has been visualized a needle is inserted through the overlying perforation, under local anaesthetic. The site of skin entry is located at the shortest distance between the skin and the lesion. The direction of the needle is parallel to and never at right angles to the chest wall.

Once the lesion is apparently impaled the compression is released, a film taken at right angles and the tip of the needle adjusted until it abuts on the abnormality. After stabilization of the wire the needle is removed, so that the x-barb expands to fix the tip. Craniocaudal and lateral views are taken and the wire clamped at the skin puncture site (Figures 3.6 and 3.7).

Surgical technique

All biopsies after needle localization are performed under general anaesthesia. Skin-crease incisions are used and usually based around the site of needle puncture. A limited

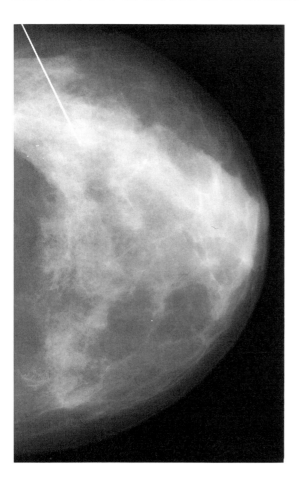

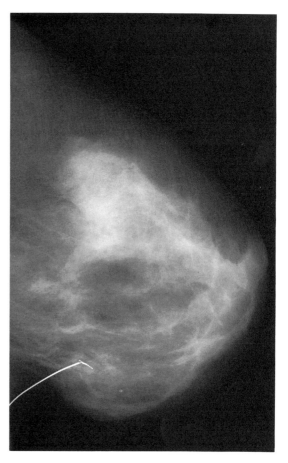

Figure 3.6   Cranio-caudal view showing Reidy needle inserted.

Figure 3.7   Medio-lateral view showing Reidy needle inserted.

excision is performed based on palpation of the needle tip and its relation to the lesion as preoperative marker mammograms. The biopsy with the wire in situ is then sent to the histopathology laboratory.

Histological technique

Specimen radiology is performed in the histopathology laboratory and the films immediately sent to the operating theatre so

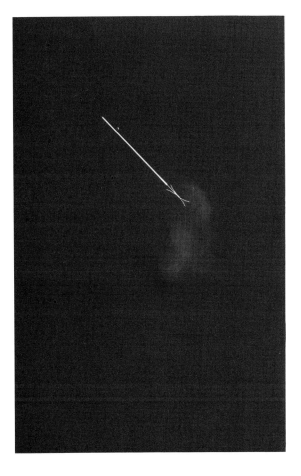

Figure 3.8   Radiograph of specimen showing presence of microcalcification.

mens are processed by paraffin section. Frozen section plays no role in the evaluation of impalpable lesions. So far the Reidy needle has been used for 50 biopsies and in every case the mammographic lesion was successfully excised. On two occasions, in patients with multiple abnormalities, it has been necessary to perform a second biopsy.

Stereotactic needle localization and cytology

Using a stereotactic system it is possible to insert a needle into the lesion and aspirate cells for cytological examination.[47,48] Azavedo et al recently reported on results of 2594 stereotactic fine-needle biopsies (SFNB) in 2594 patients, 567 of whom had an excision biopsy.[49] The sensitivity was 66 per cent and the specificity 90 per cent. Considering the cost of such equipment, which has an accuracy of only 72 per cent, this may not be the optimal way to make a diagnosis, particularly since a diagnosis of malignancy will not differentiate between in situ and invasive lesions.

Obviously, if SFNB can avoid unnecessary operations on patients with benign lesions this will be of greater benefit. However, if one in three cancers will not be correctly diagnosed, some patients and their doctors will question whether apparently benign lesions should be left unbiopsied.

that the surgeon can check that the suspect lesion of interest has been excised (Figure 3.8). The specimen is marked with Indian ink so that margins can be verified and then serially sliced and each slice X-rayed. Speci-

Staging investigations

Once the diagnosis of malignancy has been made, which particular preoperative staging investigations are necessary before proceeding to definitive therapy? In many centres it is customary to perform a full blood count, biochemical screen, chest X-ray, bilateral

Table 3.7 Value of preoperative staging tests in patients with breast cancer.[50]

Test	Sensitivity (%)	Specificity (%)	PPV (%)
Chest X-ray	31	99	44
Skeletal survey	35	99	32
Bone scan	48	95	15
Liver ultrasound	29	99	33
Liver scintigraphy	20	97	8

PPV = Positive predictive value.

mammography, liver ultrasound and isotopic bone scan. Are these investigations justified in patients with clinically localized breast cancers?

This question was studied prospectively by the Italian National Task Force for Breast Cancer (FONCaM)[50] The tests evaluated were chest X-ray, skeletal survey, bone scintigraphy, liver ultrasound and liver scintigraphy. A total of 3627 patients was studied, not all of whom were subjected to all the tests. The results are shown in Table 3.7, which indicates the low sensitivity (less than 50 per cent) for all the tests. When the analysis was restricted to those patients with Stages 1 and 2 disease the detection rate was 0.19 per cent for chest X-rays, 0.17 per cent for bone scans and there was an almost negligible detection rate for either liver ultrasound or scintigraphy.

Thus, unless patients are being entered into specific research protocols studying bone or liver metastases, preoperative bone and liver scans are a waste of both money and time in women with normal blood biochemistry. Apart from this, the only essential preoperative investigation in a patient with breast cancer is bilateral mammography in order to detect multifocal or bilateral breast carcinoma.

Steroid receptors

When considering the management of a patient with operable breast cancer, apart from information concerning the tumour type and grade and the quantitative extent of axillary nodal involvement, the question is often asked 'What is the receptor status?'. From being an assay which was only performed in research laboratories, it is now an investigation which can be carried out in any hospital laboratory because of the development of monoclonal antibody kits.

However, the commercially available kits are expensive and thus it is necessary to justify the diversion of resources to measurement of oestrogen-receptor (ER) and progesterone-receptor (PR) status. A recent review which addressed this question concluded that there was no value in the routine measurement of ER/PR.[51] The conclusion was based on several relevant observations. Originally, ER status was used in patients with advanced disease to determine likelihood of response to endocrine surgery such as oöphorectomy, adrenalectomy and hypophysectomy. The latter two procedures are now rarely used. Even oöphorectomy, which was the first-line endocrine therapy for premenopausal women, can be replaced by ovarian irradiation, tamoxifen[52,53] or LHRH agonists.[54] A trial of such agents would be justified even in patients with ER-negative tumours since one in ten would respond to these relatively non-toxic therapies.

In elderly patients with early breast cancer, tamoxifen is now being used as first-line treatment.[55] It is not necessary to know the receptor status since most of these women have ER-positive tumours and response is probably determined by factors other than ER positivity.[56]

For patients with axillary nodal involvement who have been given adjuvant tamoxifen, benefit is gained by those with both ER-positive and ER-negative tumours.[57,58] Thus receptor status does not determine suitability for adjuvant tamoxifen.

An experienced pathologist, who is used to grading infiltrating ductal carcinomas, can give information to the clinician concerning steroid sensitivity which is as accurate as that derived from steroid-receptor assays.[59] Patients with poorly differentiated (Grade III) tumours are unlikely to respond to endocrine therapy and tend to have short disease-free intervals. Medullary cancers, despite their relatively benign behaviour, tend to be ER-negative. Receptor-positive tumours display less stromal lymphoplasmacytic reaction and more stromal elastosis. Thus the combination of tumour type, grade and elastosis will predict for response to endocrine therapy.

Appropriate decisions on primary adjuvant and palliative treatment of breast cancer can be made based on histopathological data rather than ER status. Measurement of ER/PR should be restricted to research laboratories which are studying the biology of breast cancer and the interaction of steroid hormone receptors with other growth-factor receptors.

References

1 Warren SL, A roentgenologic study of the breast, *Am J Roentgenol Rad Ther* (1930) **24**:113–24.

2 Leborgne RA, *The breast in Roentgen diagnosis*, (Impresora Uraguaya: Montevideo 1953).

3 Egan RL, Experience with mammography in a tumour institute. Evaluation of 1000 studies, *Radiology* (1960) **75**:894–900.

4 Strax P, Control of breast cancer through mass screening, *JAMA* (1976) **235**:1600–1602.

5 Feig SA, Schwartz GF, Nerlinger R et al, Prognostic factors of breast neoplasms detected on screening by mammography and physical examination, *Radiology* (1979) **133**:577–82.

6 McClow MV, Williams AC, Mammographic examination (4030): ten year clinical experience in a Community Medical Centre, *Ann Surg* (1973) **177**:616–19.

7 Lesnick GJ, Detection of breast cancer in young women, *JAMA* (1977) **237**:967–9.

8 Egeli RA, Urban JA, Mammography in symptomatic women 50 years of age and under and those over 50, *Cancer* (1979) **43**:878–87.

9 Edeiken S, Mammography and palpable cancer of the breast, *Cancer* (1988) **61**:263–5.

10 Kobayashi T, Takatani O, Hattori N, Differential diagnosis of breast tumours. The sensitivity graded method of ultrasonotomography and clinical evaluation of its diagnostic accuracy, *Cancer* (1974) **33**:940–51.

11 Jellins J, Kossoff G, Reeve TS, Detection and classification of liquid-filled masses in the breast by gray scale echography, *Radiology* (1977) **125**:205–12.

12 Jellins J, Reeve TS, Croll J et al, Results of breast echographic examinations in Sydney, Australia 1972–1979, *Semin Ultrasound* (1982) **3**:58–62.

13 Schmidt W, van Kaick G, Muller A et al, Ultrasonic diagnosis of malignant and benign human breast lesions, *Ultrasound Med Biol* (1983) Supp 2:407–14.

14 Egan RL, Egan KL, Detection of breast carcinoma: comparison of automated water-path whole-breast sonography, mammography and physical examination, *Am J Radiol* (1984) **143**:493–7.

15 Hayashi N, Tamaki N, Yonekura Y et al, Real-time sonography of palpable breast masses, *Br J Radiol* (1985) **58**:611–15.

16 Warwick DJ, Smallwood JA, Guyer PB et al, Ultrasound mammography in the management of breast cancer, *Br J Surg* (1988) **75**:243–5.

17 Sickles EA, Filly RA, Callen PW, Breast cancer detection with sonography and mammography: comparison using state-of-the-art equipment, *Am J Radiol* (1983) **140**:843–5.

18 Franzen S, Zajicek J, Aspiration biopsy in diagnosis of palpable lesions of the breast, *Acta Radiol* (1968) **7**:241–62.

19 Zajdela A, Ghossein NA, Pilleron JP et al, The value of aspiration cytology in the diagnosis of breast cancer: experience at the Fondation Curie, *Cancer* (1975) **35**:499–506.

20 Bell DA, Hajdu SI, Urban JA et al, Role of aspiration cytology in the diagnosis and management of mammary lesions in office practice, *Cancer* (1983) **51**:1182–9.

21 Frable WJ, Needle aspiration of the breast, *Cancer* (1984) **53**:671–6.

22 Somers RG, Young GP, Kaplan MJ et al, Fine-needle aspiration biopsy in the management of solid breast tumours, *Arch Surg* (1985) **120**:673–7.

23 Wanebo HJ, Feldman PS, Wilhelm MC et al, Fine needle aspiration cytology in lieu of open biopsy in management of primary breast cancer, *Ann Surg* (1985) **55**:569–78.

24 Smallwood J, Herbert A, Guyer P et al, Accuracy of aspiration cytology in the diagnosis of breast disease, *Br J Surg* (1985) **72**:841–3.

25 Smith C, Butler J, Cobb C et al, Fine needle aspiration cytology in the diagnosis of primary breast cancer, *Surgery* (1988) **103**:178–83.

26 Kline TS, Joshi LP, Neal HS, Fine needle aspiration of the breast: diagnosis and pitfalls, *Cancer* (1979) **44**:1458–64.

27 Pilotti S, Rilke F, Delpiano C et al, Problems in fine needle aspiration biopsy cytology of clinically or mammographically uncertain breast tumours, *Tumori* (1982) **68**:407–12.

28 Ulanow RM, Galblum L, Canter JW, Fine needle aspiration in the diagnosis and management of solid breast lesions, *Am J Surg* (1984) **148**:653–7.

29 Roberts JG, Preece PE, Bolton PM et al, The trucut biopsy in breast cancer, *Clin Oncol* (1975) **1**:297–303.

30 Elston CW, Cotton RE, Davies CJ et al, A comparison of the use of the trucut needle and fine needle aspiration cytology in the pre-operative diagnosis of carcinoma of the breast, *Histopathology* (1978) **2**:239–54.

31 Fentiman IS, Millis RR, Hayward JL, Value of needle biopsy in outpatient diagnosis of breast cancer, *Arch Surg* (1980) **115**:652–3.

32 Gonzalez E, Grafton WD, Morris DR et al, Diagnosing breast cancer using frozen sections from trucut needle biopsies, *Ann Surg* (1985) **202**:696–701.

33 Bradbeer JW, Outpatient diagnosis of breast cancer, *Br J Surg* (1985) **72**:927–8.

34 Minkowitz S, Moskowitz R, Khafif RA et al, Trucut needle biopsy of the breast. An analysis of its specificity and sensitivity, *Cancer* (1986) **57**:320–3.

35 Baildam AD, Turnbull L, Howell A et al, Extended role for needle biopsy in the management of carcinoma of the breast, *Br J Surg* (1989) **76**:553–8.

36 Fentiman IS, Millis RR, Chaudary MA et al, Effect of the method of biopsy on the prognosis of and reliability of receptor assays in patients with operable breast cancer, *Br J Surg* (1986) **73**:610–12.

37 Shabot MM, Goldberg IM, Schick P et al, Aspiration cytology is superior to trucut needle biopsy in establishing the diagnosis of clinically suspicious breast masses, *Ann Surg* (1981) **196**:122–6.

38 Fentiman IS, Cuzick J, Millis RR et al, Which patients are cured of breast cancer? *Br Med J* (1984) **289**:1198–11.

39 Schwartz GF, Feig SA, Rosenberg AC et al,

Staging and treatment of clinically occult breast cancer, *Cancer* (1984) **53**:1379–86.

40 Skinner MA, Swain M, Simmons R et al, Non-palpable breast lesions at biopsy, *Ann Surg* (1987) **208**:203–8.

41 Silverstein MJ, Gamagami P, Rosser RJ et al, Hooked-wire directed breast biopsy and over-penetrated mammography, *Cancer* (1987) **59**:715–22.

42 Rubin E, Visscher DW, Alexander RW, Proliferative disease and atypia in biopsies performed for non-palpable lesions detected mammographically, *Cancer* (1988) **61**:2077–87.

43 Graham NL, Bauer TL, Early detection of occult breast cancer: the York experience with 678 needle localisation biopsies, *Am Surg* (1988) **54**:234–9.

44 Sigfusson BF, Andersson I, Aspegren K et al, Clustered breast calcifications, *Acta Radiol* (1983) **24**:273–81.

45 Abbes M, Vergnet, F, Aubanel D, Practical importance of breast microcalcification: report on 112 cases, *Eur J Surg Oncol* (1988) **14**:651–61.

46 Tinnemans JGM, Wobbes T, Lubbers EJC et al, The significance of microcalcifications without palpable mass in the diagnosis of breast cancer, *Surgery* (1986) **99**:652–7.

47 Nordenstrom B, Azjicek J, Stereotaxic needle biopsy and preoperative indication of non-palpable mammary lesions, *Acta Cytol* (1977) **21**:350–7.

48 Svane G, Stereotaxic needle biopsy of non-palpable breast lesions. A clinical and radiological follow up, *Acta Radiol (Diagn)* (1983) **24**:385–90.

49 Azavedo E, Svane G, Auer G, Stereotactic fine-needle biopsy in 2594 mammographically detected non-palpable lesions, *Lancet* (1989) **i**:1033–5.

50 Ciatto S, Pacini P, Azzini V et al, Preoperative staging of primary breast cancer. A multicentre study, *Cancer* (1988) **61**:1038–40.

51 Barnes DM, Fentiman IS, Millis RR et al, Who needs steroid receptor assays? *Lancet* (1989) **i**:1126–7.

52 Buchanan RB, Blamey RW, Durrant KR et al, A randomised comparison of tamoxifen with surgical oöphorectomy in premenopausal patients with advanced breast cancer, *J Clin Oncol* (1986) **4**:1326–30.

53 Ingle JN, Krook JE, Green SJ et al, Randomised trial of bilateral oöphorectomy versus tamoxifen in premenopausal women with metastatic breast cancer, *J Clin Oncol* (1986) **4**:178–85.

54 Nicholson RI, Walker KJ, Turkes A et al, Endocrinological and clinical aspects of LHRH action (ICI 118630) in hormone dependent breast cancer, *J Steroid Biochem* (1985) **23**:843–9.

55 Preece PE, Wood RAB, Mackie CR et al, Tamoxifen as initial sole treatment of localised breast cancer in elderly women: a pilot study, *Br Med J* (1982) **284**:869–70.

56 Fentiman IS, Caleffi M, Tutt P, Consequences of the administration of an anti-oestrogen to women with mastalgia and breast cancer, *Rev Endocrinol Rel Cancer* (1987) **20** (suppl):25–8.

57 Nolvadex Adjuvant Trial Organisation. Controlled trial of tamoxifen as single adjuvant agent in management of early breast cancer, *Lancet* (1985) **i**:836–40.

58 Breast Cancer Trials Committee, Scottish Trials Office. Adjuvant tamoxifen in the management of operable breast cancer: the Scottish Trial, *Lancet* (1987) **ii**:171–5.

59 Millis RR, The relationship between the pathology of breast cancer and hormone sensitivity, *Rev Endocrinol Rel Cancer* (1987) **20**(suppl):13–18.

CHAPTER 4
SCREENING

Venienti occurrite morbo.

Persius

There has been a gradual accretion of evidence, barnacle-like upon the keel of the craft of surgery, concerning the benefits of mammographic screening for breast cancer. This has been responsible for a change of direction and a drift towards the largely uncharted waters of mass screening. Are we sailing towards the rich shores of a new world where cases of advanced breast cancer will become extinct, or are we about to become becalmed in the doldrums of failure with disappointment for patients, physicians and politicians alike?

The assumptions upon which screening is based, together with the evidence of benefit, will be examined. In addition the arguments against screening, together with its disadvantages, will be considered, along with the problems inherent in setting up any nationwide system of detection for early breast cancer.

The theory

The syllogism runs thus: screening will detect small breast cancers; prognosis is related to size of tumour; therefore screening will save lives. Does this argument hold? It is undeniable that screening can detect small cancers. What is more questionable is the proportion of small cancers within the total population at risk that will be detected. Thus, unless the total group at risk is invited for screening, there will be a proportional loss of cases. On the Forrest recommendations for instance, where women will be screened between the ages of 50 and 65, approximately half the at-risk population will be excluded.[1]

In the second place, in order to detect early breast cancers women must be convinced of the benefits obtained and must also be sufficiently well-treated at their first attendance to be motivated to return for subsequent screening rounds. With the exception of Sweden, where the populations tend to be compliant in regard to public health matters, the reported take-up of screening invitations has been between 50 and 75 per cent, with the lowest rates in the largest cities. On the basis of these figures, possibly as few as one-quarter of those at risk may attend for screening. Thus the question of how non-compliant women can be persuaded to attend for screening needs to be addressed as a matter of urgency.

Do small infiltrating cancers carry a better prognosis? The 10-year survival for patients with T_1, N_0, M_0 tumours is approximately 80 per cent, with a significant proportion of deaths from metastatic carcinoma. Infiltrating carcinoma means potentially metastastatic carcinoma, and the concept of minimal breast cancer has served only to give false reassurance to both doctors and patients with regard to prognosis in these so-called minimal cases. Thus if all that mammographic screening can achieve is to diagnose smaller infiltrating carcinomas it will not achieve the level of success that its protagonists predict, and will merely prolong the lead-time with no real effect on the prognosis.

Of course, it will be argued that screening will diagnose not only small infiltrating carcinomas but also non-infiltrating cancers, particularly ductal carcinomas in situ (DCIS). This seems a much more promising prospect, but again a note of caution should be made. Not all infiltrating cancers have a premalignant radiologically detectable phase. Certainly, only 80 per cent of infiltrating carcinomas have an in situ component present and not all of these in situ components will show evidence of microcalcification. The 10–20 per cent of interval cancers are an indication of the proportion of undetectable cancers. Furthermore, not all non-infiltrating cancers will progress to frank malignancy, since post-mortem studies have shown the presence of such lesions in asymptomatic women. Finally, although DCIS would appear to be incompatible with metastasis, nevertheless 1–3 per cent of patients have axillary nodal metastases, illustrating the difficulty in exclusion of the earliest changes of infiltration through the basement membrane.

Trials of screening

The Hospital Insurance Plan (HIP) trial with its simple yet elegant design avoided the pitfalls of lead-time and length bias and has shown a long-term survival benefit for those offered screening.[2] Unlike the majority of subsequent trials, the screening involved both clinical examination and mammography. This latter resulted in a relatively high radiation dosage (30 rads for the four sets of X-ray photographs) and was of low sensitivity, with 60 per cent of the cancers being diagnosed by clinical examination without any apparent mammographic abnormality. The overall numbers of cases of breast cancer were 295 in the control group and 225 among the screened women. This similarity would argue against any overdiagnosis of malignancy in the screened group within this trial, albeit with suboptimal mammography.

After 18 years of follow-up there have been 163 deaths from breast cancer among the control group and 126 in the study group, representing a 23 per cent reduction in breast-cancer mortality in the screened population.[3] Although this study has confirmed that screening using equipment less sophisticated than that now available can save lives, nevertheless, despite the impressive percentage reduction, the absolute numbers of lives saved are modest, namely 37 out of a study group of 31 000. The more recent Swedish two-county study which employed single oblique-view mammograms showed a similar effect at 7 years to that seen in the HIP study, in that there was a 31 per cent reduction in mortality within the study group.[4] The comparative features of the four randomized trials of screening that have been carried out are shown in Table 4.1.[3–6] This includes the UK trial, which was not strictly randomized but was actually a comparison of screened and non-screened areas. It can be seen that there were differences in terms of age range, use of clinical examination, interval of mammography and length of follow-up of all these studies. The numbers of breast cancer and the mortality rates are shown in Table 4.2, together with the odds ratio of dying from breast cancer for the control and study groups.

The most recent analysis of the HIP study

Table 4.1 Comparative features of 4 randomized trials of screening.

Study	Age	Mammography (no of views)	Clinical examination	Intervals	Study group	Control group	Follow-up (years)	Reference
HIP	40–64	2-view	Yes	1 year × 4	31 000	31 000	18	3
Two-county	>40	1-view	No	2–3 years	78 085	56 782	7	4
UK trial	45–64			2 years		127 117	7	5
Edinburgh		2-view	Alternate		23 194			
Guildford		1-view	Alternate		22 647			
Malmo	>45	2-view	No	1.5–2 years	21 088	21 195	8	6

Table 4.2 Breast-cancer cases and mortality in randomized trials of screening.

Study		Breast cancer incidence		Breast-cancer deaths		Relative risk (95% CI)	Reference
		Study	Control	Study	Control		
HIP	<50	151	145	61	77	0.79	3
	>50	220	226	92	119	0.77	
Two-county	<50	222	123	25	18	1.26 (0.56–2.86)	4
	>50	1073	645	180	135	0.61 (0.44–0.84)	
UK Trial		748	1472	102	362	0.54 (0.36–0.81)	5
Edinburgh		360		51			
Guildford		388		51			
Malmo	<55	123	91	28	22	1.29 (0.74–2.25)	6
	>55	458	356	35	44	0.79 (0.51–1.24)	

with 18 years of follow-up does show a benefit in terms of reduction of the odds ratio in those under 50 years of age at first entry to the study. To date, the other studies have not yet shown such a benefit; indeed the Malmo study found an increased mortality from breast cancer in women under 55 in the study group. Figure 4.1 shows the mortality from breast cancer within the HIP study, and indicates that the benefits from screening do not emerge until year 5. Similarly, in the UK trial a significant reduction in relative risk of dying from breast cancer was only found after 7 years of follow-up. Thus results at 7 years may give artificially low indications of the overall effect on mortality. The Malmo

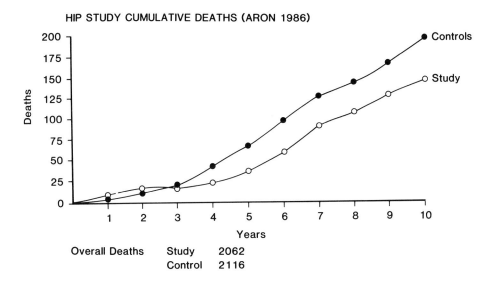

HIP STUDY CUMULATIVE DEATHS (ARON 1986)

Overall Deaths   Study   2062
                  Control   2116

Figure 4.1   Cumulative deaths in the study and control groups of the HIP trial.

Table 4.3 Results of case-control studies of screening.

Study	No of cases	Mammography (no of views)	Clinical examination	Relative risk (95% CI)	Reference
Nijmegen	62 000	1-view	Yes	0.48 (0.23–1.0)	7
DOM	20 555	2-view	Yes	0.3 (0.13–0.7)	8
Florence	24 813	2-view	No	0.53 (0.29–0.95)	9

study reported an over-representation of Stage II/III/IV cases among the non-attenders in the invited group. This does suggest that those who do not accept screening are likely to be those that will also delay in presenting with symptomatic breast lumps.

Table 4.3 lists the case-control studies of screening together with the numbers of cases, type of mammography, whether clinical examination was used and the odds ratio of reduction of mortality.[7–9] All these showed significant reductions in mortality. It is of interest that the greatest reduction was shown in the study which employed both two-view mammography and also clinical

61

Table 4.4 Acceptance rates for screening.

Study	1st Screen (%)	2nd Screen (%)	3rd Screen (%)	4th Screen (%)	Reference
HIP	65	52	48	45	3
Two-county	89	83	–	–	4
Nijmegen	85	65	57	53	7
DOM	72	58	50	42	8
Florence (CSPO)	60	–	–	–	9
UK trial					
Guildford	72	–	–	65	5
Edinburgh	60	–	–	53	
Malmo	74	70	70	70	6

Table 4.5 Pick-up rates for cancer in screening studies.

Study	Prevalent rate per 1000 cases	Reference
HIP	2.7	3
Two-county	5.6	4
Nijmegen	3.9	7
DOM	2.5	8
CSPO	3.2	9
UK		
Edinburgh	2.5	5
Guildford	2.6	

Table 4.6 Interval cases missed by screening.

Study	No of cases	Percentage of all cancers	Reference
HIP	92	42	3
Two-county	261	22	4
Nijmegen	31	10	7
DOM	17	24	8
CSPO	11	39	9
UK			5
Edinburgh	47	13	
Guildford	68	18	
Malmo	100	17	6

examination, that is the DOM study from Utrecht.

One of the major obstacles to the use of population screening is the lack of acceptance of the offer of screening by many women. The percentages accepting first screen together with follow-up screens are shown in Table 4.4. The highest acceptance rate was achieved in Sweden, the lowest rates in Edinburgh and Florence. By the fourth round of screening the greatest percentage of patients still attending was 65 per cent, reported in the Guildford component of the UK screening trial. Pick-up rates for cancers in the prevalent screen are shown in Table 4.5, which indicates that 2.5–5.6 cases per 1000 would be expected. These results need to be taken in conjunction with numbers of interval cases, that is those diagnosed within one year of a so-called negative screening. In the HIP study the interval cases comprised 42 per cent of all cancers diagnosed, but this fell to 10 per cent in the Nijmegen study. The absolute numbers and percentages of interval cases are shown in Table 4.6.

These therefore represent the results of the enthusiasts, the pioneers in this field who with evangelical style have developed screening and by obsessional attention to minor abnormalities on mammograms have reduced the mortality from breast cancer. Will these studies be translatable into successful trials of screening on a national and international basis? At present, one has doubts.

Dissent

As soon as one group of doctors propounded the theory of breast screening, and favourable results were emerging from the HIP study, others raised a voice of dissent. Bailar made several important points questioning the value of screening.[10] Apart from the various detection biases he also pointed out that selection might occur with those women most likely to be health-aware being those who would come forward for screening. Thus among the non-attenders there would be greater numbers of unfavourable cases with more advanced cancers probably related to delay, as was seen within the Malmo study.

Radiation risk

Another issue, which was of great importance but has now receded, relates to radiation dosage. In the HIP study the average skin dose was 8 rads.[11] If mammography were performed between the ages of 45 and 75, every 3 years, this would result in a cumulative exposure of 800 rads which would certainly lead to at least a doubling in the incidence of breast cancer. Follow-up studies of women subject to multiple fluoroscopies have certainly shown an increased risk of subsequent breast carcinoma developing 20 years after radiation exposure.[12] Technical improvements have led to a significant reduction in radiation dosage which is now 0.001 gray (0.1 rad), so that the cumulative dosage for 10 screening cycles would be 1 rad. Such a low dose would be very unlikely to lead to any significant increase in radiation-induced cancers among the screened population. It has been calculated that a breast dose of 0.1 rad would lead to an excess of four cancers/million women aged over 35, after a 10-year latency period.[13] This represents a very small likelihood which has been described as of similar risk to a 10-mile car journey, smoking one-eighth of a cigarette or living for 3 minutes at the age of 60.[14]

Breast self-examination

Detection of malignancy in the HIP study was achieved more frequently by clinical examination than by mammography and it was postulated that clinical examination and breast self-examination (BSE) might be as effective as mammography, without the risk or cost. This hope has proved to be false. In the first place, modern mammography is much more sensitive and can detect many more small infiltrating and non-infiltrating lesions so that the reduction in mortality reported by the HIP study has been mirrored in the Swedish two-county study, where no clinical examination was routinely performed.

The role of BSE remains contentious. It has been argued that its only achievement is to worry healthy women needlessly and that it does not lead to any reduction in mortality among those who regularly examine themselves.[15] However, a recent overview of BSE studies has suggested that there may be a small benefit.[16] Hill et al calculated the odds ratios, using logistic regression analysis to examine the relationship between BSE and two indices of the stage of cancer, namely tumour size and axillary nodal histology. Data were pooled from 12 studies comprising a total of 8118 patients. When the relationship between premorbid practice of BSE was studied in terms of axillary nodal status, the odds ratio was 0.66 (95 per cent confidence interval (CI) 0.59–0.74). This reduction in odds ratio shows a significant benefit for those practising BSE. A separate analysis was conducted looking at the circumstances of detection – that is, accidental against whilst performing BSE—and the calculated odds ratio was 0.85 (CI 0.69–1.03), which did not achieve statistical significance. It was postulated that this apparent lack of association might have been observed because of some patients who practised regular BSE and yet found the cancer by accident between routine examinations.

Similar results were reported in relation to BSE practice and tumour size, dichotomized as 2 cm or less. In relation to previous practice of BSE, the odds ratio was 0.56 (CI 0.38–0.81). The odds ratio for circumstances of detection was 0.89 (CI 0.51–1.57). The former result achieved statistical significance. In these studies the effect on mortality was not measured, merely the relationship to prognostic factors associated with risk of relapse and indirectly with mortality from breast cancer. Since patients were ques-

tioned about BSE practice prior to biopsy, attribution bias would not have been responsible for the increased number of histologically node-negative cases found among those also practised BSE.

As part of the UK trial of screening, two centres, Nottingham and Huddersfield, examined the role of BSE. The relative risk of death from breast cancer for the two centres was 1.10 (CI 0.92–1.32). When these rates were adjusted for pretrial breast-cancer mortality, the relative risk was 1.04 (CI 0.86–1.26). Thus these results do not suggest any effect on mortality in relation to practice of BSE on a population basis.

Whatever the merits of BSE alone in reducing cases of advanced breast cancer, with or without a reduction in overall mortality, it is likely that BSE will have to be introduced as part of national screening projects. Contact with screening units will provide a unique opportunity to teach the correct forms of BSE. It is likely that 10–20 per cent of women will have interval cancers which will not be detectable or will be missed by mammography. It will be necessary to make it clear to screened women that mammography is not an absolute test for breast cancer. Thus they will not merely be able to attend for X-ray scans every 3 years and then pay no further attention to their breasts until the next visit. They will need to be warned that a few cancers could be missed and any lumps which they themselves detect should not be ignored but will require rapid assessment.

Of course, there will always be some women who will be unhappy to examine their own breasts or will have difficulty differentiating between the normal and abnormal, but nevertheless the proportion of those unwilling to carry out BSE could be reduced by skilful education. A balance needs to be drawn between the responsibility of the State to provide mammography and education, and the responsibility of the individual to take sensible steps in health care, including regular BSE. If dental propaganda can lead to major improvements in dental hygiene, is there any reason why health education should not also lead to the adoption of a system of BSE that does not lead to cancerophobia, and that also does not put an undue strain on assessment clinics to which patients with self-detected lumps will report?

Further dissent

Skrabanek has been one of the most vocal critics of the principles and practice of screening for breast cancer.[17] One of his main arguments is that breast cancer is an invariably incurable condition and therefore that early diagnosis will play no role in diminishing the number of deaths from the disease. This represents an overly pessimistic reading of the literature. Probably up to one-third of patients with operable breast cancer are cured by effective local treatment. Skrabanek questioned whether all cancers detected by screening would become clinically apparent and also whether the benefits from treatment of detectable cancers might be counteracted by the more aggressive nature of the non-detectable interval cancers. More recently, Skrabanek pointed out that there was no overall reduction in mortality in the Swedish two-county study because of deaths from other causes being more frequent in the screened group.[18] This is not really an argument against breast screening, unless it could be demonstrated that somehow the effect of screening was to increase the incidence of other conditions—suicide as a result of depression, or coronary heart disease secondary to stress. An analysis of the HIP results, using the theory of competing risks, showed no effect on the rate of mortality from other causes.[19] Thus the total of deaths would have been

greater if the screened group had not taken part in the study.

The Forrest Committee suggested that 5–10 per cent of cancers would be undetectable and therefore present as interval cases. Skrabanek argued that in most series the incidence of interval cancers was higher than this. On the results of the Canadian National Breast Cancer Screening Project, the positive predictive value of mammography was 5–10 per cent, that is 90–95 per cent of abnormal mammograms were false positives. Translated to a national study in a country the size of Great Britain, this would result in 65 000 false-positive mammograms annually. Skrabanek also pointed out that there was a doubling in numbers of breast biopsies that resulted from the two-county study, together with the problems of pathological interpretation of borderline lesions, so that an overdiagnosis was occurring. Skrabanek's most telling point was the difficulty of translating the results from either University centres or specialized units to the wider field of national screening, with a likely dilution of benefit and amplification of harm resulting from both false-positive and false-negative results.

The Breast Cancer Detection and Demonstration Project (BCDDP) arose as a response to the encouraging HIP results. This multicentre study represented the loss of a great opportunity to validate prospectively the HIP results in randomized trials and was in part responsible for the worldwide delay in implementation of screening. Wright analysed the data collected in the first year and drew some interesting conclusions.[20] A total of 268 114 women were screened. Of these 14 851 (5.5 per cent) had an abnormal mammogram. Biopsy was performed in 9702 (3.6 per cent) and cancers were detected in 1460 (0.5 per cent). Thus 13 391 (5 per cent) of women had false-positive mammographic results. Wright argued that if a benign biopsy represented harm, that is unnecessary surgery, then the harm/benefit ratio was 5.6 : 1. Taking into account the mortality for breast cancer even among the screen-detected group, together with the inclusion of non-infiltrating cancers (22 per cent), Wright presented a revised harm/benefit ratio of 6.2 : 1. He therefore suggested that breast screening should be reserved for those at high risk, such as women with a strong family history. Although laudable in intent, this is unlikely to be practicable since the benefits of breast cancer screening in women under the age of 50 are marginal, whereas the majority of familial breast carcinomas will present before the age of 50.

scan it is imperative that she be seen promptly by a sympathetic experienced clinician who will be able to order appropriate investigations or interventions to confirm that the lesion is benign. Alternatively, the breast physician will need to arrange for a prompt biopsy to determine the histological nature of the suspicious lesion. The failure to achieve this target in private, so-called screening clinics, which are in reality selling mammography, has been responsible for a large amount of unnecessary worry for many unfortunate women.[21]

Training of screening personnel

The breast physician

To achieve a successful expansion of screening from the few centres that are at present operating will require the education of large numbers of medical and paramedical personnel. Central to this will be the training of breast physicians. These statusless persons, recognized by no college or association, have been major contributors to the success of screening programmes. With their diagnostic acumen allied to empathetic counselling skills they have increased both the sensitivity and specificity of screening and have also diminished the psychological morbidity associated with the discovery of an asymptomatic mammographic abnormality. Their appointments occurred largely through chance rather than any professional training scheme and it is essential now, with an extension of screening under consideration, that the structured training of breast physicians should be a priority in the budget for education.

Once the screened woman has been informed that she has an abnormal X-ray

The radiologist

The quality of mammograms depends upon close attention to detail by the radiographer to ensure that all breast tissue is included on the films and that appropriate exposure and processing gives optimal clarity and a minimal radiation dose to the screened women. If these criteria are fulfilled the radiologist will then be presented with the best opportunity to identify abnormal mammograms. With singular foresight, the College of Radiographers has established a training system for accreditation in mammography. This contrasts with the utterly haphazard system of training for medical personnel taking part in breast screening. In order to maintain the high standards of the pioneering centres some system of accreditation will be necessary.[22] This idea was originally suggested in relation to the licensing of radiologists to read screening mammograms. However, it might be more appropriate if screening assessment units were to require licences, and this would mean accreditation of surgeon, breast physician, pathologist and radiologist.

The achievement of acceptable sensitivity

and specificity requires not only the traditional radiological skills of pattern recognition and comparison, but also the capacity to maintain attention, whilst searching for the grains of microcalcification among the mountains of mammograms that must be read. Such skills are inducible, particularly among younger radiologists, although it has been claimed by Lundgren that some radiologists may be ineducable.[23] Although in principle there is no difference between the radiological approach to symptomatic or screening mammograms, in practice the recognition of the subtle changes in the asymptomatic that signal malignancy may be problematic. As an example, with experience it is possible to differentiate between significant and non-significant microcalcification. Whilst this experience is being gained there will be more false positives with no underlying malignant lesions and more false negatives, thereby increasing the numbers of interval cancers.

The surgeon

The assessment team reviewing those screened women with abnormal mammograms will comprise a clinician, who is either a surgeon or a breast physician, a radiologist with an interest in mammography and ultrasonography, and a pathologist who, in a perfect world, also has experience in fine-needle aspiration (FNA) cytology. The role of the surgeon will vary according to local developments. In some centres the clinician carrying out assessment will be a general surgeon. However, many surgeons are at present either too busy or temperamentally unsuited to the difficult task of dealing sympathetically with anxious women, most of whom have no underlying malignancy.

The particular role of the surgeon will be to carry out accurate excision of impalpable,

X-ray-detected lesions. The surgeon should work together with the radiologist who performs the localization; the objective is to remove sufficient tissue to make an accurate diagnosis, without removing an excessive amount of surrounding normal tissue which would result in cosmetic deformity. From the psychological and practical standpoint, it is essential that the procedure be performed as promptly and as efficiently as possible. However, this is not an argument in favour of over-hasty histological diagnosis (that is, frozen section). It may be very difficult to distinguish between a radial scar and a small carcinoma, and this difficulty will be compounded if attempts are made to report on a suboptimally fixed specimen.

The effect of screening does produce a temporary increase in surgical workload. In the Swedish two-county study there was a doubling of numbers of operations for breast cancer during the initial (prevalent) screen which subsequently fell to the prescreening level.[24] In parallel, there was a two-fold increase in biopsies for benign conditions.

Once the histological diagnosis of malignancy has been made it is the surgeon's responsibility to advise on appropriate therapy. Treatment will play an important role both in terms of patient satisfaction and prognosis. It is to be hoped that the majority of surgeons treating screen-detected lesions will not resort to inappropriately aggressive surgery. What is more likely is that there will be a drift towards minimalism. The hard lesson should have been learnt that inadequate treatment, such as the failure to irradiate the breast after apparent complete excision of small infiltrating carcinomas, will lead to unacceptably high rates of local relapse. Will this lesson need to be relearnt in relation to screen-detected cancers? For many borderline lesions there cannot be clear guidelines at present, and the only appropriate treatment will be to enter the patient into well-designed national clinical trials.

Fine-needle aspiration (FNA) cytology for screen-detected lesions

To obtain FNA cytology specimens from patients with impalpable lesions depends upon the combined skills of radiologist and cytologist, using stereotactic equipment, but this is too expensive for most screening assessment units. Fine-needle aspiration cytology is practicable when screened women are found to have palpable lesions. Lamb et al have described the experience of the Edinburgh Breast Screening Project where FNA was performed on 562 women, of whom 397 had a biopsy with 173 cases of breast cancer being diagnosed.[25] When the cytologist reported the presence of malignant cells the absolute sensitivity was 50 per cent, where a suspicious report claimed a complete sensitivity of 70 per cent. The specificity was 90 per cent. The predictive value for a suspicious report was 85 per cent and for a malignant report 99 per cent.

Acellular aspirates were obtained in 33 per cent of attempts. The major factors influencing sensitivity, specificity and predictive value are the size of the lesion and the experience of the individual carrying out aspirations.

These data would argue against the use of FNA by occasional operators, and with the present shortage of trained cytologists this technique will not play a major role in assessment of impalpable lesions. The final diagnosis will rest with the histopathologist, since tissue architecture is necessary to distinguish between borderline lesions.

Histopathology in diagnosis of screen-detected lesions

The interface between atypical change and in situ carcinoma is blurred. It becomes better defined with experience, but many of the histopathological patterns in specimens from screening biopsies will not have been encountered previously by the general pathologist. There is a small number of specialized pathologists who have made a particular study of breast lesions. These rare individuals will be called upon to train other pathologists to recognize subtle clues which help to make the diagnosis. In addition, they will be needed to act as referees for the many suspicious lesions arising from assessment-clinic-directed biopsies. Patchevsky et al reported histological results from 407 biopsies resulting from screening.[26] After review by the specialist pathologist it was found that there was one false-positive diagnosis (0.2 per cent) and five false-negative ones (1.2 per cent).[27] Anderson et al reviewed the histopathological findings from biopsies in both the prevalent and the incident-screening rounds from the Edinburgh project.[27] Of the 17 prevalent cancers, 8 (47 per cent) were non-invasive, compared with 8 out of 24 (33 per cent) incident cases. Few patients had axillary nodal metastases which were present in 12 per cent of prevalent and 13 per cent of incident cases. Anderson found an under-representation of poorer prognosis tumours among prevalent cases (37 per cent versus 58 per cent) and suggested that this was consistent with the length bias predicted for screen-detected cancers.

The unanswered questions

An effect has been demonstrated that even the most sceptical would accept as real. However, the argument has shifted towards questioning the magnitude of that effect, who will benefit, and therefore who should be screened and how often should this process be performed? Finally, with escalation of costs, is it possible to identify a high-risk group so that the 11 out of every 12 women who will never develop breast cancer might be spared the worry and inconvenience of screening and the State might reduce the cost of the service?

modest in population terms. Any reduction in sensitivity of screening, or lowering of acceptance rates or inadequate treatment of detected cancers could lead to an obliteration of benefit.

The magnitude of benefit

For women aged 50 years or over, one-third reductions in mortality have been demonstrated consistently in the screened groups. This saving of lives takes 5–7 years to manifest. However, it is not possible directly to translate this one-third reduction in the screened group into a similar reduced mortality in the general population.

Knox used an interactive computer-modelling process and, with data from the HIP and Swedish two-county studies, made predictions of the outcome of screening in Britain, as proposed by the Forrest Committee.[28] The model assumed that the course of breast cancer from detection to death could be separated into two periods. In period A the disease is detectable and curable, whereas in period B the disease is incurable and therefore detection will have no effect on mortality. Included within the model were the time course of disease stages, sensitivity and specificity of detection, together with acceptance rates in the various age groups invited. Knox calculated that if the HIP model were applied to Britain the reduction in mortality from breast cancer would be only 4 per cent, whereas the two-county model would produce a 20 per cent reduction.

When the Forrest report proposals were simulated in the model the predicted mortality reduction was 8 per cent, that is 901 lives saved annually from an expected total of 11 877. The approximate cost per life saved over a 7-year period would be £40 000 ($74 000). Thus the likely benefits of national screening as presently conceived are rather

Screening interval

The majority of screening studies have carried out rescreening every 2 years, but in the Swedish two-county study there was a 24–33-month interval. Of the total of 124 cancers, 5 (4 per cent) were diagnosed between randomization and invitation, 47 (38 per cent) were diagnosed at screening, 33 (27 per cent) as interval cancers and 39 (31 per cent) among non-responders.[29] When the study and control groups were compared it emerged that among women aged 40–49, 60 per cent of cancers that would have presented in the 12 months after screening were detectable by mammography, and that only 33 per cent of those presenting up to 24 months after would be detectable. Thus among younger women with 2-yearly screening intervals, two-thirds of cancers would be interval cases. This contrasted with older women, where screening detected 85 per cent of cancers that would have presented in less than 12 months, 70 per cent of those presenting in 12–24 months and 55 per cent of those presenting by the third year after screening. Tabar et al concluded that a 2-year screening interval was adequate for older women, but that in younger women annual mammography should be performed in order to minimize the number of interval cancers.[29]

This proposal would have major financial implications since if women under 50 were invited they would be the group most likely to attend. The provision of annual mammograms for, say, 5 years would be very expensive on a cost/benefit basis. In Britain this issue has been evaded since it is not planned to offer screening to women under the age of 50.

Number of mammographic views

In the early days of mammography two views, namely craniocaudal and mediolateral, were taken in order to localize any abnormality. Recently, in many centres the latter view has been replaced by an oblique projection. Lundgren and Helleberg developed the use of the oblique view for screening purposes and have shown that the technique has a low absorbed-radiation dosage (70 mrad) and reduces cost and increases throughput for screening.[30] The sensitivity of a single oblique view was 93 per cent compared with 95 per cent for a triple-view mammogram in the same centre. Thus a 2 per cent gain in sensitivity is achieved at an increase in cost of 60 per cent for two extra views. With a limited budget available for screening, single oblique films represent the best bargain.

Identification of a high-risk group

So far, the search for a high-risk group marker has been unsuccessful. The most obvious marker is a family history. However, the majority of women giving a family history will not be at any increased risk. It is only the rare group, with more than one first-degree relative who developed unilateral or bilateral breast cancer before the age of 50, that are truly at increased risk. As has been discussed, mammography may be of such low specificity in younger women that its effect on mortality is marginal. Even if screening were successful it would only be helping

possibly 5 per cent of those who would eventually develop breast cancer.

Benign breast conditions are not markers of premalignancy. The majority of biopsied patients carry no greater risk, and the premalignant changes of atypical hyperplasia with or without a family history are rare.

The parenchymal pattern of mammograms categorized by Wolfe grade has a relationship to risk of cancer carried by the DY and P2 grading. However, Wolfe grades change with age and are not sufficiently specific to be used as a marker of risk and therefore as selection criteria for entry to a high-risk group.

Studies are under way to examine whether the hormone profile, in particular plasma binding of oestrogens, can serve as a marker of a high-risk group.

No good marker has yet emerged, which means that at present it is necessary to screen the entire population at risk. For all the marginal changes that may be effected by improvements in the sensitivity of mammography, with further views and with shorter screening intervals, probably the most significant improvement would be an increase in not only the acceptance rate but also the re-attendance rate for breast screening. Only in this way will the maximal benefits of screening be seen with minimal offsetting from the damage done to women whose tests gave false-negative or false-positive results.

References

1 Working Group (Chairman APM Forrest) *Breast cancer screening. Report to the Health Ministers of England, Wales, Scotland, and Northern Ireland*, HM Stationery Office: London 1987).

2 Shapiro S, Evidence on screening for breast cancer from a randomised trial, *Cancer* (1977) (Suppl 6):2772–82.

3 Shapiro S, Venet W, Strax P, Venet L, Roeser R, Ten to fourteen year effect of screening on breast cancer mortality, *JNCI* (1982) **69**:349–53.

4 Tabar L, Fagerberg CJG, Gad A et al, Reduction in mortality from breast cancer after mass screening with mammography, *Lancet* (1985) **i**:829–32.

5 UK trial of early detection of breast cancer group. First results on mortality reduction in the UK trial of early detection of breast cancer, *Lancet* (1988) **ii**:411–16.

6 Andersson I, Aspegren K, Janzon L, Landberg T, Lindholm K et al, Mammographic screening and mortality from breast cancer. The Malmo mammographic screening trial. *Lancet* (1988) **ii**:943–8.

7 Verbeek ALM, Hendriks JHCL, Holland R et al, Reduction of breast cancer mortality through mass screening with modern mammographs, *Lancet* (1984) **i**:1222–4.

8 Collette HJA, Day NE, Rombach JJ et al, Evaluation of screening for breast cancer in a non-randomised study (the DOM project) by means of a case-control study, *Lancet* (1984) **i**:1224–6.

9 Palli D, Del Turco MR, Buiatli E et al, A case-control study of the efficacy of a non-randomised breast cancer screening programme in Florence (Italy), *Int J Cancer* (1986) **38**:501–4.

10 Bailar JC, Mammography: a contrary view, *Ann Intern Med* (1976) **84**:77–84.

11 Strax P, Venet L, Shapiro S, Value of mammography in reduction of mortality from breast cancer in mass screening, *Am J Roentgenol Radium Ther Nucl Med* (1973) **112**:686–9.

12 Delarue NC, Gale G, Ronald A, Multiple fluoroscopy of the chest: carcinogenicity for the female breast and implications for breast cancer screening programmes, *Can Med Assoc J* (1975) **21**:1405–13.

13 Feig S, Radiation risk from mammography: is it clinically significant? *AJR* (1984) **143**:469–75.

14 Pochin EE, *Why be quantitative about radiation risk estimates?* Lecture 2, Lauriston S Taylor lecture series in radiation protection and measurements (National Council on Radiation Protection and Measurements: Washington DC 1978).

15 Frank JW, Mai V, Breast self examination: more harm than good? *Lancet* (1985) **ii**:654–7.

16 Hill D, White V, Jolley D, Mapperson K, Self examination of the breast: is it beneficial? Meta-analysis of studies investigating breast self examination and extent of disease in breast cancer, *Br Med J* (1988) **297**:271–5.

17 Skrabanek P, False premises and false promises of breast cancer screening, *Lancet* (1985) **ii**:316–19.

18 Skrabanek P, The debate over mass mammography in Britain. The case against, *Br Med J* (1988) **297**:971–2.

19 Aron JL, Prorok PC, An analysis of the mortality effect in a breast cancer screening study, *Int J Epidemiol* (1986) **15**:36–43.

20 Wright CJ, Breast cancer screening: a different look at the evidence, *Surgery* (1985) **100**:594–8.

21 Fentiman IS, Pensive women, painful vigils: consequences of delay in the assessment of mammographic abnormalities, *Lancet* (1988) **i**:1041–2.

22 Witcombe JB, A licence for breast cancer screening, *Br Med J* (1988) **296**:909–11.

23 Lundgren B, Breast screening in Britain and Sweden, *Br Med J* (1988) **297**:1266.

24 Holmberg L, Adami H, Persson I et al, Demands on surgical in patient services after mass mammographic screening, *Br Med J* (1986) **293**:779–82.

25 Lamb J, Anderson TJ, Dixon MJ et al, Role of fine needle aspiration cytology in breast cancer screening, *J Clin Pathol* (1987) **40**:705–9.

26 Patchetsky AS, Shaber GS, Schwartz GF et al, The pathology of breast cancer detected by mass population screening, *Cancer* (1977) **40**:1659–70.

27 Anderson TJ, Lamb J, Alexander F et al, Comparative pathology of prevalent and incident cancers detected by breast screening, *Lancet* (1988) **i**:519–22.

28 Knox EG, Evaluation of a proposed breast cancer screening regimen, *Br Med J* (1988) **297**:650–4.

29 Tabar L, Faberberg G, Day NE et al, What is the optimum interval between mammographic screening examinations? An analysis based on the latest results of the Swedish 2 County breast cancer screening trial, *Br J Cancer* (1987) **55**:547–51.

30 Lundgren B, Helleberg A, Single oblique-view mammography for periodic screening for breast cancer in women, *JNCI* (1982) **68**:351–5.

CHAPTER 5

BREAST CONSERVATION

'We have left undone those things which we ought to have done,
And we have done those things which we ought not to have done.'

The Book of Common Prayer

Whereas the acceptance of complex and radical surgery may be rapid, the move away from such procedures marches to a slower drum. That change has begun, with a significant shift towards breast-conserving treatment. In 1929, the art historian and surgeon Geoffrey Keynes published his results of radium-implant treatment for primary breast cancer.[1] Although he convinced himself and a few others of the value of this technique, nevertheless 60 years later mastectomy is still regarded as the treatment of choice for the majority of breast cancers.

The current problem is to focus attention on the most appropriate treatment for particular types and stages of operable breast cancer. Blinkered total acceptance of breast-conserving treatment will lead to its use in the wrong patients, who will suffer the trauma of local relapse and subsequent inadequate control of disease.

What breast-conserving treatment has achieved for patients is paralleled by its success in changing the attitude of clinicians, many of whom have now come to realize that a team rather than an individual approach is necessary for the optimal treatment of patients. It will be by the dovetailing of appropriate and cosmetically acceptable surgery with accurate and effective radiotherapy that the best results will be obtained in the primary treatment of the disease. Any mismatch may lead to the patient paying a penalty both in terms of local control and cosmetic outcome. Aside from affecting mortality, chemotherapy also plays a role in local disease control in selected cases, and might, in time, extend the indications for breast conservation.

History

Geoffrey Keynes became sceptical about the dogma of lymphatic permeation being the only means by which breast cancer metastasized. In addition, he doubted the wisdom of dissection of the heavily infiltrated axilla. At the prompting of the then Professor of Surgery at St Bartholomew's Hospital, George Gask, he started to use implanted radium needles, at first to treat local relapse after mastectomy. Subsequently indications were extended and the technique was used to treat locally advanced cases and then women with primarily operable disease. Needles were implanted around the primary tumour, within the axilla, supraclavicular fossa and within the intercostal spaces to treat internal mammary nodes. Because of the associated pleural reaction and pain this latter aspect was omitted in later cases.

Of the 75 cases with the disease apparently restricted to the breast, the 5-year survival was 71 per cent, as compared with 69 per cent for historical controls treated by radical mastectomy.[2] For the 66 women with clinical involvement of axillary nodes the 5-year survival was 29 per cent compared with 30 per cent among historical controls. Because of difficulties with availability of radium, together with handling problems and inaccuracies of dosage and subsequent fibrosis, radium implants were not widely used for the primary treatment of breast cancer. A more widely applicable alternative was the use of relatively low-energy external radiotherapy and Pfahler reported a series of 53 women with early breast cancer treated in this way.[3] They had either refused mastectomy or were unfit for anaesthesia, and yet the overall survival at 5 years was 80 per cent. Pfahler was the first to suggest that results might be improved with the combined use of both implant and external radiation.

French radiotherapists deserve much of the credit for the development and acceptance of the use of radiotherapy as a replacement for radical surgery in the primary treatment of early breast cancer. Baclesse, at the Institute Curie, demonstrated that local control of relatively large tumours could be achieved using radiation dosages of 66–70 Gy given over up to 3 months.[4] Pierquin extended this work and used a combination of external radiotherapy together with iridium (^{129}Ir) implants.[5] This technique was introduced to the USA by Hellman, who popularized its use and stimulated others to test its value in clinical trials.[6]

The worldwide move away from mastectomy has profoundly affected attitudes to the disease. Surgeons once regarded any treatment other than Halsted mastectomy as gross negligence. Nowadays, many have adopted a fatalistic approach in which minimal surgery is used because it is believed that no local therapy can affect the course of the disease. Patients are better informed about options nowadays, but unfortunately some have adopted an antagonistic stance towards those treating them, feeling that it is 'every woman's right' to keep her breast, irrespective of the variety of breast cancer from which she is suffering, because it is wrongly suspected that mastectomy signifies 'mutilating surgery carried out by uncaring male surgeons'. The States of California and Maine in the USA require by law that options for treatment be explained to all patients with breast cancer.

It will never be possible to separate completely the emotional and biological aspects of breast cancer. None the less, the evidence is now available from clinical trials to enable sensible decisions to be made with regards to indications for breast-conserving treatment.

Trials of breast conservation

Hedley Atkins and his colleagues from Guy's Hospital were the first to conduct a prospective randomized trial which set out to determine whether a breast-conservation technique yielded results which were similar to those following radical mastectomy. The surgical procedure comprised removal of the tumour together with a minimum of 3 cm normal surrounding tissue. This was dubbed 'extended tytectomy' by Sir Hedley Atkins, but the appellation has since lapsed into desuetude. The studies became known as the Guy's wide-excision trials.

Guy's wide-excision trials

In the first trial, which accrued patients between 1961 and 1971, a total of 376 cases was entered. All had operable breast cancer (T_1, T_2, T_3, N_0, N_1, M_0), and were aged 50 years or above. They were randomized to primary treatment by either radical mastectomy or wide excision. Both groups received postoperative radiotherapy. The mastectomy group received 30 Gy to the gland fields. The wide-excision group were given 38 Gy (maximum) to the breast and internal mammary chain by megavoltage radiotherapy with bolus and 30 Gy to the axilla and supraclavicular fossa by orthovoltage radiotherapy. Thus treatment to the axilla for the mastectomy group comprised surgical clearance and radiotherapy, whereas the wide-excision group had no surgery, and an inadequate dosage of radiotherapy (by present-day standards).

By the time that the first report on the trial was written, it was apparent that all was not well with the breast-conserving technique.[7] Among those cases with clinically involved axillary nodes there was a significantly increased rate of local relapse (68 per cent versus 14 per cent) for those treated by wide excision compared with mastectomy. This in turn affected 10-year overall survival which fell from 60 per cent in the mastectomy group to 28 per cent in the wide-excision group. However, for patients who had no clinical evidence of axillary nodal metastases the relapse-free and overall survival rates did not differ significantly for the two treatment arms.

The second wide-excision trial was limited to cases without clinical evidence of axillary involvement, but comprised women of any age. Between 1971 and 1975, 252 patients were entered. The treatment techniques remained unchanged. To the surprise of the investigators, even after establishing these more restrictive criteria for entry, the group treated by breast conservation fared worse.[8] Both relapse-free and overall survival were significantly reduced in the wide-excision group. This occurred not because the wide-excision groups in the two trials showed any

difference in relapse-free survival or overall survival, but because the group treated by radical mastectomy fared significantly better in the second trial.

This was difficult to explain. It was unlikely that changes in surgical personnel could have led to such major changes in the results of mastectomy. In all other respects treatment had remained the same. The answer came from a re-analysis of the clinical data which showed that there were more small (T_1) tumours in the second study.[9] It was among those patients with small tumours that the differences emerged. Thus women with T_1 tumours treated by radical mastectomy in the second trial had better relapse-free survival and overall survival than those treated by wide excision. Patients with T_2 tumours fared similarly after both forms of treatment.

These studies can teach us many lessons. First, inadequate local treatment of small tumours lends to increased incidence of local and distant relapse. This may be masked in patients with larger tumours because of the presence of pre-existing micrometastases. Second, the use of historical controls as a means of assessment of a new treatment can lead to serious mistakes. The pattern of disease in patients presenting to even one institution may change with time and thus give a misleading picture if compared with a cohort treated differently at a later date. Third, these trials with relatively few cases succeeded in demonstrating inadequacies of treatment after long follow-up. Preliminary reports, even of very large trials, may suggest conclusions which may not necessarily hold up with time. Finally, the aim of breast conservation is to achieve good cosmesis. This was patchy within these two trials. The combination of extensive tissue excision, the use of bolus and orthovoltage radiotherapy is not a recipe for good cosmesis. Skin marbling, telangectases and fibrosis were common sequelae of radiation treatment. Many patients, particularly those with smaller breasts, finished up with a distorted asymmetric treated breast, as a result of wide excision of tissue.

successful local control of disease in those treated by this particular breast-conservation technique.

Milan trial

After this inauspicious start, it was evident that more radical approaches to breast conservation would be required. The Milan group carried out a trial between 1973 and 1980 to examine breast conservation for patients with tumours up to 2 cm diameter.[10] This latter referred to the pathologically measured size of the tumour in the biopsy specimen rather than a preoperative clinical measurement which would have usually overestimated the actual size. Eligible patients were aged up to 70 years and had no clinical evidence of axillary nodal involvement. They were randomized to treatment by either a radical mastectomy without postoperative irradiation, or a quadrantectomy (removal of the quarter of the breast containing the cancer) axillary clearance and subsequent radiotherapy to the breast (50 Gy). After 1976, all patients with axillary nodal involvement received adjuvant chemotherapy (CMF) for 12 cycles.

Of the 701 evaluable patients, 352 were treated conservatively and 349 by mastectomy. After 5 years of follow-up, both relapse-free survival and overall survival curves for the two groups were identical. This was maintained after a median follow-up of 8 years.[11] Cosmetic results were described as satisfactory in 70 per cent of cases. Thus almost 1 in 3 had less than satisfactory cosmesis. This is not surprising since removal of a breast quadrant may lead to deformity similar to that after wide excision, particularly in those with medially or centrally located lesions. This cosmetic failure is the disadvantage of extensive surgery, but represents a major factor in the

Villejuif trial

A different technique, using local excision followed by external irradiation, was tested at the Institute Gustave-Roussy.[12] Eligible cases had single tumours which were mammographically or pathologically measured as no greater than 2 cm diameter. They were randomized to treatment by either local excision or total mastectomy. All cases had a low-level axillary dissection (to the lower border of pectoralis minor). Those with proven axillary metastases had a full axillary clearance and were then re-randomized to receive or not receive axillary irradiation. The local excision group received cobalt irradiation to the breast (45 Gy) with an external boost to the tumour site (15 Gy).

Only 179 cases were entered into this study (88 breast conservation, 91 mastectomy), so that the trial lacked statistical power to confirm adequately the null hypothesis. With this major drawback, the finding of no difference between relapse-free survival and overall survival of the two groups has to be interpreted with caution. What this study did achieve was a cosmetically acceptable result in 92 per cent of cases, indicating the aesthetic improvement obtained by more localized surgery.

NSABP B-06 trial

The National Surgical Adjuvant Breast Project (NSABP) conducted a multicentre trial B-06 which, at a stroke, confirmed the results of both the Guy's wide-excision trial and the

Milan quadrantectomy trial.[13] Eligible cases had primary tumours up to 4 cm diameter, that is the majority of cases presenting to breast clinics rather than the selected group with 2 cm lesions. Patients were aged up to 70 years and were randomized to one of three options. The first (standard) option comprised total mastectomy and full axillary clearance without postoperative irradiation. The second treatment arm was a segmental mastectomy, that is a wide excision of the tumour. Pathological confirmation was obtained that the tumour had been completely excised and, if not, the patient had an immediate total mastectomy. The third option comprised a segmental mastectomy, again with pathological control, followed by external radiotherapy to the breast (50 Gy). All patients with confirmed axillary-nodal metastases received chemotherapy.

In all, 2163 patients were entered into the study but for reasons of ineligibility or refusal to take part only 1843 (85 per cent) were assessable. Of the 1257 randomized to segmental mastectomy, with or without irradiation, 1131 (90 per cent) had histologically clear excision biopsy margins. The extent of axillary nodal involvement and the likelihood of biopsy margin positivity were related. Of those with 10 or more nodes involved, one-third had positive biopsy margins and were reassigned to treatment by total mastectomy.

One clear message from the NSABP trial was that inadequate local treatment leads to an increased rate of local relapse, irrespective of whether patients were given adjuvant chemotherapy. The incidence of relapse among those treated by segmental mastectomy is shown in Table 5.1. Overall 10 per cent of the non-irradiated group developed relapse, almost invariably in the same quadrant, compared with only 4 per cent of the irradiated cases. Life-table analysis indicated that 7 per cent of the irradiated group would relapse by 5 years, compared with 28 per cent of the non-irradiated women. This rose

Table 5.1 Breast relapse in NSABP trial B-06.

	Segmental mastectomy	Segmental mastectomy + radiotherapy
Total	565	566
Relapse	54 (10)	22 (4)
Node-negative	358	373
Relapse	15 (4)	19 (5)
Node-positive	207	193
Relapse	39 (19)	3 (2)

Percentages in parentheses.

to 36 per cent among the non-irradiated node-positive cases.

The NSABP did not consider that relapse within the breast represented treatment failure. This is at variance with the views of most patients and doctors. After exclusion of these cases, the local failure rates are shown in Table 5.2, as are the results when ipsilateral breast relapse is added, indicating that with relatively short follow-up almost 1 in 5 of those women treated by segmental mastectomy without radiation had relapsed.

More recently the 8-year follow-up has been reported.[14] Even excluding relapse in the breast (which occurred in 37 per cent of those treated by tumourectomy without irradiation), a significantly better relapse-free survival occurred among the group treated by tumourectomy and irradiation. Both distant disease-free and overall survival were lower in the non-irradiated group, but these differences have not yet reached statistical significance.

Table 5.2 Loco-regional relapse in NSABP B-06.

	Total mastectomy	Segmental mastectomy	Segmental mastectomy + radiotherapy
No of cases	586	632	625
Local (axilla)	27 (5)	25 (4)	4 (0.5)
Regional	18 (3)	20 (3)	10(1.5)
Breast	0	54 (9)	22 (4)
Total	45 (8)	99 (16)	36 (6)

Percentages in parentheses.

Table 5.3 Eight-year survival data after adequate local treatment in NSABP B-06.

	Total mastectomy (%)		Segmental mastectomy + radiotherapy (%)	
	N−	N+	N−	N+
Relapse-free survival	66	45	66	47
Overall survival	79	60	83	68

The NSABP results do support the Milan data in that among those treated by adequate local treatment, either mastectomy or segmental mastectomy and radiotherapy, there were no differences in terms of relapse-free or overall survival, as shown in Table 5.3.

Meanwhile, at Guy's Hospital a new approach was formulated. Convinced by the data from the wide-excision studies that inadequate local treatment leads to increase of both loco-regional and distant relapse, it was determined that an aggressive breast-conserving technique was required. This criterion appeared to be met by the combined use of surgery and interstitial radiotherapy.

Guy's combined breast-conservation technique

It was agreed that any technique of breast conservation needed to fulfil several requirements.

1 It had to achieve local control and overall survival which was as good as that following modified radical mastectomy
2 It had to give good cosmetic results
3 It had to be compatible with either cytotoxic or endocrine adjuvant therapy
4 It had to yield full prognostic information including axillary nodal status, tumour histology and tissue for flow cytometry and receptor measurements
5 If possible, it should be a single-anaesthetic procedure.

The reader may judge how well those criteria have been met.

The information yielded by a modified radical mastectomy has come to be taken for granted, as have the effects on local control of disease. These features need to be considered separately for breast-conserving techniques.

Treatment of primary tumour

It was decided that it would be worthwhile to use the advantages of both surgery and radiotherapy to achieve maximum benefit. Thus for selected tumours—those no greater than 4 cm diameter, which were unifocal and had no evidence of metastases—tumour excision was performed. The aim was to take the least amount of surrounding normal tissue, thereby keeping tissue deficit to a minimum. A study of such cases in whom a modified radical mastectomy was performed indicated that residual carcinoma was present at the biopsy site in up to 50 per cent of cases.

In order to eradicate this residual tumour, a peroperative iridium implant was performed by the radiotherapist who was present in the operating theatre. Flexible plastic tubes were implanted which were after-loaded with iridium (^{192}Ir), approximately 24–48 hours later. Usually a two-plane implant was used.

Treatment of axilla

In order to obtain the greatest amount of prognostic information, it is necessary to clear the axilla in order that the histopathologist can report on the number and levels of nodes with and without metastases. Technical details of axillary clearance are given in Appendix 1.

When a patient had the histological diagnosis made by needle biopsy, the axillary clearance was followed by excision of the tumour. A redivac drain was invariably inserted at the biopsy site in order to minimize the risk of haematoma formation, which can greatly prejudice the cosmetic outcome. The radiotherapist then performed the implant as described in Appendix 2.

Usually the biopsy site drain can be removed within 48 hours, but the axillary drain was left in situ during the entire iridium implant, 20 Gy, given over 48 hours.

Once the patient's nodal histology was available those with nodal involvement were advised to have adjuvant therapy, which comprised chemotherapy for both premenopausal and postmenopausal patients during the time of the trial. The first cycle of chemotherapy was given on the tenth to twelfth postoperative day. External radiation was started 2–3 weeks postoperatively and was given on a 4 MeV linear accelerator giving a total breast dose of 46 Gy (minimum), using wedged opposed tangential fields. The axilla and supraclavicular regions were not irradiated in either the node-positive or node-negative groups. Relapse in the axilla after meticulous surgical clearance was rare.

This technique was piloted at Guy's and the preliminary results were encouraging.[15] Following this, a prospective randomized clinical trial was set up. Other workers in Amsterdam, Leuven and Capetown had similar ideas, and joined together to conduct EORTC Trial 10801 into which 903 patients were entered. Of these, just under half were from Guy's Hospital.

Guy's component of EORTC 10801

Eligible patients were aged under 70 years and had a single breast carcinoma measuring clinically no greater than 4 cm diameter. Bilateral mammography was performed to exclude multifocal and contralateral disease. Staging investigations, including a bone scan, were performed to exclude metastatic disease. Those fulfilling these criteria were randomized to primary treatment by either modified radical mastectomy or alternatively by the combined conservation technique,

Table 5.4 Relapses in Guy's cases entered into EORTC 10801 trial.

	Loco-regional			Distant
	Breast	*Chest wall*	*Other*	
Breast conservation (214 cases)	14 (7%)	–	21 (10%)	28 (13%)
Mastectomy (185 cases)	–	13(7%)	20(11%)	29(16%)

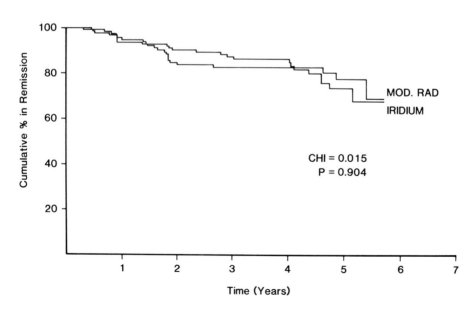

Figure 5.1 Relapse-free survival of node-negative patients treated by either modified radical mastectomy or iridium implant.

OVERALL SURVIVAL NODE NEGATIVE PATIENTS

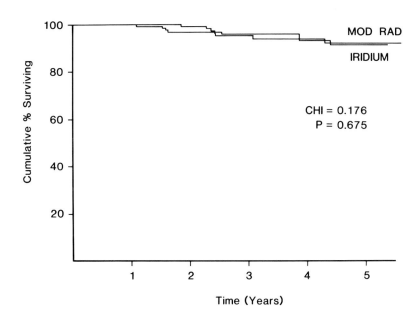

Figure 5.2   Overall survival of node-negative patients treated by either modified radical mastectomy or iridium implant.

comprising tumourectomy, axillary clearance, iridium implant (20 Gy) and external radiotherapy (46 Gy).

Between 1981 and 1986, 399 patients were entered, of whom 214 were treated by iridium implant and 185 by mastectomy. The reason for the slight imbalance was a temporary computer lapse in which a 2:1 rather than 1:1 randomization was used. So far, loco-regional relapse has occurred in 35 (17 per cent) of the iridium group and 35 (18 per cent) of the mastectomy group, and details are given in Table 5.4. The relapse-free survival and overall survival are given in

Figures 5.1 and 5.2, which show no significant difference between the two groups.

Thus after a median follow-up of 5 years the breast-conserving technique is as effective as mastectomy in achieving local control. Obviously these results are still preliminary, but it is encouraging since after this time of follow-up in the wide excision trials a difference in relapse rate was already seen. Equally encouraging are the cosmetic results which were observer rated as good/excellent in over 80 per cent of patients. Cosmesis was rated by patients as good or excellent in over 90 per cent. There were differences between both surgical and radiotherapy techniques in Amsterdam and London. At Guy's a tumourectomy rather than a wide excision was performed. In Amsterdam, patients with upper outer quadrant lesions usually had an *en-bloc* resection of tumour and axillary nodes. The dosage of external radiation was 50 Gy in Amsterdam and 46 Gy in London. This led to significantly improved cosmetic results in London, with as yet no difference in terms of loco-regional relapse rates.

At Guy's, patients with involved axillary nodes were randomized to receive either adjuvant chemotherapy (CMF) or no further treatment, and results of this are given in Chapter 7. Essentially, irradiated cases received less CMF but so far this has not been found to affect loco-regional or distant relapse rates.

Lessons from the Guy's iridium trial

The most important finding was that for a substantial proportion of patients with early breast cancer a safe alternative to mastectomy was available. Unlike many of the previous attempts at breast conservation, the cosmetic results were good or excellent in the majority of patients, due to the dovetailing of surgery and interstitial radiotherapy. Tumourectomy yielded sufficient pathological material, except in the case of very small cancers, so that not only were tumour type and grade available but also sufficient tissue was left for measurement of oestrogen and progesterone receptors, and often for subsequent measurement of flow cytometry. Total axillary clearance proved to be an effective way of achieving local control, provided accurate staging information and did not compromise the cosmetic outcome.

The successful results of adjuvant chemotherapy were found to extend not just to those treated by mastectomy, but also to those given radiotherapy, even if some dosage reduction was necessary.

The local relapse rate was the same after mastectomy, with similar numbers developing chest-wall recurrence in the mastectomy group and ipsilateral breast relapse in the irradiated group. Thus it is likely that there is a group of patients with aggressive tumours who will relapse locally after either mastectomy or adequate radiotherapy.

So far approximately 1 per cent of patients undergoing conservative treatment have developed ipsilateral breast relapse every year, and this is consistent with other reports of successful breast-conserving therapy. As in the NSABP B-06 trial, the majority of breast relapses in the irradiated group occurred in the same quadrant which contained the primary tumour. Salvage mastectomy was carried out without any increased morbidity.

The need for external radiotherapy, which must be given over a 5–6-week period, is a limitation on this treatment in that the elderly would be reluctant to undergo so many visits to hospital for treatment.

The requirement for a radiotherapist and physicist to be on site for loading of iridium and treatment planning restricts the applicability of this treatment to centres with on-site radiotherapy facilities.

Ten-year results

It will always be argued that, because of the long-term propensity for relapse in patients with breast cancer, early results of treatment may not adequately reflect the eventual outcome. At present, long-term results are not available for any of the apparently successful trials of breast conservation but some groups, particularly the French, who have been enthusiastic about this technique

Table 5.5 Ten-year relapse-free survival after breast conservation.

No of cases	Stage I (%)	Stage II (%)	Stage III (%)	Reference
304	89	52	29	16
258	90	53	30	17
314	74	56	30	18
263	59	39	–	19
300	72	59	39	20

for some decades, have reported their 10-year results which are summarized in Table 5.5.[16–20] All the data from the French centres are remarkably similar, with an average 81 per cent relapse-free survival for Stage I cases at 10 years, and 55 per cent for patients with Stage II disease. Of those patients with Stage III breast cancers, only 32 per cent were free from disease at 10 years.

Only the British reported atypical results.[19] This was a long-term follow-up of cases treated at the Royal Marsden Hospital by wide excision of tumour, without axillary clearance. Patients received orthovoltage external radiotherapy (45 Gy) to breast and gland fields, subsequently boosted with a further 10 Gy. For patients without clinical evidence of axillary nodal involvement, the 10-year relapse-free survival was 59 per cent for cases with T_1 tumours, and 49 per cent among those with T_2 tumours. However, for those with clinical evidence of axillary nodal metastases the 10-year relapse-free survival fell to 29 per cent. It was recommended by Osborne et al that orthovoltage therapy was inadequate treatment for a patient with clinically involved axilla.[19]

Relapse within the breast after conservative treatment

At present, on an international basis, it is likely that the commonest cause of relapse within the breast after attempted conservation is inadequate treatment. Despite histological confirmation of the completeness of excision of both primary tumour and surrounding in situ component, up to one-third of patients who have not received radiotherapy will develop relapse within the breast, particularly among those with axillary nodal involvement.[13] Thus a major advance in the local control of breast cancer would be to persuade recalcitrant surgeons that their patients will benefit from local irradiation and that this will not invariably lead to telangectasia, fibrosis, radiation necrosis and brachial plexopathy.

However, even after an adequate course of radiotherapy, some patients will subsequently develop relapse in the treated breast. Can such cases be identified in order that they and their doctors can be better informed of the results of breast conservation? At present the answer is a qualified 'no'.

Stage of tumour

The majority of trials of breast conservation have been restricted to patients with Stage I and Stage II tumours. However, in France the tradition of breast irradiation has been such that many patients with larger Stage III cancers have been treated, often without any attempt to remove the large primary tumour. Results of these studies are given in Table 5.6.[17,18,21] What these indicate are that patients with Stage III carcinomas have a high rate of loco-regional relapse (53 per cent) and that only 21 per cent of these patients will have an intact breast 5 years after treatment. These figures should be

Table 5.6 Five-year results of irradiation treatment for Stages I, II and III breast cancer.

	Stage I			Stage II			Stage III			Reference
	n*	DFS†	B+	n*	DFS†	B+‡	n*	DFS†	B+‡	
	120	102	96	203	156	63	191	112	46	17
	550	420	368	553	325	243	341	126	77	18
	89	83	82	235	177	169	74	48	7	21
TOTAL	759	605	546	991	658	475	606	286	130	
(%)		80	72		66	48		47	21	

*n = total number of patients.
†DFS = number of patients disease-free.
‡B+ = number with conserved breasts.

Table 5.7 Age and breast relapse after irradiation.

Follow-up	<30	31–50	>51	Reference
5 years	7/20 (35%)	11/163 (7%)	0/131	22
2 years	10/72 (14%)	15/133 (11%)	9/173 (5%)	23
5 years	26/47 (55%)	14/251 (6%)	10/309 (3%)	24
1 year	4/20 (20%)	88/675 (13%)	55/687 (8%)	25
TOTAL	47/159	128/1222	74/1300	
AVERAGE	(30)	(10)	(6)	

taken into account by anyone planning breast-conserving trials for patients with larger, operable cancers.

Age and relapse

Nature has played a cruel trick. The available data suggest that one of the major determinants of breast relapse is young age—that is, the group of women most anxious to retain their breasts. The results of series in which breast relapse has been examined in relation to age at treatment are shown in Table 5.7.[22–5] Overall, the group aged under 30 have a 30 per cent breast relapse rate. The study with the shortest follow-up has shown the least effect, but all show a consistently increased breast-relapse rate in the younger group treated by radiotherapy. Nevertheless, this does not represent an absolute contraindication to breast conservation. Approximately 70 per cent of those aged under 30 will have successful breast conservation. No evidence is yet available to suggest that the overall survival of these younger women who develop breast relapse is compromised. Faced with this information it is likely that many would still wish to be considered for breast-conserving treatment.

Completeness of excision of the primary tumour

This is a particular problem for radiotherapy centres treating referred patients who have been subjected to a variety of surgical biopsy procedures, with specimens examined by equally varied pathologists. This aspect has been particularly studied by the Joint Center for Radiation Therapy in Boston, where the aforementioned circumstances applied.[26] Among those patients who were originally diagnosed by a less than excisional biopsy, the breast-relapse rate was 35 per cent which fell to 7 per cent in those who had undergone an excision biopsy. This is another argument in favour of close cooperation between surgeons, pathologist and radiologist. For this reason, the Boston group have adopted a policy of re-excision in dubious cases, prior to iridium implantation.[27]

Histopathological prediction of relapse

Since the histological differentiation of a primary tumour does bear a relationship to the subsequent behaviour of the breast cancer it would seem likely that this might

also predict for response to radiotherapy and thus for likelihood of local relapse. Clarke et al reported a breast-relapse rate of 1/139 (1 per cent) for patients with Bloom grade I cancers, compared with 8/66 (12 per cent) for those with grade III lesions.[28] Although this does represent a substantial statistical increase in relative risk, it suggests that the majority of poorly differentiated carcinomas of the breast can be adequately treated by irradiation. The Boston group also found that there was an over-representation of grade III carcinomas among those patients who relapsed within the breast.[29] However, a more important determinant of risk appeared to be the patterns of intraductal carcinoma. Where there was extensive intraductal carcinoma (EIC) present within the tumour itself, or around the tumour, which occupied more than one-quarter of the primary biopsy, this led to a doubling in the risk of local relapse.

In subsequent work the problem of EIC was examined in 607 cases treated by tumourectomy and radical radiotherapy, of which 50 (8 per cent) had relapsed within the

Table 5.8 Age, intraductal carcinoma component and relapse after irradiation.[24]

Age	5-year breast recurrence (%)	
	EIC−	EIC+
<34	22	38
35–50	4	29
51–65	4	16
>66	0	12

EIC = Extensive intraductal carcinoma.

breast. Cases were subdivided into those with EIC (>25% intraductal component) and those with EIC (<25% intraductal component) and the results are given in Table 5.8. This shows that there is an increased relapse rate in all groups with EIC. However, whereas this difference is significant for the older age groups, this is not so for the younger patients (under 30) in whom there is also a high incidence of breast relapse in the absence of EIC.

Thus although the problem of intraductal carcinoma may be partially predictive in older women, it is of less value in younger patients. The conclusion must be that with adequate radiotherapy there is a low risk of breast relapse and no clinical or pathological features are presently known that can be used specifically to exclude patients from breast conservation (provided that they have Stage I or II tumours).

Detection of relapse within the breast

The very act of surgery, followed by radiotherapy, marks the breast with signs normally associated with cancer, that is the presence of a mass (scar tissue), tethering and skin thickening, which both clinically and radiologically can be perplexing. It has become customary to carry out annual bilateral mammography in patients who have been treated by breast conservation. This may be of value in the early detection of contralateral lesions, but it is of much less use in the early detection of relapse. Confronted with a palpable mass deep to the biopsy site, often with skin fixation, tenderness and sometimes skin erythema, most clinicians are reluctant to observe such a case and therefore a biopsy is performed. Approximately 50 per cent of such patients have fat necrosis, rather than relapse.[30]

At Guy's, out of 214 patients treated by breast conservation, 17 developed lumps in the treated breast.[31] Of these, 10 were found to be benign (7 fat necrosis, 2 foreign body granulomas and 1 scar tissue). Mammographic findings of trabecular distortion, skin oedema and breast asymmetry were equally distributed between those with benign and malignant lumps. Spiculated lesions were more commonly found in those with relapse (five versus one). Microcalcification was seen in three of those who had relapsed and none of those whose biopsy was benign.

Mahoney examined both mammography and thermography as methods to detect relapse and concluded that the latter was valueless.[32] Out of 51 patients who relapsed, this was detected originally by mammography alone in only one case. However, Stomper et al reported from JCRT in Boston that of 23 patients with breast relapse the reason for the biopsy was a mammographic abnormality in eight (35 per cent). The usual finding was microcalcification, occasionally with a spiculated mass.

It has to be concluded that regular examination by an experienced clinician is the basis for follow-up of patients treated by breast irradiation. Mammography provides some back-up, but the decision on whether to biopsy or not will largely depend upon unquantifiable clinical judgments.

References

1 Keynes G, The treatment of primary carcinoma of the breast with radium, *Acta Radiol* (1929) **10**:393–402.

2 Keynes G, Conservative treatment of cancer of the breast, *Br Med J* (1937) **2**:643–47.

3 Pfahler GE, Results of radiation therapy in 1022 private cases of carcinoma of the breast, *Am J Roentgenol Rad Ther* (1932) **27**:497–508.

4 Baclesse F, Roentgen therapy as the sole method of treatment of cancer of the breast, *Am J Roentgenol Rad Ther* (1949) **62**:311–318.

5 Pierquin B, Owen R, Maylin C et al, Radical radiation therapy of breast cancer. *Int J Radiat Oncol Biol Phys* (1980) **6**:17–24.

6 Hellman S, Harris JR, Levene MB, Radiation therapy of early carcinoma of the breast without mastectomy, *Cancer* (1980) **46**:;988–94.

7 Atkins HJ, Hayward JL, Klugman DJ et al, Treatment of early breast cancer: a report after ten years of a clinical trial, *Br Med J* (1972) **2**:423–9.

8 Hayward JL, Trials of wide excision and radiation therapy at the Breast Unit, Guy's Hospital, London. In: Zander JBJ, ed. *Early breast cancer.* (Springer-Verlag: Berlin, Heidelberg 1985).

9 Hayward JL, Caleffi M, The significance of local control in the primary treatment of breast cancer, *Arch Surg* (1987) **122**:1244–47.

10 Veronesi U, Saccozzi R, Del Vecchio M et al, Comparing radical mastectomy with quadrantectomy, axillary dissection, and radiotherapy in patients with small cancers of the breast, *N Engl J Med* (1981) **305**:6–11.

11 Veronesi U, Banti A, Del Vecchio M et al, Comparison of Halsted mastectomy with quadrantectomy, axillary dissection and radiotherapy in early breast cancer: long-term results, *Eur J Cancer Clin Oncol* (1986) **22**:1085–9.

12 Sarrazin D, Le M, Rouesse J et al, Conservative treatment versus mastectomy in breast cancer tumours with macroscopic diameter of 20 millimetres or less, *Cancer* (1984) **53**: 1209–13.

13 Fisher B, Bauer M, Margolese R et al, Five-year results of a randomised clinical trial comparing total mastectomy and segmental mastectomy with or without radiation in the treatment of breast cancer, *N Engl J Med* (1985) **312**:665–73.

14 Fisher B, Redmond C, Poisson R et al, Eight year results of a randomised trial comparing total mastectomy and lumpectomy without irradiation in the treatment of breast cancer, *N Engl J Med* (1989) **320**:822–8.

15 Hayward JL, Winter PJ, Tong D et al, A new combined approach to the conservative treatment of early breast cancer, *Surgery* (1984) **95**:270–4.

16 Schottenfeld D, Nash AG, Robbins GF et al, Ten year results of the treatment of primary operable breast carcinoma. A summary of 304 patients evaluated by the TNM system, *Cancer* (1976) **38**:1001–7.

17 Calle R, Pilleron JP, Schlienger P et al, Conservative management of operable breast cancer. Ten years experience at the Foundation Curie, *Cancer* (1978) **42**:2045–53.

18 Amalric R, Santamaria F, Robert F et al, Radiation therapy with or without primary limited surgery for operable breast cancer. A 20 year experience at the Marseilles Cancer Institute, *Cancer* (1982) **49**:30–4.

19 Osborne MP, Ormiston N, Harmer CL et al, Breast conservation in the treatment of early breast cancer, *Cancer* (1984) **53**:349–55.

20 Pierquin B, Raynal M, Otmezguine Y et al, Le traitement conservateur des cancers du sein. Resultats à 10 ans, *La Presse Medicale* (1986) **15**:375–7.

21 Pierquin B, Otymezguine Y, Lobo PA, Conservative management of breast carcinoma. The Creteil experience, *Acta Radiol Oncol* (1983) **22**:101–7.

22 Vilcoq JR, Calle R, Stacey P et al, The outcome of patients with operable breast cancer. *Int J Radiat Oncol Biol Phys* (1981) **7**:1327–37.

23 Matthews RH, McNeese MD, Montague ED et al, Prognostic implications of age in breast cancer patients treated with tumourectomy and irradiation or with mastectomy, *Int J Radiat Oncol Biol Phys* (1988) **14**:659–63.

24 Recht A, Connolly JL, Schnitt SJ et al, The effect of young age on tumour recurrence in the treated breast after conservative surgery and radiotherapy, *Int J Radiat Oncol Biol Phys* (1988) **14**:3–10.

25 Kurtz JM, Spitalier J-M, Amalric R et al, Mammary recurrences in women younger than forty, *Int J Radiat Oncol Biol Phys* (1988) **15**:271–6.

26 Recht A, Silver B, Schnitt S et al, Breast relapse following primary radiation therapy for early breast cancer. I. Classification frequency and salvage, *Int J Radiat Oncol Biol Phys* (1985) **11**:1271–6.

27 Schnitt SJ, Connolly JL, Khettry U et al, Pathologic findings on re-excision of the primary site in breast cancer patients considered for treatment by primary radiation therapy, *Cancer* (1987) **59**:675–81.

28 Clarke DH, Le MG, Sarrazin D et al, Analysis of local-regional relapses in patients with early breast cancers treated by excision and radiotherapy: experience of the Institut Gustave-Roussy, *Int J Radiat Oncol Biol Phys* (1985) **11**:137–45.

29 Schnitt SJ, Connolly JL, Harris JR et al, Pathologic predictors of early local recurrence in Stage I and II breast cancer treated by primary radiation therapy, *Cancer* (1984) **53**:1049–57.

30 Clarke D, Curtis JL, Martinez A et al, Fat necrosis of the breast stimulating recurrent carcinoma after primary radiotherapy in the management of early stage breast carcinoma, *Cancer* (1983) **52**:442–5.

31 Chaudary MA, Girling A, Girling S et al, New lumps in the breast following conservation treatment for early breast cancer, *Breast Cancer Res Treat* (1988) **11**:51–8.

32 Mahoney L, Methods for detecting locally recurrent and contralateral second primary breast cancer, *Can J Surg* (1986) **29**:372–3.

33 Stomper PC, Recht A, Berenberg AL, Mammographic detection of recurrent cancer in the irradiated breast, *Am J Roentgenol* (1987) **148**:39–43.

Appendix 1 to Chapter 5

Surgical Technique of Axillary Clearance

The patient is placed in the supine position with a small sandbag under the ipsilateral latissimus muscle in order to compress and display its lateral margin. Skin preparation includes the entire breast and extends medially over the midline inferiorly to the costal margin, superiorly to the supraclavicular fossa and laterally to include the latissimus dorsi and arm down to the elbow. The arm is draped in stockinette and then tied over a sterile draped armboard with a crepe bandage, in order that it can be moved during the procedure. Final draping is as shown in Figure 5.5.

It is usually easiest if the assistant stands on the same side as the operator, on the other side of the patient's outstretched arm. The proposed skin crease incision, which lies just posterior to the lateral border of pectoralis major, is marked. The length of this incision will depend upon the experience of the operator and the build of the patient. It is possible to perform the procedure through a 4 cm incision.

Before surgery is commenced the skin is infiltrated with 1:200 000 adrenaline in normal saline, in order to reduce subcutaneous haemorrhage.

After the skin incision has been made the edges are undercut. Anteriorly, the dissection extends down to the fibres of pectoralis major and the lateral margin of the muscle is freed from its covering fat (Figure 5.6). Similarly the posterior flap is extended to the anterior border of latissimus dorsi and these

two are joined at the lateral end. With a combination of sharp and blunt dissection the suspensory ligament of the axilla is divided and the lateral border of pectoralis minor is exposed. The muscle is encircled 3 cm below its insertion on to the coracoid process. Until recently it has been customary to divide the insertion of pectoralis minor in order to facilitate access to high nodes. Recently, in thinner patients it has been possible to retract the muscle, which is therefore conserved.

The axillary vein is exposed by gentle blunt dissection with Lahey swab-holding forceps. Tributaries of the axillary veins joining its infero-medial side are dissected and diathermied. Only rarely is it necessary for these to be ligated. The dissection proceeds apically. The apex of the axilla is best displayed by abduction and external rotation of the shoulder with the elbow flexed. A marker suture is inserted in the fat at the lower border of pectoralis minor and another at the apex. The tissue is then swept downwards by finger direction with or without division of the origin of pectoralis minor. As the finger sweeps downward, so intercostal perforators will be encountered which require diathermy. In the fold of fat the nerve to serratus anterior is usually evident and is freed by incision along its lateral wide. It can then be swept medially with a gauze dissecting swab. The fold of fat to which it was attached is grasped with artery forceps and gently retracted whilst diathermy is

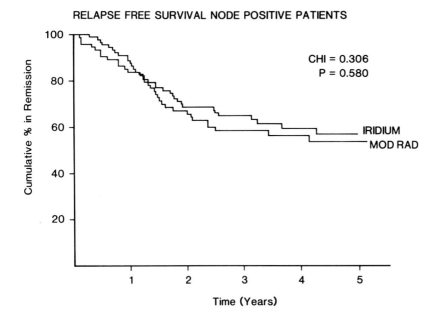

Figure 5.3　　Relapse-free survival of node-positive patients treated by either modified radical mastectomy or iridium implant.

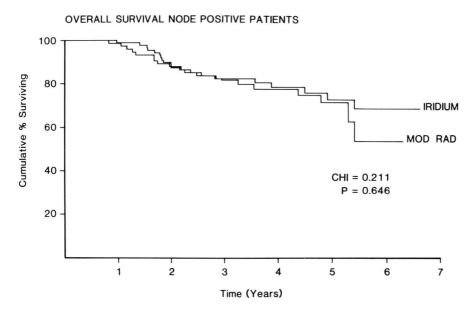

Figure 5.4　　Overall survival of node-positive patients treated by either modified radical mastectomy or iridium implant.

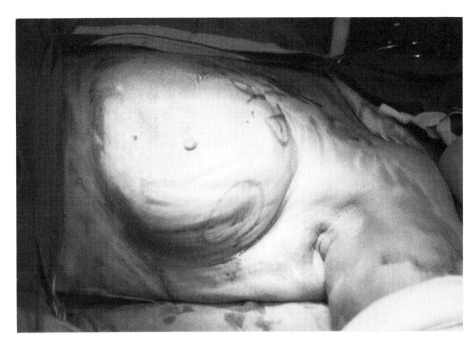

Figure 5.5   Draping of patient for axillary clearance procedure has been marked preoperatively on patient's skin.

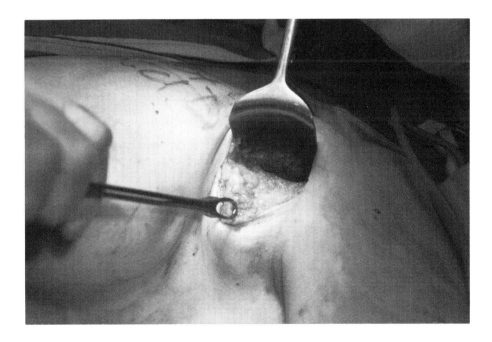

Figure 5.6   Axillary clearance retraction displays edge of pectoralis minor. Forceps on axillary fat.

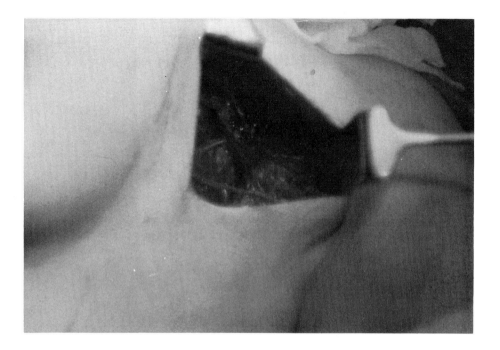

Figure 5.7   Completion of axillary dissection shows nerves to serratus anterior and latissimus dorsi which have been preserved.

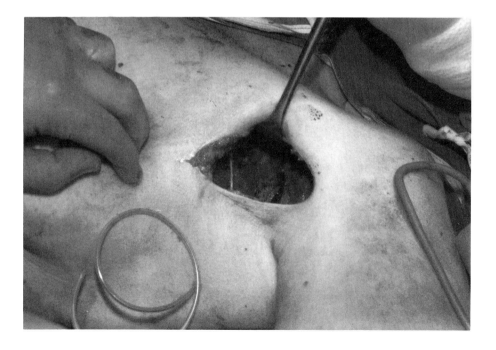

Figure 5.8   Insertion of drain to axilla.

applied to small vessels. The fold is freed until the nerve to latissimus dorsi is identified after which the fold can be swept downwards with gauze dissection. Fat and nodes are cleared from the subscapular vessels. Only rarely, when the nerve is infiltrated by a metastatic node, is it necessary for it to be sacrificed. Fat is then cleared from the fibres of latissimus dorsi until the specimen is attached only by a pedicle formed by the axillary tail of the breast. This is divided with a knife, after which on or two medium-sized vessels in the axillary tail require coagulation (Figure 5.7).

After a preliminary check of haemostasis, the wound is irrigated with sterile water at 47°C and final haemostasis is checked paying attention to the apex, the divided origin and pectoralis minor and the axillary tial. A single suction drain is inserted and sutured to fibres of serratus anterior with a catgut suture. The skin is then closed and the drain fixed to the skin with non-absorbable sutures, after which the drain is attached to suction (Figure 5.8).

Postoperatively, shoulder exercises are not started until the drainage has reduced sufficiently for the axillary drain to be removed. This minimizes the length of time during which drainage occurs, and yet does not lead to any increase in shoulder stiffness. It was the policy at Guy's to leave the axillary drain in situ until the daily drainage was less than 20 ml on two successive days. However, recently a trial has been conducted which has shown that there are no disadvantages in taking the drain out after 5 days, irrespective of volume of fluid drained. Some patients will need to return for outpatient aspiration but this does not lead to any increase in infection, nor any depreciation in either shoulder movement or cosmetic outcome.

Appendix 2 to Chapter 5

Technique of Iridium Implant

Once the axillary clearance has been completed and the tumour has been excised through a skin-crease incision, the cavity is drained with a closed vacuum drain (Figures 5.9–5.11) after which the radiotherapist performs the implant. After measurement and marking of the proposed entry and exit sites on the skin, a series of hollow steel introducers are inserted (Figure 5.12). A single-, double- or very rarely a triple-plane implant is performed. Through the steel introducers plastic tubes are inserted, after which the steel tubes are removed. Marker wires (non-active) are inserted and crimped in

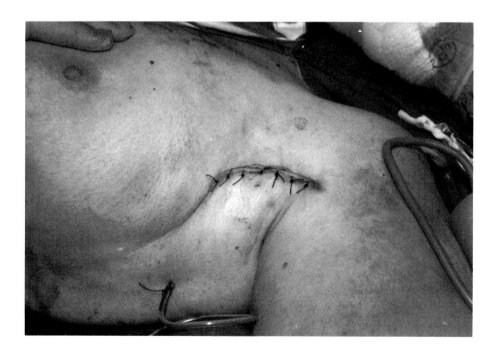

Figure 5.9   Completion of axillary clearance.

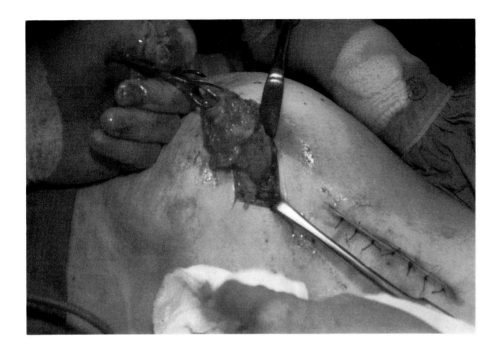

Figure 5.10   Excision of carcinoma.

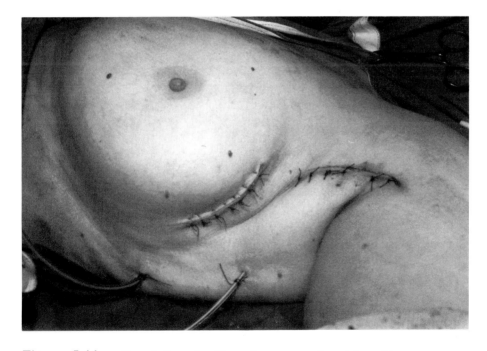

Figure 5.11   Completion of axillary clearance and excision of tumour with drain to both biopsy site and axilla.

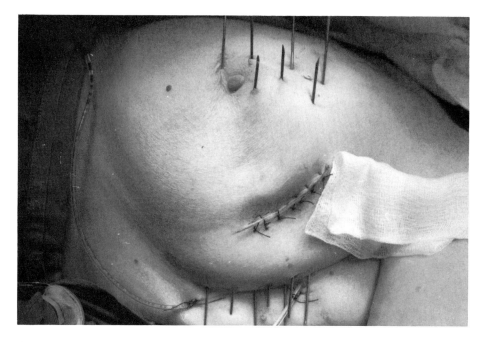

Figure 5.12   Insertion of needles through biopsy site.

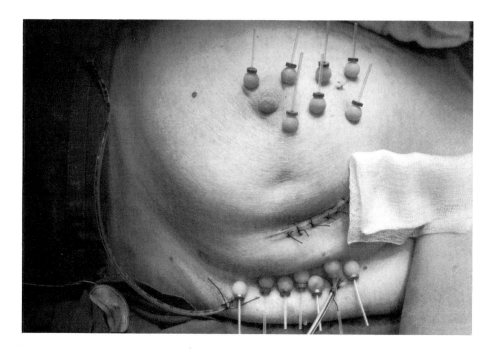

Figure 5.13   Two-plane implant showing plastic tubes with inert wires.
Plastic beads are held in place with lightly crimped lead discs.

place with lead discs and nylon balls to hold the flexible tubes in place. Another marker wire is taped along the skin incision (Figure 5.13). The entire implant is dressed with cotton wool.

The following day, orthogonal radiographs are taken in order to determine the geometry of the implant and then the required lengths, activity and location of the iridium wires are computed in order to deliver a mid-phase dose of 20 Gy. This implant remains in situ for approximately 48 hours, after which both the active wires and the plastic tubes are removed. This is a virtually painless procedure.

CHAPTER 6
THE ROLE OF MASTECTOMY

These statistics are so remarkably good that we are encouraged to hope for a much brighter, if not a very bright future for cancer of the breast.

William Halsted

In 1894, Halsted published the results of his new radical operation for breast cancer.[1] He had been fairly successful in treating 50 patients with tumours that were so advanced that nowadays they would not be considered for surgery. Some of his reasoning can now be seen as fallacious, and his statistical techniques and assessment of response were primitive, but nevertheless they were in accordance with the *Zeitgeist*.

Regrettably, his memory has been besmirched with revelations of opiate addiction and the implication that this clouded his judgment, so negating his achievement. Now that we have the opportunity to treat patients with much smaller breast cancers it is still important that the lessons that Halsted taught are not forgotten.

A move from radical towards minimal surgery may lead to an increase in local relapse rate and a loss of important prognostic information upon which subsequent treatment can be planned. As smaller tumours are treated by conservation, so cases with larger cancers may amplify the inadequacy of procedures such as total (simple) mastectomy.

History

As part of the background for his work, Halsted reviewed the published results of surgical treatment for breast cancer.[2] Largely emanating from the Austro-Hungarian Empire they make sorry reading (Table 6.1). This indicates that the majority of patients developed loco-regional relapse after these procedures, because of their irradical nature. Halsted reversed this trend and managed to achieve loco-regional control in over 80 per cent of his patients, even though three-quarters had Stage III cancers. Interestingly, loco-regional relapse occurred more frequently in Stage II than in Stage III tumours (23 per cent versus 14 per cent).

Halsted recognized that unless clearance of the malignant field was achieved local relapse would be inevitable. Thus the concept of *en bloc* resection was introduced with extension of the operative field not only to the axilla, but also to the supraclavicular fossa. The theory of lymphatic spread is now regarded as an oversimplification. However, to disregard a radical approach, which need not necessarily be surgical, will be to risk the

Table 6.1 Local control after mastectomy by Halsted and his peers.

Surgeon	Number of cases	Local relapse-free survival (%)
Bergmann	114	45
Billroth	170	18
Czerny	102	38
Fischer	147	25
Gussenbauer	151	36
König	152	40
Kuster	228	40
Lucke	110	34
Volkmann	131	40
Halsted	50	84

high rates of local relapse which so appalled nineteenth-century surgeons.

One problem remains the same. The reason why Halsted saw so few early breast cancers was not just because patients presented with more advanced cancers, but also because physicians were reluctant to refer cases of breast cancer, because they regarded the condition as incurable. This nihilistic predeterminist philosophy still prevails among many clinicians.

In the same year, Meyer published the results of his similar radical operation in which both the pectoralis major and minor muscles were invariably excised.[3] The operation, separately devised by Halsted and Meyer, became the standard surgical treatment for breast cancer. In this way surgery came to be regarded as the treatment of choice for early breast cancer, although gradually the ascendancy of radical mastectomy came to be challenged.

It was apparent that lymphatic dissemination was not the only route of metastasis and that many patients with apparently early disease had blood-borne micrometastases. In addition, radiotherapy techniques improved so that McWhirter took the apparently heretical step of treating patients by total mastectomy without axillary surgery but using external radiotherapy to treat the axilla.[4] The sky did not descend upon the earth. Results of this lesser surgical procedure appeared to be as good as those following radical mastectomy.

Patey responded in a different way. Arguing that local spread was more likely to be lymphatic, and that fascia did provide a barrier in early stages, he modified Halsted's operation.[5] Pectoralis major was left intact, but pectoralis minor was excised in order that the axilla could be cleared. The local relapse-free survival of 42 patients treated by radical mastectomy was 76 per cent compared with 82 per cent for the 40 patients treated by the modified operation. Many surgeons changed to the modified operation which avoided chest-wall indentation produced by removal of pectoralis major. This was taken one stage further by Madden who described another modification in which both pectoral muscles were conserved.[6]

Meanwhile, the flame of radical surgery was still burning at the Memorial Hospital in New York. As a result of the work of Handley which had shown that lymphatic spread occurred not only laterally to the axilla but also medially to the internal mammary nodes,[7] Urban designed the extended radical mastectomy.[8] This represented the ultimate in surgical endeavour to extirpate breast cancer, with an *en bloc* resection of ribs, costal cartilages and internal mammary nodes.

Then the fragmentation of surgical confidence began. As results of long-term follow-up became available it was apparent that only 1 in 5 of patients treated by mastectomy would be alive 20 years later and this diminished surgeons' belief in their ability to cure breast cancer. Another cause of confusion was the proliferation of clinical trials which, far from clarifying the appropriate options, actually led to a higher state of uncertainty and a drift away from radical surgery.

Finally, other disciplines proved their ability to contribute to the treatment of patients with apparently early breast cancer. Because of this some surgeons felt that their leading role had been usurped by thrusting radiotherapeutic and chemotherapeutic pretenders to the throne.

Can the confidence of surgeons be restored? Can the multiple strands derived from clinical trials be united in a common thread to fix firmly the appropriate role for the appropriate mastectomy?

Clinical trials of mastectomy options

The prime determinant of the success of mastectomy must be its effect on local control. This will in turn have some bearing on survival, contrary to the view of the predeterminist school. Two important events have forced a recommendation of the most appropriate form of mastectomy. The first is the overwhelming evidence that some small cancers can be treated by breast conservation (as discussed in Chapter 5). The second is the proof that systemic adjuvant therapy can improve both relapse-free and overall survival rates. Since at present axillary nodal status is the major prognostic determinant and therefore indicator of need for adjuvant treatment, this information has to be acquired as part of the primary procedure.

Thus control of disease and prognostic feedback have to be jointly considered in the evaluation of any technique of mastectomy.

Merits of a variety of available procedures have been ignored. Unfortunately, the neologistically designated 'total mastectomy' has hijacked the position of treatment of choice. The nomenclature 'total mastectomy' has been pressed upon the oncological world and, like the euphemisms of the copywriter, 'total' is deemed synonymous with 'complete', that is an adequate procedure. It is assumed that all forms of mastectomy achieve equal end-results. The following myths are current:

1 Total mastectomy = total mastectomy + radiotherapy
2 Total mastectomy = radical mastectomy
3 Modified radical mastectomy = radical mastectomy
4 Extended radical mastectomy = radical mastectomy.

The present *laissez faire* attitude is not justified by a critical examination of the results of clinical trials. Subgroups of patients require different forms of treatment. The lowest common denominator, total mastectomy, will if employed ubiquitously result in the lowest rate of local control and subsequent diminution of survival for some patients.

Total mastectomy versus radical mastectomy

Only one trial has directly compared total mastectomy with radical mastectomy and this was aborted prematurely because the investigators became aware of the inadequacy of total mastectomy.[9] The study was conducted at Groote Schuur Hospital in Capetown and 95 patients were entered, all of whom had Stage I or II disease.

All were aged less than 70 years and had primary tumours no greater than 5 cm diameter which had a histological diagnosis

Table 6.2 Loco-regional relapse in trial of total (TM) versus radical mastectomy (RM).[9]

	TM	RM
No of cases	51	44
Flap recurrence	7	1
Axilla	5	0
Total no of relapses	12 (24%)	1 (2%)

Table 6.3 NSABP trial B-04 comparing radical mastectomy (RM), total mastectomy + radiotherapy (TMR) and total mastectomy (TM) for node-negative cases.

	RM	TMR	TM
No of cases	362	352	365
Axillary relapse	5 (1)	11 (3)	65 (18)
Supraclavicular node relapse	4 (1)	1 (0.3)	11 (3)
10-year overall survival	165 (46)	169 (48)	151 (41)

Percentages in parentheses.

made by frozen section. Details of loco-regional relapse are given in Table 6.2, which shows the very high rate of 24 per cent in those treated by total mastectomy as compared with only 2 per cent for those treated by radical mastectomy. This result

demonstrating a tenfold increase should be engraved upon the scalpels of all surgeons who treat breast cancer.

The NSABP trial B-04 investigated the respective merits of radical mastectomy, total mastectomy and total mastectomy with post-operative radiotherapy for patients with clinically node-negative operable breast cancer.[10,11] The 10-year results are given in Table 6.3. In the group treated by total mastectomy alone tumour relapse occurred in the axillae of 65 patients (18 per cent). This was treated by delayed axillary clearance. Supraclavicular fossa node recurrence was the first site of treatment failure in 11 of the group treated by total mastectomy as compared with only one of the irradiated group and four of the group treated by radical mastectomy. This does imply that a few patients went on to develop regional relapse that would not have occurred if the axilla had been adequately treated at the time of diagnosis. Supraclavicular fossa node relapse carries a dire prognosis, being almost invariably associated with subsequent distant relapse.[12]

Although there was no statistically significant difference between the overall survival rates of the three groups, there were fewer survivors in the group treated by total mastectomy. Even with marginal survival benefits, it is most important for patients' quality of life that optimal local control is obtained, which total mastectomy alone signally fails to achieve. Trial B-04 indicates that even patients with clinically negative axilla have a 20 per cent relapse rate within the axilla which will require salvage treatment.

In the Cardiff trial, patients with clinically negative axillary nodes were randomized to treatment by either total or radical mastectomy.[13] As is shown in Table 6.4, there was a 19 per cent rate of relapse within the untreated axillae of the total mastectomy group. Despite the lack of statistical significance, again the overall survival of the

Table 6.4 Cardiff trial comparing radical mastectomy (RM) with total mastectomy (TM) for clinically node-negative cases.

	RM	*TM*
No of cases	66	64
Axillary relapse	1 (2%)	12 (19%)
Scar relapse	10 (15%)	9 (13%)
10-year overall survival	44 (66%)	37 (58%)

radical mastectomy group was better (66 per cent versus 56 per cent).

Radical versus total mastectomy and radiotherapy

Within the NSABP B-04 trial, patients with clinically positive axillae were randomized to either radical mastectomy or total mastectomy with irradiation of axilla, internal mammary nodes and supraclavicular fossa (45 Gy). Similar entry criteria were used within the Cardiff trial and patients were similarly irradiated, but to a dose of 40 Gy. Both studies reported no significant differences in terms of relapse-free or overall survival, as shown in Table 6.5. However, the overall survival of the radical mastectomy group was better than the total mastectomy group in both trials.

The Manchester regional trial also allocated clinically node-positive cases to treatment by either radical mastectomy or total mastectomy with irradiation.[14] No differences were found in terms of relapse-free survival, but after 10 years 13 per cent more of those treated by radical mastectomy were alive.

In a multicentre trial conducted in southeast Scotland, women aged 35–69 with operable breast cancer were treated by either radical mastectomy or total mastectomy with postoperative radiotherapy.[15] The results of this trial, given in Table 6.5, were that both relapse-free and overall survival were significantly better in the group treated by radical mastectomy. This survival benefit was largely enjoyed by those with Stage I tumours.

The results of both this study and the Guy's Hospital trials provide a powerful argument in favour of adequate local treatment.[16] Thus failure to control the primary disease complex can not only result in an increased local relapse rate but may also diminish the patient's chances of survival.

Total mastectomy with or without axillary irradiation

Several trials have examined the value of immediate axillary irradiation compared with subsequent irradiation, or surgery, at the time of clinical relapse and these are shown in Table 6.6. The Southampton study included patients aged up to 70 years and all had a total mastectomy with an axillary lymph-node biopsy.[17] Irrespective of the axillary nodal histology they were randomized to immediate radiotherapy or observation. A significantly increased rate of axillary nodal relapse was reported in the observation group, but no effect on overall survival was seen.

Table 6.5 Trials comparing total mastectomy and axillary irradiation (TMR) with radical mastectomy (RM).

	Follow-up	TMR			RM			
		No	Local relapse (%)	Overall survival (%)	No	Local relapse (%)	Overall survival (%)	References
NSABP	10 years	294	13	26	292	15	30	11
Cardiff	10 years	39	31	38	31	9	41	13
SE Scotland	12 years	242	17	50	256	12	55	15
Manchester	10 years	159	38	31	149	39	35	14

Table 6.6 Results of trials comparing total mastectomy (TM) with total mastectomy and radiotherapy (TMR).

	Follow-up	TM			TMR			
		No	Axillary relapse (%)	Overall survival (%)	No	Axillary relapse (%)	Overall survival (%)	References
Southampton	3 years	76	28	81	74	9	78	17
CRC	10 years	1140	10	70	1103	2	73	18
Manchester	10 years	359	37	55	355	19	62	14
NSABP	10 years	365	18	41	352	3	48	11

The Cancer Research Campaign (CRC) supported a British trial which set out to compare a watch policy with immediate axillary irradiation.[18,19] Although the trial aimed to accrue patients with both clinically positive and negative axillae, there was an under-representation of the former group within the study. Of the total of 2243 evaluable cases, 1140 were treated by the watch policy and 1103 had immediate post-operative irradiation. Significantly more of the watched patients developed axillary relapse, but overall survival rates were not significantly different, although more of the watched group died of breast cancer. Broadly similar results were reported by both the Manchester Regional study[14] and the NSABP.[11] In every study, the survival of the irradiated group was slightly better than that of the total mastectomy cases.

Modified versus radical mastectomy

There is a tacit agreement between most surgeons to accept that the Patey and Halsted operations are equally effective in terms of local disease control and overall survival. Few have deemed it necessary to subject the two procedures to a clinical trial. However, two studies have specifically addressed this question.[20,21] The outline results are given in Table 6.7. Although neither study found any statistically significant difference between the results of the two operations, nevertheless the overall survival of patients treated by the Halsted operation was greater in both trials. In addition, local control was better for those treated by the Halsted procedure.

When the subset of patients with larger tumours (T_2T_3) was examined separately there was a significantly increased relapse-free survival rate for those treated by radical mastectomy (59 per cent versus 38 per cent). As mastectomy becomes the exclusive therapy for patients with larger primary tumours, so these trials may need to be repeated, to make sure that such cases are not being deprived of the maximal chance of local control of disease.

Radical versus extended radical mastectomy

A large international study has compared patients treated by Halsted mastectomy with those who received an extended operation with dissection of the internal mammary nodes.[22] Collaborating centres were the Institut Gustave-Roussy Paris, National Cancer Institute (NCI) Milan, Regina Elena Institute Rome, NCI Warsaw and NCI Lima. A total of 1580 cases was entered and the 5-year results are given in Table 6.8.

Table 6.7 Trials comparing modified radical mastectomy (MRM) with radical mastectomy (RM).

n	Follow-up	Local RFS (%)		Overall survival (%)		Reference
		MRM	RM	MRM	RM	
534	5 years	78	75	78	85	20
311	10 years	89	94	64	71	21

RFS = Relapse-free survival.

Table 6.8 Five-year survival rates of patients in trial comparing radical mastectomy (RM) with extended radical mastectomy (ERM).[22]

	RM	ERM
No of cases	811	769
Overall survival (%)	69	72
Node negative		
Outer T_1T_2 (%)	87	78
Inner/central T_1T_2 (%)	89	88
Node positive		
Outer T_1T_2 (%)	63	68
Inner/central T_1T_2 (%)	52	71

Although there was no significant difference between the overall survival of the two groups, when a subset analysis was conducted there did appear to be a benefit for patients with medial/central T_1/T_2 tumours in whom there was axillary nodal involvement.

The 10-year results again showed no significant difference between the outcome of patients treated by the two operations.[23] In addition, it was apparent that there were wide differences between the centres in terms of the numbers of axillary nodes examined and the percentage of involved internal mammary nodes. Thus the group postulated to benefit may have been a statistical artefact, particularly since the groups were not well defined.

Meier has argued that the extended radical mastectomy used in the international trial was not the operation designed by Urban.[24]

Thus an *en bloc* resection of ribs and internal mammary nodes was not performed. For this reason a trial was run at the University of Chicago, comparing the Halsted radical with the Urban extended-radical operation, with 56 patients treated by the former and 56 treated by the latter procedure. After 10 years, the overall survival of the Halsted group was 74 per cent compared with 62 per cent for those treated by the Urban procedure. Survival was similar for those with laterally located tumours treated by both procedures. However, for those with central/medial lesions, the overall survival was 85 per cent for those treated by extended radical compared with only 60 per cent for those treated by radical mastectomy. Thus Meier and colleagues recommend an extended radical mastectomy for patients with T_1/T_2 medially located tumours.

A Danish study compared extended radical mastectomy with total mastectomy followed by radiotherapy to the gland fields including the internal mammary chain.[25] After 5 years the relapse-free and overall survival of the two groups were identical. This does suggest that irradiation of the internal mammary chain, which is an intrinsic part of breast-conserving treatment, will obviate the need for extended surgery.

Indications for mastectomy

Total mastectomy is a totally inadequate procedure for both the local treatment and prognostic staging of operable invasive breast cancer. It is an appropriate operation for patients with proven multifocal ductal carcinoma in situ (DCIS), where the probability of axillary nodal metastasis is less than 0.02. For patients who have had breast conservation including axillary clearance and irradiation, total mastectomy is the correct salvage procedure following operable relapse within the treated breast.

Additionally, total mastectomy is the operation of choice for patients with breast sarcomas where there is no likelihood of axillary nodal involvement. Finally, total mastectomy may have a place when a salvage procedure is necessary under local anaesthetic because the patient is too ill to withstand a general anaesthetic. Such cases are rare and, with the high standards of present-day anaesthesia, are likely to become even rarer, particularly if their pre-existing medical conditions are optimally treated.

Total mastectomy should not be used as the standard operation for elderly women. If a patient can tolerate a general anaesthetic and requires a mastectomy, this should include an axillary clearance. For a surgeon trained in this procedure, the increase in operating time is likely to be less than 15 minutes, but with a disproportionate increase in probability of local disease control.

This is not the time to argue for a return to the Halsted mastectomy, even though the procedure may give slightly better local control for some patients with larger tumours. The approximately equivalent Patey operation should be regarded as the most appropriate procedure for patients with invasive breast cancer who need a mastectomy. Trials still need to be conducted to elucidate whether patients with larger tumours, without nodal involvement, will derive more or similar benefit from radiotherapy rather than the systemic adjuvant therapy which is now being advocated.

If the classical mastectomy is unpopular, then the extended radical mastectomy probably ranks as public enemy number one in the view of most surgeons. The possible benefits for probably less than 5 per cent of patients are outweighed by the prolongation of operative time (which may be as long as 5 hours) with the consequent postoperative morbidity. As a site of local relapse, internal mammary nodes rarely produce a clinical problem, which can usually be treated by subsequent radiotherapy.

It is important that the benefits from breast conservation for the majority are not counterbalanced by the more widespread acceptance of total mastectomy (without axillary clearance) as the treatment of choice for larger breast cancers. Since clinical trials of different forms of mastectomy are likely to be regarded as *passé*, it may take many years before surgeons are able to appreciate the patient morbidity caused by the inadequate and inaccurately titled total mastectomy.

Breast reconstruction after mastectomy

Some of the arguments concerning breast reconstruction after mastectomy have lost their heat. Many of the patients (particularly younger women) can now be treated by conservation that, when performed correctly, is capable of yielding much better cosmetic results than even the most carefully performed plastic surgery. This is not intended as a slight on plastic surgeons, but their task is made very difficult following the preliminary attack by a general surgeon, together with the propensity of the subcutaneous tissue of the breast to form a constricting capsule around an implanted prosthesis.

Despite these difficulties, plastic surgeons have been very ingenious in devising a variety of techniques to replace lost skin, missing breast tissue and an absent nipple. Skin flaps may be based on the subscapular artery (latissimus dorsi flap),[26] or on the superior epigastric artery (transverse or longitudinal rectus abdominus flap).[27] More recently, subcutaneous expanders have been inserted and gradually inflated with sterile fluid in order to stretch the skin of the mastectomy flaps.[28] Following this a sub-pectoral implant of a silicone prosthesis can be achieved. Subcutaneous placement of the prosthesis has been largely superseded since the cosmetic results were less satisfactory because of capsule formation. The nipple/areola complex can be reconstructed either by a splitting of the contralateral nipple, or alternatively with a labial or auricular graft.[29,30] These procedures are now being performed by many breast surgeons, keen to exercise their operative skills in an environment where major procedures are being eschewed as primary treatment.

It is important that enthusiasm for breast reconstruction is tempered by consideration of its value for individual patients. Thus some women are rather bludgeoned into accepting a reconstructive procedure as part of their primary treatment, despite being prepared to accept the change of body image implicit in mastectomy. Absent or altered skin sensation, with or without capsule formation, may lead to equally serious changes in body image with dissatisfaction concerning the reconstructive procedure.

Apart from the subjective problems associated with immediate reconstruction, it is also important to question whether this has any effect on outcome after local relapse, and particularly on overall survival. At present there are no data available to answer this question, which has not been subjected to a prospective trial.

Skin relapse after mastectomy can be divided into two subtypes, multiple and single, and patients with these different patterns of local relapse carry a different prognosis.[31] Multiple recurrences are associated with a dire prognosis and all such cases will be dead within 5 years. In contrast, single skin recurrence has a slightly better outlook with 20 per cent being alive without further relapse 10 years later, provided that these receive adequate local treatment (excision and radiotherapy).

Of the local relapses the majority will occur within 2 years of mastectomy. Thus the conservative advice would be to defer breast reconstruction for a minimum of 2 years after primary treatment, particularly in node-positive cases. However, this may be longer than many patients will tolerate being without one of their breasts. For the woman who needs a mastectomy, but refuses this procedure unless immediate reconstruction is performed, it is kinder to concur with her wishes, providing that she accepts that there may be problems of subsequent relapse within a reconstructed field. This is much less of a risk in patients with multifocal DCIS where immediate reconstruction is unlikely to be compromised by subsequent local relapse.

A trial that needs to be carried out is a randomized comparison of radiotherapy to the breast for patients with multifocal DCIS compared with total mastectomy and immediate reconstruction.

References

1 Halsted WS, The results of operations for the cure of cancer of the breast performed at the Johns Hopkins Hospital from June 1889 to January 1894, *Arch Surg* (1894) **20**:497–501.

2 Halsted WS, The results of operations for the cure of cancer of the breast performed at the Johns Hopkins Hospital from June 1889 to January 1894, *Johns Hopkins Hospital Reports* (1895) **4**:297–349.

3 Meyer W, An improved method for the radical operation for carcinoma of the breast, *Med Rec* (1894) **46**:746–51.

4 McWhirter R, The value of simple mastectomy and radiotherapy in the treatment of cancer of the breast, *Br J Radiol* (1948) **21**:599–605.

5 Patey DH, Dyson WH, The prognosis of carcinoma of the breast in relation to the type of operation performed, *Br J Cancer* (1948) **2**:7–13.

6 Madden JL, Kandalaft S, Bourque R, Modified radical mastectomy, *Ann Surg* (1972) **175**:624–34.

7 Handley RS, Thackray AC, Invasion of the internal mammary lymph glands in carcinoma of the breast, *Br J Cancer* (1947) **1**:15–20.

8 Urban JA, Radical excision of the chest wall for mammary cancer, *Cancer* (1951) **4**:1263–9.

9 Helman P, Bennett MB, Louw JH, Interim report on trial of treatment for operable breast cancer, *S Afr Med J* (1972) **46**:1374–5.

10 Fisher B, Montague E, Redmond C et al, Comparison of radical mastectomy with alternative treatments for primary breast cancer. A first report of results from a prospective randomised clinical trial, *Cancer* (1977) **39**:2827–39.

11 Fisher B, Redmond C, Fisher ER et al, Ten year results of a randomised clinical trial comparing radical mastectomy and total mastectomy with or without radiation, *N Engl J Med* (1985) **312**:674–81.

12 Fentiman IS, Lavelle MA, Kaplan D et al, The significance of supraclavicular fossa node recurrence after radical mastectomy, *Cancer* (1986) **57**:908–10.

13 Forrest APM, Roberts MM, Stewart HJ, Selection of local therapy for primary breast cancer by lower axillary node histology, *Eur J Cancer* (1980) suppl 1, 237–42.

14 Lythgoe JP, Palmer MK, Manchester regional breast study—5 and 10 year results, *Br J Surg* (1982) **69**:693–6.

15 Langlands AO, Prescott RJ, Hamilton T, A clinical trial in the management of operable cancer of the breast, *Br J Surg* (1980) **67**:170–4.

16 Hayward JL, Caleffi M, The significance of local control in the primary treatment of breast cancer, *Arch Surg* (1987) **122**:1244–7.

17 Turnbull AR, Turner DTL, Chant ADB, Treatment of early breast cancer, *Lancet* (1978) **ii**:7–9.

18 Cancer Research Campaign Working Party, Management of 'early' cancer of the breast. Report on an international multicentre trial supported by the CRC, *Br Med J* (1976) **i**:1035–8.

19 Cancer Research Campaign Working Party, Cancer Research Campaign (King's/Cambridge) trial for early breast cancer. A detailed update at the tenth year, *Lancet* (1980) **ii**:55–60.

20 Turner L, Swindell R, Bell, WGT et al, Radical versus modified radical mastectomy for breast cancer, *Ann R Coll Surg Engl* (1981) **63**:239–43.

21 Maddox WA, Carpenter JT, Laws HT et al, Does radical mastectomy still have a place in the treatment of primary operable breast cancer? *Arch Surg* (1987) **122**:1317–20.

22 Lacour J, Bucalossi P, Caceres E et al, Radical mastectomy versus radical mastectomy plus internal mammary dissection. Five year results of an international cooperative study, *Cancer* (1976) **37**:206–14.

23 Lacour J, Le M, Caceres E et al, Radical mastectomy versus radical mastectomy plus internal mammary dissection. Ten year results of an International Cooperative Trial in breast cancer, *Cancer* (1983) **51**:1941–3.

24 Meier P, Ferguson DJ, Karrison T, A controlled trial of extended radical versus radical mastectomy, *Cancer* (1989) **63**:188–95.

25 Kaae S, Johansen H, Breast cancer. Five year results: two random series of simple mastectomy with postoperative irradiation versus extended radical mastectomy, *AJR* (1962) **87**:82–8.

26 Bostwick J, Vasconez LO, Jurkiewicz MJ, Breast reconstruction after a radical mastectomy, *Plast Reconstr Surg* (1978) **61**:682–93.

27 Tai Y, Hasegawa H, A transverse abdominal flap for reconstruction after radical operations for recurrent breast cancer, *Plast Reconstr Surg* (1974) **53**:52–5.

28 Radovan C, Breast reconstruction after mastectomy using a temporary expander. *Plast Reconstr Surg* (1982) **69**:195–208.

29 Adams WM, Labial transplant for loss of nipple, *Plast Reconstr Surg* (1949) **4**:295–7.

30 Brent B, Bostwick J, Nipple–areola reconstruction with auricular tissues, *Plast Reconstr Surg* (1977) **60**:353–61.

31 Fentiman IS, Matthews PN, Davison OW et al, Survival following local skin recurrence after mastectomy, *Br J Surg* (1985) **92**:14–16.

CHAPTER 7

ADJUVANT THERAPY

Then unbelieving priests reformed the nation
And taught more pleasant methods of salvation

Alexander Pope

Viewed simplistically, the concept of adjuvant treatment for breast cancer is an extension of the rationale for *en bloc* resection. This postulates that the more extensive the treatment, the greater the probability of both control and cure of disease. It is of course now fashionable to discount the Halstedian approach and eschew radical attempts at local control whilst leaning on the crutch of systemic therapy to 'control' both local and micrometastatic disease.

Is this justified? What is the relative efficacy of systemic adjuvant therapy after inadequate local control compared with effective combined approaches to local control? Are there subsets of patients for whom more aggressive local treatments, such as adjuvant radiotherapy, may be of value? How great is the survival benefit of adjuvant therapy and who is gaining this advantage?

Has the shift in management of early disease from mastectomy towards breast conservation, with radiotherapy forming an intrinsic part, affected the probability of delivering adequate adjuvant chemotherapy? Finally, is it now meet and right to recommend that all patients with operable breast cancer should receive some form of systemic adjuvant therapy? An attempt will be made to address these questions and to identify signs of promising approaches which will require testing in controlled clinical trials.

Who needs adjuvant therapy?

The most important known prognostic indicator of disease relapse in patients with operable breast cancer is the number of axillary nodes containing metastases. Almost all adjuvant trials have used axillary nodal involvement as an entry criterion. The validity of this approach is demonstrated in a combined study reported by the Royal Marsden Hospital, London, and the National Cancer Institute, Milan.[1] Five-year relapse-free survival data were examined from patients treated by radical mastectomy who did not receive any adjuvant therapy, and have been summarized in Table 7.1. Of those patients without axillary-nodal involvement, after 5 years of follow up, 2–3 out of every 10 had relapsed as compared with 6 out of 10 in the node-positive group. On this basis, adjuvant treatment would be of no benefit to 70 per cent of node-negative and possibly 40 per cent of node-positive cases. Within the

Table 7.1 Five-year relapse-free percentage survival rates of patients treated by mastectomy in London and Milan.

	Milan		London	
	N−	N+	N−	N+
No of patients	(769)	(540	(188)	(258)
Entire group	81	44	69	44
1–3 nodes positive		53		51
> nodes positive		31		32
Age				
<40	71	32	86	20
40–49	83	45	77	43
50–59	80	43	68	55
60–69	82	47	67	30
>70	83	65	63	41
Menopausal status				
Pre	82	46	75	52
Peri/Post	81	43	68	40
Tumour site				
Medial	80	45	81	27
Central	80	42	61	33
Lateral	82	42	66	48
Tumour size (cm)				
<1	90	61	76	59
1.1–2	83	46	73	50
2.1–5	75	36	64	36

subset with only 1–3 nodes involved, 50 per cent had developed relapse of disease at 5 years.

It would be useful to identify the subset of node-negative patients most likely to develop relapse. This study suggests that clinical variables such as age, menopausal status, tumour size and tumour site do not delineate a high-risk group.

Five-year relapse rates give an incomplete picture of the pattern of recurrence since both loco-regional and distant metastatic events may occur for at least 20 years after first treatment. At Guy's Hospital Breast Unit a review was conducted of patients treated by radical mastectomy to compare 20-year survivors with those who had died prior to 20 years.[2] In this study the most powerful indicators of survival were axillary-nodal status, tumour size and tumour grade. However, these predicted for relatively early events during the first 10 years. Thereafter these lost prognostic power and subsequently age alone (that is the risk of dying or other diseases) was the most powerful indicator of survival.

Of the 20-year survivors, one-third had axillary-nodal involvement and one-third had poorly differentiated (grade III) cancers. One-quarter of survivors had tumours which were greater than 5 cm in diameter. Thus it is important to recognize that even amongst those cases with apparently the most dire prognostic features, there is a subset of women who will survive after adequate local treatment, without any adjuvant systemic therapy. If these could be prospectively identified they could be saved the potential toxicity of unnecessary adjuvant treatment.

In an attempt to refine prognostic grouping, the Nottingham group have proposed a prognostic index (I) based upon tumour size, stage and grade and applied to patients treated by total mastectomy, after triple-node biopsy:[3]

$$I = 0.2 \times \text{size} + \text{stage} + \text{grade}$$

Size was clinically derived and measured in cm. Stage was derived not from an axillary clearance but by means of a triple-node biopsy (low axillary, apical axillary and internal mammary). This is a discontinuous variable, 1, 2 or 3, based on stages A, B and

C. In Stage A none of the nodes contained metastases, in B the low axillary node was involved and in C either the apical or internal mammary node contained tumour. Grade is a discontinuous variable 1–3, based on a modification of the Bloom and Richardson grading system to encompass tumours other than infiltrating ductal carcinomas.

These numbers yield a prognostic index of between 2 and 7. The lower the index, the better the prognosis. In the original retrospective study from which the index was derived it was shown that those cases with an index <3.4 had a good prognosis, whereas those women with an index >5.4 carried a poor prognosis. Subsequent follow-up showed that the prognostic index continued to predict for relapse in the original group for up to 10 years after first treatment. In addition, a prospective evaluation of the index showed that it could be applied not only to patients treated by total mastectomy, but also as an indicator of prognosis among those treated by breast conservation (tumourectomy, triple-node biopsy and external radiotherapy).[4]

It may not be possible for this particular index to be used widely since most centres do not carry out internal mammary node biopsy as a routine staging procedure. Furthermore, some pathologists may be unwilling to grade all cancers. Nevertheless, this combined approach to formulation of a prognostic index and its potential for selection of cases for adjuvant therapy is an important concept and should form the basis of future prospective studies.

In a comprehensive study, Fisher et al have examined the relative prognostic power of oestrogen (ER) and progesterone receptor (PR) status compared with histological grade of primary tumours in patients with node-negative breasta cancer.[5] These patients were entered into NSABP Protocol 06, in which they were randomized to one of three treatments: total mastectomy with axillary clearance, partial mastectomy or partial mastectomy with radiotherapy. Within this study, 1157 patients had proven histologically negative axillary nodes. The histological slides were reviewed by one experienced pathologist. The values of ER and PR were measured using the sucrose-density-gradient method. Life tables were calculated and a Cox multivariate regression analysis was performed.

When the four variables, ER status, PR status, nuclear grade and histological grade, were entered into the Cox regression model, only nuclear grade predicted significantly for relapse-free survival. However, both nuclear grade and histological grade predicted for distant metastatic relapse-free survival. In terms of overall survival only nuclear grade was significant. Thus tumour differentiation is a better predictor of relapse than steroid-receptor status in node-negative patients. McGuire has argued that the reproducibility of receptor status may be better than that of nuclear grade, since it is more objective than assessment of the latter, where there may be great disagreement between pathologists.[6] This problem might be overcome with the use of flow cytometry to measure S-phase fraction as another indicator of tumour growth and differentiation, but this question remains unanswered at present.

Adjuvant postoperative radiotherapy

The present dogma asserts that adjuvant radiotherapy will decrease the risk of post-operative loco-regional relapse, but will not affect overall survival and indeed may lead to a long-term increased chance of death from coronary heart disease as a result of fibrosis due to radiation. Although this is true when the entire group of patients with early breast cancer is considered, there may be a subset who will benefit from intensified local treatment. Long-term follow-up is presently available only for patients treated by orthovoltage radiotherapy, which has now been superseded by megavoltage therapy. Problems of myocardial irradiation are much less likely to occur in patients who have been treated by more accurately delivered megavoltage radiation.

A recent meta-analysis of trials in which adjuvant radiotherapy was given after radical mastectomy has apparently confirmed the current prejudices.[7] Thus overall there was no survival benefit for the irradiated group during the first 10 years after treatment. Indeed, after longer follow-up (10–15 years) there was an increased mortality among the irradiated cases. However, when the data are re-examined with regard to numbers of women alive at 10 years, subdivided by axillary-nodal status, an interesting trend emerges (Table 7.2). Whilst there is no consistent effect in node-negative cases, there is a small (3–7 per cent) reduction in mortality among those with axillary-nodal

involvement. For this small benefit to have achieved statistical significance would have required much larger trials than those considered within the overview. Interestingly the Stockholm trial, which showed no apparent survival benefit, has recently reported not only a reduced loco-regional relapse rate among node-positive irradiated cases, but also a reduction in distant metastases which would normally manifest as an improvement in overall survival.[8]

Because updated data were unavailable from the NSABP trial B-02 this was not directly considered in the overview. In this study, patients treated by radical mastectomy were randomized to either observation or to receive irradiation. Relapse-free survival rates were increased in node-positive (1–3) patients who were irradiated (28 versus 18 per cent).[9] It has been suggested that the radiotherapy may have been less than optimal for some cases,[10] and a non-randomized study from MD Anderson Hospital comparing apparently similar cases showed an even better 10-year relapse-free survival rate (33 versus 13 per cent).[11]

Table 7.2 Ten-year survival rates from trials of radical mastectomy with or without postoperative irradiation (XRT).[7]

	Node-negative		Node-positive	
	Control	With XRT	Control	With XRT
Manchester Q	86/142 (61)	57/105 (54)	67/251 (27)	69/222 (31)
Manchester P	86/142 (61)	79/139 (57)	75/217 (35)	77/243 (32)
Oslo I	131/173 (76)	133/174 (76)	40/94 (43)	55/111 (50)
Oslo II	89/187 (48)	74/178 (42)	27/98 (28)	31/100 (31)
Heidelberg	16/131 (12)	20/44 (45)	5/27 (19)	11/40 (28)
Stockholm	39/189 (21)	50/184 (27)	30/132 (23)	27/139 (19)

Percentages in parentheses.

Need for more aggressive local therapy

Fowble has recently reviewed the loco-regional relapse rates in patients treated by mastectomy followed by adjuvant chemotherapy in an Eastern Co-operative Oncology Group (ECOG) trial.[12] The original aim of the trial was to compare two combined endocrine and chemotherapy regimens, namely CMF plus prednisone (CMFP) versus CMF plus prednisone plus tamoxifen (CMFPT). With a median follow-up of 4.5 years, 225 patients out of 627 had relapsed. Of these relapsers, 70 were loco-regional without evidence of distant metastases.

A series of prognostic variables were examined both individually and in a logistic regression model. No treatment factors emerged as significant for prediction of local relapse. The only significant clinical variable was tumour size, in that patients with cancers less than 5 cm in diameter had a 9 per cent local relapse rate compared with 19 per cent for those with tumours >5 cm. The pathological factors predicting for recurrence were tumour necrosis, pectoral fascia invasion and the number of involved axillary nodes.

In a multivariate analysis, tumour size and nodal status emerged as the most important variables. The loco-regional relapse rates for the subgroups are shown in Table 7.3. For those patients with tumours >5 cm and with 4–7 axillary nodes involved, 1 in 3 developed loco-regional relapse. Of these patients with recurrence, no distant metastases were detectable in 62 per cent. Thus adjuvant chemotherapy does not prevent loco-regional relapse in this subgroup and therefore a good case could be made for setting up a multicentre study to examine the role of adjuvant radiotherapy combined with chemotherapy in patients with tumours greater than 5 cm, treated by mastectomy with more than four nodes involved with metastases.

This type of combined approach has been

Table 7.3 Loco-regional relapse percentage in relation to primary tumour size and nodal status.[12]

No of nodes involved	Tumour <5 cm	Tumour >5 cm
1–3 nodes	6	12
4–7	10	31
>7	15	15

advocated by Edland, who has emphasized that either chemotherapy or tamoxifen may represent less than optimal therapy for the subset of patients with moderate or heavy axillary nodal involvement.[10]

Supportive evidence for the selective use of radiotherapy and chemotherapy has been provided as part of the study reported by Cooper et al.[13] All patients had been primarily treated by radical mastectomy and had histologically confirmed axillary metastases. After a four-way randomization they received either L-phenylalanine mustard (L-PAM) or L-PAM plus radiotherapy (RT). Alternatively they were given cyclophosphamide, methotrexate and fluorouracil (CMF) or CMF plus RT. Overall, the relapse rate was higher among those receiving radiotherapy and chemotherapy, but the lowest relapse rate of 8 per cent was reported among those with more than four nodes involved who had been treated with both CMF and RT. This compared in the same subset with a 61 per cent relapse rate for L-PAM alone, 22 per cent for L-PAM + RT and 15 per cent for CMF alone.

This sort of subset analysis can of course lead to spuriously significant results, but nevertheless these findings are consistent with those of Fowble et al,[12] and all point towards a benefit for a particular group of patients. Thus it is premature to speak of the demise of radiotherapy as an adjuvant treatment. It may only be of benefit for a small subset of patients, but nevertheless within this group it could make the difference between the disease relapsing locally or being controlled. This improved local control of disease might in turn lead to an overall survival benefit.

The magnitude of the benefit of adjuvant treatment

For many years an argument has been under way between the proponents of systemic adjuvant therapy, convinced of an effect on both relapse-free and overall survival, and the opponents, sceptical of any benefit and certain of the toxicity of chemotherapy and expense of treatment by tamoxifen. At last this particular argument can be extinguished. This enlightenment is due in large part to the overview of trials that has been conducted by the Early Breast Cancer Trialist's Collaborative Group (EBCTCG).[14] The overview represented the pooling of data from 28 randomized trials of adjuvant tamoxifen, comprising a total of 16 513 patients, and 40 chemotherapy trials into which 13 442 cases had been entered.

Criteria of eligibility for the overview analysis were that the patients were randomly assigned to their adjuvant therapy and also that they differed from one another within a particular trial only in terms of receiving or not receiving the adjuvant treatment of interest. Thus trials comparing tamoxifen with no treatment were eligible, as were trials in which chemotherapy alone was compared with chemotherapy and tamoxifen. Studies in which an untreated control arm was compared with combined chemotherapy and endocrine therapy were not included.

Mortality figures were obtained from all the trialists and the differences between the number of observed and expected deaths in the treated and control groups within each trial were calculated, as were the variance and standard deviations of these values. This enabled the calculation of an odds ratio of mortality for the treated compared with the control group, together with the 95 per cent confidence intervals of this odds ratio. The overview results derived from trials of adjuvant chemotherapy are shown in Table 7.4. For patients aged less than 50 years, 35 per cent of the control group had died, compared with 30 per cent in the treated groups. This gives an odds ratio of 0.78, that is, 22 per cent fewer of the treated group had died. The lowest odds ratio was found among the patients treated by CMF, where there was a one-third reduction in mortality.

Single-agent chemotherapy was less effective than polychemotherapy, but the addition of other agents to CMF did not lead to any detectable extra reduction in mortality. Indeed, the percentage reduction was only 20 per cent. For women aged above 50 years there was no significant effect on mortality overall in those receiving adjuvant chemotherapy. This inefficacy was seen among all of the individual therapy regimes including CMF. Thus any effect of adjuvant chemotherapy in postmenopausal women is so small as to be of no clinical value. Of course a benefit in particular subgroups with axillary nodal metastases cannot be excluded as a result of this particular overview analysis.

The results of tamoxifen treatment trials are summarized in Table 7.5. Interestingly this shows that there is no detectable effect on mortality when tamoxifen was given to women aged less than 50 for periods up to 2 years. In contrast, an overall reduction in mortality of 20 per cent is seen in women

Table 7.4 Mortality rates and odds ratios from overview of trials of adjuvant chemotherapy.[14]

	Mortality rates		Odds ratio ± 95% CI
	Control (%)	Treated (%)	
Age < 50 years	35	30	0.78 ± 0.06
Single agent	41	37	0.89 ± 0.10
CMF	34	25	0.63 ± 0.09
CMF + other	32	27	0.80 ± 0.17
Age >50 years	32	31	0.96 ± 0.05
Single agent	46	47	1.04 ± 0.10
CMF	27	26	0.91 ± 0.09
CMF + other	35	32	0.91 ± 0.03

Table 7.5 Mortality rates and odds ratios from overview of trials of adjuvant tamoxifen.[14]

	Mortality rates		Odds ratio ± 95% CI
	Control (%)	Treated (%)	
Age <50 years	21	22	1.1 ± 0.08
>2 years treatment	21	21	0.99 ± 0.09
<1 year treatment	23	22	1.07 ± 0.15
Age >50 years	25	21	0.80 ± 0.03
>2 years treatment	22	21	0.77 ± 0.04
<1 year treatment	33	29	0.85 ± 0.06

aged over 50, which increased to 23 per cent in those receiving 2 years of treatment.

These results have clear implications for the routine postoperative management of breast cancer. All patients with proven axillary nodal metastases should receive adjuvant systemic therapy. The nature of this therapy will be dependent upon the patient's age (and almost certainly her menopausal status). There is little benefit for women under 50 being given tamoxifen, nor for those over 50 being treated with cytotoxic chemotherapy. An untreated control arm should not be included in future adjuvant trials of patients with proven axillary nodal metastases. Thus the overview has provided a firm basis from which to plan further trials of both endocrine and cytotoxic adjuvant therapy. However, even though the question of an effect and its magnitude have been answered, many new questions have emerged with regard to the most appropriate form and scheduling of systemic adjuvant treatment.

Adjuvant chemotherapy

Bonadonna and Valagussa have suggested that the apparent lack of effect of adjuvant chemotherapy observed among postmenopausal women could be due to dosage reduction resulting in inadequate treatment.[15] The question of dose intensity of cytotoxics has broad implication for the planning of adjuvant chemotherapy. First, within the normal therapeutic range, what evidence is there to suggest that dosage reduction leads to worsening of disease-free and overall survival? Viewed conversely, will dosage escalation lead to improvement in results of adjuvant therapy? Third, as radiotherapy is used with greater frequency as part of the combined management of early breast cancer, what effect will its action of bone-marrow suppression have on the ability to deliver adequate dosages of adjuvant chemotherapy? In addition, if dose reduction is not the explanation for the inefficacy of adjuvant cytotoxics in older women, does this mean that the action of chemotherapy is dependent largely upon an endocrine-mediated mechanism?

Evidence for dose response of breast cancer

This topic has recently been extensively reviewed by Henderson.[16] He suggested that although there are indications from experimental work that some agents do display a dose-response effect with certain rodent tumours, that this may have little relevance to the dosages used and tumours encountered in humans. No direct data are available from studies of CMF dose intensity in patients with advanced breast cancer. The closest approach was a study which used the FAC regimen (fluorouracil, adriamycin and cyclophosphamide), in which patients were either treated with standard FAC or alternatively with a schedule in which the dosages of both adriamycin and cyclophosphamide were escalated.[17] Patients receiving higher dosages were nursed in a protected environment and given prophylactic antibiotics to prevent life-threatening infections due to bone-marrow suppression. In this study there was no difference between response rate or duration of response of patients treated by either regimen.

In the context of adjuvant therapy, Bonadonna et al re-analysed data from the trials carried out in Milan and found evidence of a dose-response effect.[15] The optimal dosage was that calculated for the first course based upon the patient's surface area. Subsequent reductions were the result of either haematological or gastrointestinal toxicity. The optimal cumulative dose was the original dosage multiplied by either 6 or 12, and the actual delivered dosage was given as a percentage of the optimal dose. Differences in terms of both relapse-free and overall survival emerged when patients were subdivided into three groups: those receiving >85 per cent of optimal dose, those given 65–84 per cent, and those who received <65 per cent. The latter group displayed a significantly worse outcome, and within this subset there was an over-representation of older women. Two different trials of CMF have also displayed evidence of a dose-response effect,[18,19] whereas two other studies found no difference in relapse-free or overall survival for those receiving high or low dosages of CMF.[20,21]

Henderson has pointed out that retrospective analyses of this type may introduce a variety of confounding biases.[16] In particular, patients who relapse whilst receiving adjuvant therapy will not be given their full predicted dosage and will of course have a poor prognosis. Other confounding factors include patient age and performance status.

Hryniuk and Levine have adopted a different approach to examination of dose intensity, albeit still based upon retrospective analysis.[22] Instead of taking total dosages, the proportion of the dosage administered was taken as a percentage of that originally described by Cooper.[23] Patients in the control arm of trials were described as having 0 per cent. In order to include trials of patients given L-PAM, an assumption was made that 1 mg L-PAM was equal to 40 mg cyclophosphamide. Having made these assumptions, Hryniuk concluded that there was evidence of a dose-response effect in trials of adjuvant chemotherapy. Gelman and Henderson refuted this analysis, arguing that giving an equal weighting to all components of cytotoxic regimens was inconsistent with experimental evidence.[24] Furthermore, they argued that it was illogical to take no treatment as the lowest dosage of chemotherapy and finally that it was inappropriate to lump together a variety of cytotoxic regimens. Thus when those trials of CMF were re-analysed, no evidence of any correlation between dosage and response could be found.

The Cancer and Acute Leukaemia Group B (CALGB) conducted an adjuvant trial in which two different dosages of CMF were used in combination with vincristine and prednisone (CMF VP).[25] With a median follow-up of 45 months there was no difference between the relapse-free or overall survival of the two groups of patients.

Thus it appears likely that neither an escalation of dosage of CMF nor the addition of agents such as anthracyclines will result in a striking improvement in relapse-free or overall survival in patients with Stage II breast cancer. This contrasts with the improvement in both response rate and duration of response when anthracyclines are used in place of CMF in the first-line cytotoxic treatment of advanced breast cancer. Thus possibly much of the benefit of adjuvant chemotherapy may not be due to a direct cytotoxic effect.

Mechanism of action of adjuvant chemotherapy

The overview analysis of adjuvant chemotherapy demonstrated a 30 per cent reduction in mortality in women under 50 years of age, but no significant effect in older women. This finding requires explanation. A re-analysis of data from the Guy's/Manchester trial of CMF has provided some interesting suggestions.[26,27] In this study both pre- and postmenopausal women with axillary nodal metastases were randomized to treatment with CMF or to observation. Among postmenopausal cases no effect was seen in terms of relapse-free or overall survival. In contrast, a significantly improved relapse-free and overall survival was seen in the CMF-treated premenopausal cases.

Because of this striking difference between responses in the premenopausal and postmenopausal patients, a re-analysis was conducted to examine the effect of the development of amenorrhoea and steroid-receptor status of the primary tumour on relapse-free and overall survival. Permanent amenorrhoea developed in 60 per cent of patients given adjuvant CMF, and occurred more frequently among the older yet premenopausal women. Both relapse-free and overall survival were significantly increased among the group who developed amenorrhoea. When the control group was compared with the CMF-treated cases who continued to menstruate, both relapse-free and overall survival life-table curves were superimposable.

Oestrogen-receptor (ER) and progesterone-receptor (PR) assay data were available for 87 per cent of patients within the trial. After subdivision of the CMF-treated group into those with PR values >30 fmol/mg cytosol protein and those with values <30 fmol/mg, both relapse-free and overall survival were significantly prolonged in the former group. The percentages of patients free from relapse are given in Table 7.6.

Table 7.6 Relapse-free survival (RFS) rates of premenopausal patients treated with adjuvant CMF, subdivided by steroid-receptor status.[27]

Receptor status	RFS rate (%)
ER+	89
ER−	60
PR+	94
PR−	58
ER+ PR+	97
ER+ PR−	74
ER− PR+	85
ER− PR−	48

This combined observation of an effect related to both the development of amenorrhoea and the presence of a hormonally sensitive tumour would strongly support the hypothesis that the major activity of adjuvant CMF is to induce ovarian inhibition. If this is the case, ovarian ablation can be achieved in a much less toxic manner by surgeon, radiotherapist or physician using drugs such as LHRH agonists.

Further evidence which partially supports this viewpoint has been furnished by the Danish Breast Cancer Cooperative Group (DBCCG). This national group conducted a trial of adjuvant chemotherapy into which 1032 pre- and perimenopausal women were entered.[28] All had standard primary treatment comprising total mastectomy, axillary node sampling and postoperative radiotherapy. Patients were then randomized to receive either C, cyclophosphamide (130 mg/m^2 orally, days 1–14), or CMF, comprising cyclophosphamide (80 mg/m^2, days 1–14), methotrexate (30 mg/m^2 iv, days 1 and 8) and 5-fluorouracil (500 mg/m^2 iv, days 1 and 8), or to receive no systemic adjuvant therapy. Both cytotoxic regimens, C and CMF, significantly prolonged relapse-free survival. In the CMF-treated group, overall survival was increased by 14 per cent.

Amenorrhoea developed in 70 per cent of those given C and 63 per cent of those treated with CMF. Relapse-free survival was significantly prolonged among cases in the C group who developed amenorrhoea, but no effect was seen in the CMF group. Oestrogen-receptor measurements were available for only a small subset of 169 cases. Relapse-free survival in the CMF group was not influenced by ER status, but a significantly better relapse-free survival was seen in the cyclophosphamide-treated group among those patients with ER-positive tumours.

These results are not fully consistent with the Guy's/Manchester findings. However, all cases in the DBCCG trial had adjuvant radiotherapy so that a local relapse of only 9 per cent was seen in the control group. This may have obliterated part of the benefit of CMF in terms of reduction of local relapse rate.

Perioperative chemotherapy

Nissen-Meyer postulated that viable malignant cells might be disseminated as a result of primary treatment and that an intensive yet truncated course of chemotherapy might eradicate these potentially metastatic tumour emboli.[29] Based on this premise, the Scandinavian Adjuvant Chemotherapy Study Group carried out a trial in 11 different centres. The primary treatment in almost all cases was radical mastectomy followed by radiotherapy. Patients were randomized to no further treatment or to receive cyclophosphamide (30 mg/kg) given intravenously over 6 days postoperatively. One institution to which cases were referred for postoperative radiotherapy gave the treatment 3 weeks postoperatively.

After exclusion of ineligible cases, the trial comprised a total of 1026 cases, of whom 507 received cyclophosphamide and 519 served as controls. Side-effects of cyclophosphamide included nausea and alopecia in a few cases. Haematological toxicity was never severe enough for radiotherapy to be delayed. No effects were seen with regard to wound healing, skin reaction or pulmonary complications.

After 10 years of follow-up there had been 234 relapses in the controls as compared with 175 in the cyclophosphamide-treated group. In parallel, 196 of the controls had died but only 146 of the chemotherapy group.

An effect on mortality began to manifest after 5 years. By 10 years of follow-up, 11 per cent fewer of the treated group had died and by 15 years this rose to 15 per cent.[30] With more prolonged follow-up the survival curves for the two groups have started to converge because of the incidental deaths from other diseases in these aging cohorts.[31]

It is particularly interesting that these results were consistent within all the collaborating centres, except the radiotherapy institution where cyclophosphamide administration was delayed and where no benefit from perioperative chemotherapy was observed. This would suggest that the mechanism of action of this schedule is to destroy cells shed by primary surgery, thereby confirming the Nissen-Meyer hypothesis. Another possible explanation might be that micrometastases are particularly sensitive to chemotherapy immediately after surgery.

Because of the importance of this finding, many groups are conducting trials of perioperative chemotherapy, sometimes using much more toxic agents such as anthracyclines. Two groups have reported results of trials. The Cancer Research Campaign (CRC) Adjuvant Breast Trial Working Party set up a factorial 2 × 2 design study, which sought to examine the roles of cyclophosphamide and tamoxifen.[32] Primary treatments were various. Some patients were treated by total mastectomy and axillary-node sampling. Those with involved nodes received radiotherapy. Others had a total mastectomy and axillary clearance, without radiation. Finally, as the retreat from radical surgery became a rout, others were treated by tumourectomy, axillary sampling and radiotherapy. The four randomization options were: no treatment, tamoxifen 10 mg twice daily for 2 years, cyclophosphamide 30 mg/kg for 6 days postoperatively or both tamoxifen and cyclophosphamide. A total of 2230 patients was entered into the trial. Instead of presenting results in terms of relapse-free survival, the endpoint chosen was 'first event'. This included not only relapse of disease, but also new primary tumours and deaths from any cause. Analysed in this way there was a significant reduction in number of first events in the cyclophosphamide-treated group (27 versus 30 per cent after a median follow-up of 3.5 years). Not surprisingly, so far no effect on mortality has been observed. Thus the CRC trial has shown a marginal effect of cyclophosphamide after a variety of primary treatments, not all of which may have been equally effective.

The Ludwig Group used a different approach to examine the relative efficacy of early postoperative chemotherapy versus standard chemotherapy.[33] Primary treatment was either a total mastectomy with axillary clearance or a modified radical mastectomy. Cases were then randomized to one of three treatments: perioperative CMF given 36 hours postsurgery, or intravenous CMF for 6 cycles or both perioperative and intravenous CMF. As an additional complication, node-positive postmenopausal cases were also given 20 mg tamoxifen, and both pre- and postmenopausal women were given 7.5 mg prednisone daily. When the pathologist had reported on the axillary-nodal status, those with negative nodes who had been randomized to CMFP were not given that treatment. The reported analysis was restricted to node-positive cases. Perioperative CMF was given to 413 women, standard CMF to 415 and combination treatment to 401 cases. With a median follow-up of 42 months the estimated relapse rates were 60 per cent for perioperative CMF, 38 per cent for postoperative CMF and 40 per cent for the combined treatment group.

What this study has done is to demonstrate that CMF given 36 hours after surgery is inferior to 6 cycles of CMFP for premenopausal women and CMFPT in the postmenopausal. It is possible that different results might have been obtained if the CMF had been given immediately postoperatively. The addition of both tamoxifen and prednisone make the situation for the postmenopausal uninterpretable.

It is difficult to accept that the addition of more toxic agents will effect an improvement on the results of cyclophosphamide alone, given immediately postoperatively. It is probable that metastatic emboli may be at their most sensitive in the immediate postoperative phase and would be destroyed by any adequate form of chemotherapy, so that increasing the toxicity of treatment will be unlikely to lead to a detectable survival benefit.

Adjuvant chemotherapy and breast conservation

Radiotherapy forms the core of all proven techniques of breast-conserving treatment. Since radiation will induce lymphopenia and thus reduce the total white count, this could lead to dosage reduction of administered cytotoxics. A preliminary report from the National Cancer Institute (NCI) did indicate that there was some reduction of dosage among patients treated by radiotherapy as part of breast conservation.[34]

These cases were entered into a clinical trial within which patients with tumours up to 5 cm in diameter were treated by either modified radical mastectomy or tumourectomy, axillary clearance and external radiotherapy. Patients with involved axillary nodes were given adjuvant chemotherapy comprising adriamycin ($30\,mg/m^2$ on day 1) and cyclophosphamide ($150\,mg/m^2$ on days 3, 4, 5 and 6). This was given for 9 cycles and the median interval between primary surgery and the first course was 9 days. The third cycle, given during the course of external radiotherapy, comprised cyclophosphamide alone.

Twenty patients had been treated by mastectomy and 17 with breast conservation. The latter group received a slightly lower total dosage of chemotherapy, with dosage reduction being required twice as frequently as among those treated by mastectomy.

However, a subsequent expanded publication which included results from 163 cases did not show any significant difference between the dosage of chemotherapy administered to the two groups.[35]

At Guy's, two interconnected trials examined the respective roles of mastectomy and breast conservation and also the value of adjuvant chemotherapy in node-positive cases.[36] Eligible patients for the conservation trial were aged up to 70 years, with unifocal infiltrating breast cancer up to 4 cm in diameter. They were randomized to be treated by either a modified radical mastectomy or to breast-conservation treatment which comprised tumourectomy, axillary clearance, iridium implant and external radiotherapy. Those aged less than 65 years, who had axillary nodal metastases, were then randomized to either no further treatment or to receive CMF (cyclophosphamide 100 mg/m^2, days 1–14, methotrexate 32 mg/m^2, days 1 and 8 and fluorouracil 480 mg/m^2, days 1 and 8) for 12 cycles.

The first course of chemotherapy was given within 10 days of surgery, but the second was delayed in the breast-conservation group until the external radiotherapy had been completed 7–8 weeks after surgery. CMF was given to 35 patients

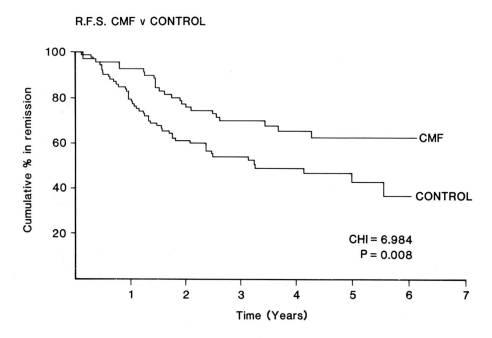

Figure 7.1   Relapse-free survival of node-positive patients who received either adjuvant CMF or were untreated controls.

treated by mastectomy and 41 treated by breast conservation. Among the latter group, significantly less CMF was administered (67 versus 77 per cent). Toxicity of treatment was similar for both groups, except that severe alopecia occurred more frequently among those treated by radiotherapy (22 versus 9 per cent).

The trial comprised both pre- and postmenopausal women and the relapse-free and overall survival were significantly better among those cases in both groups who received CMF, as shown in Figures 7.1 and 7.2. No difference was found in the relapse-free or overall survival of those cases who received CMF and were treated by either mastectomy or radiotherapy (Figures 7.3 and 7.4). Thus dosage reduction of CMF does not lead to a detectable alteration in relapse rate among node-positive cases treated by breast conservation. Thus breast-conserving techniques are compatible with the administration of an adequate dosage of adjuvant chemotherapy.

Chemotherapy given as adjuvant treatment can save lives of both pre- and postmenopausal women, when given perioperatively. When administered postoperatively for 6 cycles it can also reduce the mortality in premenopausal women with

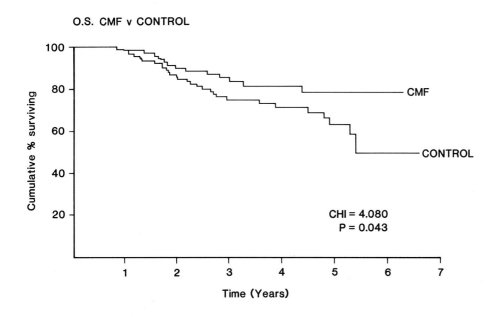

Figure 7.2 Overall survival of node-positive patients given CMF and untreated controls.

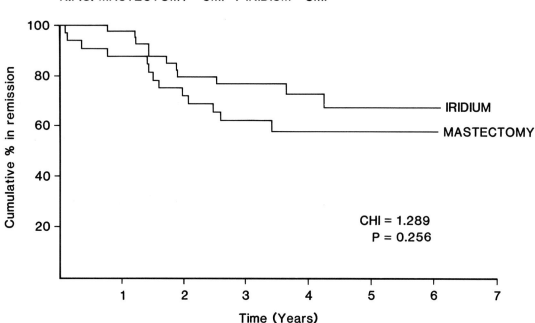

R.F.S. MASTECTOMY + CMF v IRIDIUM + CMF

Figure 7.3 Relapse-free survival of node-positive patients who received CMF and had been treated by either modified radical mastectomy or iridium implant.

Stage II breast cancers. It has yet to be determined whether all or part of this role can be replaced by endocrine treatment.

Combined adjuvant cytotoxic and endocrine therapy

Working on the principle that more is better, several groups have examined combined adjuvant treatment including both cytotoxic and endocrine treatment. The overview analysis showed that chemotherapy exerts a minimal effect in postmenopausal women and therefore it would be unlikely that the addition of chemotherapy to tamoxifen would yield better results than that of tamoxifen alone. Similarly, in the premenopausal, where therapeutic castration may be central to the action of CMF, the addition of oöphorectomy would be unlikely to achieve any significant improvement, except possibly

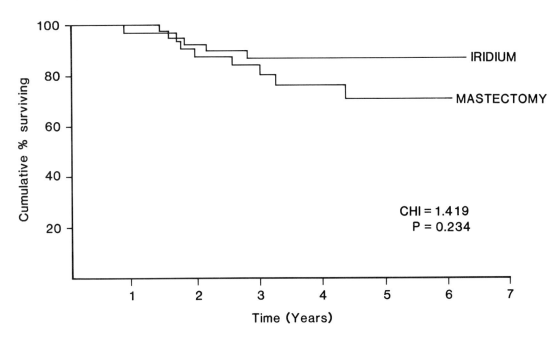

Figure 7.4 Overall survival of node-positive patients who received CMF and had been treated by either modified radical mastectomy or iridium implant.

in those not developing amenorrhoea. Essentially this is what the studies have shown.

The Ludwig Group conducted a multicentre trial into which premenopausal patients treated by total mastectomy and axillary clearance were entered.[37] Eligible cases who had four or more axillary nodes involved were randomized to either chemotherapy alone (CMFP), or to CMFP and oöphorectomy. A total of 327 patients were evaluable, of whom 161 were treated by CMFP and 166 received CMFP and oöphorectomy. With a

median follow-up of 4 years there was no difference between the relapse-free survival of the two groups, even when subdivided on a basis of extent of nodal involvement, receptor status and tumour grade.

The Eastern Co-operative Oncology Group (ECOG) conducted an adjuvant trial for postmenopausal patients who were treated primarily by modified or radical mastectomy and who had axillary-nodal involvement.[38] Patients were randomized to one of three options: control (untreated), CMFP or CMFP

125

and tamoxifen (CMFPT). On the assumption that the CMF was largely redundant, it was in effect a comparison between prednisone and prednisone + tamoxifen. With a median follow-up of 3 years, the relapse-free survival for the treated group was similar to that of untreated controls (52 versus 51 per cent).

However, at 1 year there was a significantly different relapse rate between the controls and the combined treated groups (70 versus 90 per cent). The early behaviour of the CMFP and CMFPT groups was identical and suggested that 1 year of tamoxifen conveys little benefit when added to prednisone.

In NSABP trial B-09 patients with axillary nodal involvement were randomized to receive either L-PAM and 5-fluorouracil (PF) or L-PAM, 5-fluorouracil and tamoxifen (PFT).[39] After 6 years mean follow-up the overall survival of the two groups was similar. However, relapse-free survival was increased among those receiving PFT (52 versus 47 per cent). When subdivided by ER status, survival was similar. Of the PR-negative cases, significantly fewer relapsed in the PF group (59 versus 52 per cent). This could have arisen because tamoxifen blocked a cytotoxic effect in women aged under 50.

Further subset analyses showed this disadvantage to be borne by those aged <49 years with PR-negative tumours. However, among those cases aged >50 years, PFT increased relapse-free survival in patients with ER-positive tumours (54 versus 45 per cent) and 45 to 55 per cent in those with PR-positive primaries. Overall survival was prolonged for only one subset, those women aged above 50 years with more than four nodes involved. Among this particular subset, there was a significant 28 per cent reduction in mortality for those with PR-positive tumours. This study has indirectly demonstrated the value of adjuvant tamoxifen in patients aged over 50 years.

The North Central Cancer Treatment Group and Mayo Clinic ran a joint trial in which postmenopausal women with nodal metastases were randomized to observation, or to receive cyclophosphamide, fluorouracil and prednisone (CFP) or CFP plus tamoxifen.[40] After 5 years median follow-up, relapse-free survival was 43 per cent in the control group, 61 per cent in those given CFP and 59 per cent in those given CFPT. Thus again, no additive benefit was shown for 1 year of tamoxifen and prednisone.

The Group of the University of Naples (GUN) recently reported a trial in which 125 premenopausal patients with axillary metastases were randomized to receive either CMF for 9 courses or alternatively CMF plus tamoxifen 30 mg daily for 2 years.[41] After a median follow-up of 5 years there was no difference between either relapse-free or overall survival in either group.

Thus there is little evidence to support the combined use of endocrine and cytotoxic agents as adjuvant therapy. This contrasts strongly with the impressive effects that have been demonstrated for various forms of adjuvant endocrine therapy.

Adjuvant endocrine treatment

Since the growth of many breast cancers can be modulated by hormonal influences it was natural that endocrine treatments which had been found to be effective in advanced disease would also be tested in an adjuvant role. For premenopausal women, oöphorectomy performed either surgically or radiotherapeutically has become the first-line endocrine manipulation at the time of relapse. This procedure has also been widely tested as a putative adjuvant treatment in women deemed at risk of relapse after primary therapy. A small but consistent improvement in both relapse-free and overall survival is seen in almost all the randomized trials.

Table 7.7 Controlled trials of adjuvant oöphorectomy.

Follow-up	Survival		Control (%)	Oöphorectomy (%)	Reference
15	OS	N–	68	80	43
		N+	37	43	
10	RFS	N–	85	92	44
		N+	42	54	
5	RFS		54	68	45
5	RFS	N–	90	79	46
		N+	39	45	
10	RFS		53	69	47
20	OS		44	54	48

OS = Overall survival.
RFS = Relapse-free survival.
N– = Node negative.
N+ = Node positive.

Adjuvant oöphorectomy

Taylor was the first to use oöphorectomy in a prophylactic role and concluded that the procedure conveyed no benefit.[42] This was followed by several trials testing adjuvant oöphorectomy and the message that has been received by the oncological community was overwhelmingly negative. However, a closer examination of these trials does suggest that a false impression may have been formed.

Those randomized trials which compared no systemic therapy with oöphorectomy are summarized in Table 7.7.[43–8] When the trials are subdivided on a basis of node-negative and node-positive cases, a consistent but modest increase in relapse-free survival is seen in almost all the studies for node-positive patients. Because of the relatively

small number of cases in each trial, none was of a size for this difference to have become statistically significant. These trials were conducted without the benefit of ER measurements. It is likely that up to 50 per cent of these premenopausal women may have had ER-negative tumours. Thus a bigger benefit would be likely if the studies were repeated using ER positivity as a criterion for entry.

The adjuvant endocrine study with the longest follow-up and which has shown a benefit was that conducted at the Princess Margaret Hospital in Toronto.[49] Eligible patients were premenopausal but aged 45 years or older. All received radiotherapy to the gland fields and were then randomized to one of three options: no further treatment, ovarian irradiation or ovarian irradiation followed by prednisone 7.5 mg daily for 5 years. It is important to note that all data from this trial have been independently reviewed. In the most recent report follow-up was available for between 12 and 18 years.[50]

In the control group the median time to relapse was 5 years, compared with 11 years for those treated by ovarian ablation. The median time to relapse in the group treated by ovarian ablation and prednisone has not yet been reached. In terms of overall survival, the median time was 8 years for controls, 12 for the ovarian irradiation group and again has not yet been reached by the group given additional prednisone. These significant benefits were achieved in both node-negative and node-positive cases.

Thus there is evidence of a benefit from adjuvant oöphorectomy for certain patients and also that a significant improvement can be obtained with additional prednisone. There is a pressing need to re-examine in controlled trials the respective values of oöphorectomy and cytotoxic chemotherapy with or without prednisone/prednisolone.

Adjuvant tamoxifen

Because of the low profile of both short- and medium-term toxicity following tamoxifen administration, this agent has become the most popular drug in use for the treatment of breast cancer, particularly as an adjuvant. The overview analysis provides compelling evidence of its benefit among postmenopausal women with Stage II disease. However, the overview provides little comfort for those advocating use in premenopausal node-positive cases, where no definite benefit has been demonstrated.

There are still several outstanding questions with regard to the use of tamoxifen as an adjuvant. For how long should the agent be given? Does tamoxifen benefit patients with ER-negative primary tumours? Finally,

should tamoxifen be given to all patients with early breast cancer?

Duration of treatment

The overview clearly showed that 2 years of tamoxifen treatment were superior to 1 year, with a decrease in the mortality odds ratio from 0.85 to 0.77. Thus mortality was decreased by 23 per cent rather than 15 per cent.

One of the largest studies on tamoxifen which has failed to show a mortality decrease was carried out at the Christie Hospital in Manchester.[51] Tamoxifen was given for only 1 year. In the postmenopausal group there was a reduction in the proportion of patients developing distant metastases, but no overall effect on survival.

The NSABP carried out a continuing non-randomized study after accrual ceased for trial B-09.[52] In the original trial, node-positive patients were randomized to L-PAM and fluorouracil (PF) or PF plus tamoxifen. Additional cases were all registered and given PFT. After 2 years they were asked if they wished to continue taking tamoxifen for a further 12 months, to which 72 per cent agreed. This third year of tamoxifen resulted in an increase in relapse-free survival from 65 to 75 per cent among those aged over 50 years. There was also an increase in overall survival. No benefit was seen in those aged less than 50 years.

Additional supportive data were given by the Scottish trial in which patients who received 5 years of tamoxifen had a significant prolongation of survival.[53] Thus if 5 years of tamoxifen are better than 2 years, it could be argued that the drug should be given on a lifelong basis, or until relapse. The case for prolongation of tamoxifen therapy is strengthened by laboratory experiments which have shown that tamoxifen is tumouristic rather than tumouricidal, and that relapse occurs in rodent models when the agent is withdrawn.[54]

One major argument against such an approach is the very high financial cost involved with probably only a relatively small gain in terms of lives saved. In the Stockholm trial, more prolonged adjuvant tamoxifen has been given and recent results both support and oppose such treatment.[55] The gain of tamoxifen may be not only in terms of relapse, but also there may be a reduction in second primary breast cancers. In the Stockholm study there were 32 cancers in the control group but only 18 in those given tamoxifen. Against this, there were two endometrial cancers in the control group against 13 in the treated group. This latter increase may result from the oestrogen-agonist effect of tamoxifen. Thus the prolonged administration of tamoxifen to women with an intact uterus may be problematic. Rather, as has evolved with design of hormone replacement therapy, it may be necessary to administer concomitant progestogen. This needs evaluation prospectively.

Tamoxifen and receptor status

Experience with the use of tamoxifen in patients with advanced breast cancer shows that only those patients with ER/PR-positive tumours are likely to obtain benefit. When both PR and ER are negative, the chance of a response is less than 1 in 10.

A similar response was reported by the Danish Breast Cancer Cooperative Group (DBCG).[56] In the DBCG trial, postmenopausal node-positive patients received tamoxifen 30 mg daily for 1 year, or alternatively received no additional systemic therapy. No mortality reduction has been seen within this study. Relapse-free survival was significantly increased among those patients with more

than 4 nodes involved. The relapse-free survival was 87 per cent among those with ER-positive tumours, compared with only 70 per cent among those with ER-negative cancers.

In contrast, the Nolvadex Adjuvant Trial Organisation (NATO) which compared tamoxifen 20 mg daily for 2 years with no adjuvant treatment and was the first trial to show a significant reduction in mortality, has reported that the survival benefit was unrelated to ER status of the primary tumour.[57]

At 6 years of follow-up, the overall survival was similar for both ER-negative and ER-positive cases, irrespective of a cut-off point of 5 fmol/mg or 30 fmol/mg, as shown in Table 7.8. Similar results were reported in

Table 7.8 Overall survival in NATO trial in relation to oestrogen receptor (ER) status.

	Control (%)	Tamoxifen (%)
Six years		
ER < 5 fmol/mg	61	82
ER > 5 fmol/mg	75	80
ER < 30 fmol/mg	63	78
ER > 30 fmol/mg	73	84
Eight years		
ER < 5 fmol/mg	50	74
ER > 5 fmol/mg	65	72
ER < 30 fmol/mg	54	71
ER > 30 fmol/mg	65	75

Table 7.9 Relapse-free (RFS) and overall survival (OS) in NATO trial in relation to tumour grade and treatment.

	RFS (%)	OS (%)
Grade I		
Control	54	69
Tamoxifen	72	78
Grade II		
Control	46	57
Tamoxifen	65	72
Grade III		
Control	30	37
Tamoxifen	32	34

the most recent, 8-year, analysis, where the lack of interaction between ER status and tamoxifen has persisted.[58] Histological grading was carried out on tumours from 600 patients within the NATO study.[59] Both overall and event-free survival are shown in Table 7.9. This shows that patients with well-differentiated tumours (grade I) carry a better prognosis and are more likely to respond to tamoxifen.

In the Scottish trial the maximum benefit occurred in those patients with tumours containing more than 30 fmol/mg protein, but improved survival was also seen in those with ER-negative tumours.[53]

At present a benefit for adjuvant tamoxifen cannot be excluded in patients with ER-negative tumours. In the absence of a less toxic alternative, node-positive postmenopausal patients should be given the possible benefit of adjuvant tamoxifen.

Tamoxifen and prednisone

The addition of prednisone to adjuvant oöphorectomy has been shown to prolong the lives of women aged over 45 who were premenopausal.[49] Similarly, the addition of prednisone to tamoxifen has also been shown to increase both the response rate and duration of remission in patients with advanced breast cancer.[60] It is therefore likely that the addition of prednisone or prednisolone to adjuvant tamoxifen might convey an additional benefit in postmenopausal patients with node-positive disease. This is at present under study in prospective trials.

Adjuvant treatment for node-negative patients

The majority of studies of adjuvant treatment have included patients with proven axillary metastases, partly because of their increased risk of relapse, but also because of the toxicity of chemotherapy. The balance has altered as tamoxifen has become more widely used because of its tolerability and low incidence of toxicity. Results have recently emerged from various studies which prompted the National Cancer Institute to try an experimental technique of information dissemination. A 'Clinical Alert' was sent to 13 000 doctors treating breast cancer in the USA. This included the statement 'Adjuvant hormonal or cytotoxic chemotherapy can have a meaningful impact on the natural history of node-negative breast-cancer patients'.

If the intention of the 'Alert' was to provide work for underemployed medical oncologists and lawyers, in this it has probably been successful. Furthermore, if the aim was to produce consternation among both patients and physicians, again a direct hit was scored. However, with regards to the more laudable purpose of reducing the mortality from breast cancer, what has been the potential impact of the 'Alert'?

The data which formed the core of the 'Clinical Alert' were derived from three unpublished American papers, together with three European papers. The American papers have now been published.[61-3] In a variety of ways, all these studies had examined the role of either adjuvant endocrine treatment (tamoxifen) or chemotherapy in node-negative patients.

Tamoxifen in node-negative patients

The three trials of tamoxifen were the NATO study, the Scottish trial and NSABP B-14. The NATO trial admitted node-negative post-menopausal patients, whereas both pre- and postmenopausal women were entered into the Scottish trial. Although the latter study reported similar results for all subgroups examined, the paper did not give a break-down of node-negative patients on a basis of menopausal status. NSABP trial B-14 included both pre- and postmenopausal women, who had primary treatment by total mastectomy and axillary clearance.[61] All were node-negative and had tumours which were ER-positive (>10 fmol/mg).

The results of the three studies are outlined in Table 7.10. The largest study has the shortest follow-up, and thus although a significant difference was reported in relapse-free survival, no significant effect on overall survival was seen. In contrast, both the NATO and Scottish trials showed a 7 per cent increase in overall survival for the tamoxifen-treated group.

Table 7.10 Tamoxifen trials in node-negative patients.

Group	No of patients	Follow up (years)	RFS (%)	OS (%)
Scottish trial				
Control	374	5	72	80
Tamoxifen	377		84	87
NATO trial				
Control	305	8	65	75
Tamoxifen	300		73	82
NSABP B-14				
Placebo	1318	4	77	92
Tamoxifen	1326		83	93
Placebo <50	406		73	
>50	920		79	
Tamoxifen <50	406		85	
>50	912		82	

RFS = Relapse-free survival.
OS = Overall survival.

Chemotherapy in node-negative patients

In the Milan trial, which comprised 90 patients, all with ER-negative tumours and negative axillary nodes, cases were randomized to CMF or no treatment.[64] Significant differences emerged, as shown in Table 7.11. However, the untreated ER-negative patients fared worse than would have been expected in this subgroup.

The NSABP trial B-13 recruited both pre- and postmenopausal patients who had primary treatment by total mastectomy and axillary clearance.[62] All were both node-negative and ER-negative and were randomized to either observation or to receive chemotherapy. The regimen used was a combination of methotrexate 100 mg/m^2 and fluorouracil 600 mg/m^2 followed by folinic acid rescue. This was given on days 1 and 8

Table 7.11 Chemotherapy trials in node-negative patients.

Group	No of patients	Follow up (years)	RFS (%)	OS (%)
Milan				
CMF	45	5	90	91
Control	45		45	65
NSABP B-13				
MF	339	4	80	87
Control	340		71	86
<50				
MF			74	
Control			66	
>50				
MF			89	
Control			78	
INT-0011				
CMFP	210		84	
Control	196		69	
ER− CMFP			83	
Control			71	
ER+ CMFP			87	
Control			62	

ER-negative primary tumour or an ER-positive tumour measuring at least 3 cm. After a median follow-up of 3 years, the relapse-free survival of the control group was 69 per cent compared with 84 per cent for those given CMFP. Benefit was seen for both ER-negative and positive cases. When subdivided on menopausal status, a significant effect was seen in the premenopausal but this improvement in relapse-free survival among the postmenopausal cases did not achieve statistical significance. No actual survival benefit was seen.

Should these data compel us to treat all node-negative patients with systemic adjuvant therapy? No. First, the trials comprised both pre- and postmenopausal patients. Overview analysis suggests little value for tamoxifen in premenopausal women. Thus the main options for this group would probably be either combination chemotherapy or oöphorectomy with or without prednisone. Caution should be exhibited in the consideration of the early results of chemotherapy. As an example, the earliest report of the NSABP L-PAM study suggested a benefit for all patients.[65] Subsequent follow-up showed the benefit to be more modest, and indeed the Guy's/Manchester trial of L-PAM showed no benefit whatsoever.[66] If the early report had signalled a change in policy, thousands of women would have received an ineffective treatment with a known carcinogenic activity resulting in leukaemia among those given L-PAM at a rate of 5 per 1000.[67]

Rather than give a blanket treatment of chemotherapy to all node-negative premenopausal patients it is necessary to refine prognostic tests such as tumour-labelling index or S-phase fraction and use these as a basis of controlled trials.

To give adjuvant chemotherapy to node-negative postmenopausal patients would be a pointless exercise, with minimal benefit accruing. Thus tamoxifen emerges as the

and repeated for 13 cycles. With a median follow-up of 4 years, there was a 9 per cent increase in relapse-free survival among those treated with adjuvant chemotherapy (80 versus 71 per cent), but no effect on overall survival.

The final chemotherapy trial cited by the 'Clinical Alert' was the Intergroup Study (INT-0011).[63] Node-negative pre- and postmenopausal patients were treated by CMFP or observation. Eligible cases had either an likely treatment because of its known efficacy and high acceptability to patients. However, is such a step justified? First of all, the expense is considerable. Figure 7.5 gives an approximate costing for treatment of node-positive patients, with a cost of £5000 per life saved. However, if node-negative cases were treated than this would cost £19 000 per life saved, assuming that only 2 years of treatment were given (Figure 7.6). This sum would rise to £47 500 if node-negative patients received 5 years of tamoxifen.

Another consideration, if long-term tamoxifen administration is contemplated, is that there could be an increased risk of endometrial cancer as a result of oestrogen-agonist activity. Most important of all is that the majority of node-negative patients do not require adjuvant treatment because they will never relapse. Potential reinforcement of fear of relapse may lead to increased psychiatric morbidity. Thus although plans to reduce the mortality from breast cancer are welcome, it is necessary to define more accurately those in need of treatment and then to target that

For 100 post-menopausal N− patients

	£	$
Cost per patient of 1 year's treatment	280.00	500.00
Cost per 100 per year	28 000	50 000
Cost per 100 for 2 years	56 000	100 000
Untreated, 13 will die		
With 25% reduction in mortality		
3 lives will be saved		
Cost per life saved	19 000	33 000

Figure 7.6   Cost of tamoxifen treatment of node-negative cases.

cohort. Premature adoption of adjuvant therapy for all will lead to great financial cost and unnecessary toxicity for rather borderline benefits for the majority.

For 100 post-menopausal N+ patients

	£	$
Cost per patient of 1 year's treatment	280.00	500.00
Cost per 100 per year	28 000	50 000
Cost per 100 for 2 years	56 000	100 000
Untreated, 43 will die		
With 25% reduction in mortality		
11 lives will be saved		
Cost per life saved	5 000	9 100

Figure 7.5   Cost of tamoxifen treatment of node-positive cases.

Perioperative endocrine therapy

The benefit of perioperative cytotoxic treatment has been demonstrated by Nissen-Meyer and subsequently confirmed by the CRC trial.[29,32] Since both pre- and postmenopausal patients are benefited, this suggests that perioperative treatment destroys tumour cells shed at the time of surgery.

Because therapy is instigated before axillary-nodal histology is available this means that both node-positive and node-negative cases are exposed to treatment that is unnecessary for some, and is associated with short-term toxicity in that one-third of patients will develop alopecia. Is it possible to replace perioperative cytotoxics with a gentler form of endocrine treatment?

The only consistent endocrine alteration found in patients undergoing surgery for breast cancer is an elevation of serum prolactin.[68] This is almost certainly a physiological response to the stress of both the diagnosis and treatment of malignancy. This hyperprolactinaemia has been found to be associated with a worsening of prognosis among certain groups of patients with early breast cancer, in that those with higher levels of prolactin were more likely to relapse.[69]

Prolactin is known to stimulate the growth of human breast-cancer cells, and thus the shedding of viable tumour cells into an environment rich in growth promoter might lead to the establishment of micrometastases.[70] This could have clinical significance for those patients in whom no viable tumour cells had escaped from the primary site, prior to surgery.

For these reasons a pilot study was run at Guy's to examine the feasibility and toxicity of the agent bromocriptine, a dopamine antagonist known to reduce levels of prolactin in the blood. This took the form of a double-blind, placebo-controlled randomized trial into which patients with suspected operable breast cancer were entered.[71] After they had agreed to take part, patients were randomized to receive either bromocriptine or identical placebo tablets for 5 days preoperatively and thereafter for a further 14 days if the biopsy confirmed the diagnosis of malignancy.

A total of 38 patients were entered. Eighteen received bromocriptine and 20 were given placebo. Interestingly, no side-effects were reported by either group, but a significant reduction in prolactin levels was achieved in those receiving bromocriptine. Malignancy was confirmed in 28 cases and flow cytometry was performed on disaggregated specimens from 25. There was a significant reduction in S-phase fraction of the group given bromocriptine (3 versus 10 per cent). Thus bromocriptine lowered prolactin levels without toxicity and, either directly or indirectly, inhibited the growth of the primary tumour. It is therefore conceivable that a similar effect may have been exerted on tumour cells shed by surgery. This study is being repeated at present, with measurement of S-phase fraction of tumours both before and after treatment with bromocriptine.

These preliminary results support the use of perioperative bromocriptine. It is likely that any effect on survival would be modest and might only be detectable if optimal primary treatment were given. Nevertheless, bromocriptine represents a non-toxic putative adjuvant treatment which would be compatible with subsequent endocrine or cytotoxic adjuvant therapy. The ease of administration of bromocriptine makes it a promising candidate for testing in a multicentre study.

Biological-response modifiers as adjuvant treatment

There are those who perceive breast cancer as a state in which a weakened or incompetent immune system fails to recognize tumour cells as 'non-self', thereby allowing the growth and metastasis of the carcinoma. Others suspect that the very success of tumour cells arises because they are 'self' and do not display unique tumour-specific antigens. Several trials of adjuvant treatment have been carried out using immunostimulating agents, based on the first premise, but the results yielded have tended to support the second hypothesis.

Levamisole, which normalizes the function of T-lymphocytes in immune-compromised hosts, has been tested in two trials. The Danish Breast Cancer Cooperative Group (DBCCG) treated node-positive patients with postoperative radiotherapy or radiotherapy plus levamisole (given for 48 weeks).[72]

Treatment with levamisole had to be discontinued in over 50 per cent of patients because of side-effects, including agranulocytosis, leukopenia and gastrointestinal symptoms. Recurrence rates were similar for treated and control premenopausal patients. Among the postmenopausal cases, relapse rates were higher in the levamisole-treated group.

Kay et al conducted a trial in which node-positive patients all received L-PAM, but were randomized to receive one of two dosages of levamisole or placebo.[73] No overall differences were seen between the treated and control cases. Among the premenopausal subset with less than four nodes involved, those given levamisole fared worse.

Encouraging results have been reported by Lacour et al who used as adjuvant polyadenylic-polyuridylic acid (poly A-poly U).[74] This agent stimulates natural killer (NK) cell activity and also enhances interferon synthesis. Patients were both pre- and post-menopausal, with or without axillary-nodal metastases. Postoperatively they were given either poly A-poly U (30 mg weekly) or placebo injections. After 7 years of follow-up, relapse-free survival of the treated group was 61 per cent compared with 57 per cent for the controls. Overall survival was 75 per cent in the poly A-poly U group and 65 per cent for the placebo-treated controls. No benefit was seen in node-negative cases, but overall survival was significantly increased in the node-positive group who were given poly A-poly U. This is unusual in that it would be expected that an immune stimulant would work best under conditions of minimal tumour burden, that is for node-negative patients.

At Guy's a trial was conducted to examine the value of alpha-interferon as an adjuvant treatment.[75] Rather than use node positivity as an entry criterion, a different approach was used to define a high-risk group. Eligible cases were those who had developed loco-regional relapse after primary surgery. Thus there were patients with recurrence in skin flaps, axilla or supraclavicular fossa in which recurrent disease had been obliterated by surgery and radiotherapy and where staging investigations had shown no apparent metastatic disease. Previous studies had shown that these particular patients were at very high risk of subsequent relapse of disease and therefore provided a very suitable group on which to test a putative adjuvant treatment.[76,77]

Eligible patients were randomized to receive no further treatment or to be given alpha-interferon, 3 megaunits subcutaneously daily for one year. There was a high relapse rate of over 50 per cent in both groups within 1 year and no significant differences were found, but if anything the interferon-treated group fared slightly worse. The study was stopped, partly because of the high incidence of hypothyroidism which developed in the group given interferon.[78] Subsequent work showed that the interferon or a contaminant was responsible for the production of thyroid autoantibodies.[79]

Thus, at present there is very limited evidence supporting the value of biological-response modifiers as adjuvant treatment. However, as more evidence of a value for agents such as interleukin-2 in advanced disease becomes available so it may be possible to test newer adjuvant strategies.

References

1 Moon TE, Jones SE, Bonadonna G et al, Development and use of a natural history data base of breast cancer studies, *Am J Clin Oncol (CCT)* (1987) **10**:396–403.

2 Fentiman IS, Cuzick J, Millis RR et al, Which patients are cured of breast cancer? *Br Med J* (1984) **289**:1108–11.

3 Haybittle JL, Blamey RW, Elston CW et al, A prognostic index in primary breast cancer, *Br J Cancer* (1982) **45**:361–5.

4 Todd JH, Dowle C, Williams MR et al, Confirmation of a prognostic index in primary breast cancer, *Br J Cancer* (1987) **56**:489–92.

5 Fisher B, Redmond C, Fisher ER et al, Relative worth of estrogen or progesterone receptor and pathologic characteristics of differentiation as indicators of prognosis in node negative breast cancer patients: findings from NSABP Protocol B-06, *J Clin Oncol* (1988) 1076–87.

6 McGuire WL, Estrogen receptor versus nuclear grade as prognostic factors in axillary node negative breast cancer, *J Clin Oncol* (1988) 1071–2.

7 Cuzick J, Stewart H, Peto R et al, Overview of randomised trials of post-operative adjuvant radiotherapy in breast cancer, *Cancer Treat Rep* (1987) **71**:15–29.

8 Rutqvist LE, Cedermark B, Glas U et al, The Stockholm trials on adjuvant therapy of early breast cancer, *J Clin Oncol* in press.

9 Fisher B, Slack NH, Cavanough ED, Postoperative radiotherapy in the treatment of breast cancer. Results of the NSABP clinical trial, *Ann Surg* (1970) **172**:711–30.

10 Edland RW, Does adjuvant radiotherapy have a role in the post-mastectomy management of patients with operable breast cancer—revisited, *Int J Radiat Oncol Biol Phys* (1988) **15**:519–35.

11 Tapley N du V, Spanos WJ, Fletcher GH et al, Results in patients with breast cancer treated by radical mastectomy and post-operative irradiation with no adjuvant chemotherapy, *Cancer* (1982) **49**:1316–19.

12 Fowble B, Gray R, Gilchrist K et al, Identification of a subgroup of patients with breast cancer and histologically positive axillary nodes receiving adjuvant chemotherapy who may benefit from post-operative radiotherapy, *J Clin Oncol* (1988) **6**:1107–17.

13 Cooper MR, Rhyne AL, Muss HB et al, A randomised comparative trial of chemother-apy and irradiation therapy for Stage II breast cancer, *Cancer* (1981) **47**:2833–9.

14 Early Breast Cancer Trialist's Collaborative Group, Effects of adjuvant tamoxifen and or cytotoxic therapy on mortality in early breast cancer, *N Engl J Med* (1988) **319**:1681–92.

15 Bonadonna G, Valagussa P, Dose response effect of adjuvant chemotherapy in breast cancer, *N Engl J Med* (1981) **304**:10–15.

16 Henderson IC, Hayes DF, Gelman R, Dose-response in the treatment of breast cancer: a critical review, *J Clin Oncol* (1988) **6**:1501–15.

17 Hortobagyi, GN, Bodey SP, Buzdar AV et al, Evaluation of high dose versus standard FAC chemotherapy for advanced breast cancer in protected environment units: A prospective randomised study, *J Clin Oncol* (1987) **5**:354–64.

18 Hakes T, Geller N, Petroni G et al, Confirmation of dose-survival relationship in breast adjuvant chemotherapy, *Proc Am Soc Clin Oncol* (1984) **3**:122 (abstr).

19 Howell A, Rubens RD, Bush H et al, A controlled trial of adjuvant chemotherapy with melphalan versus cyclophosphamide, methotrexate and fluorouracil for breast cancer. In: Senn HJ, ed. *Recent results in cancer research. Adjuvant chemotherapy of breast cancer* (Springer Verlag: Heidelberg 1984.)

20 Mouridsen HT, Rose C, Brincker H et al, Adjuvant systemic therapy in high risk breast cancer: the Danish Breast Cancer Cooperative Groups trials of cyclophosphamide or CMF in premenopausal and tamoxifen in postmenopausal patients. In: Senn HJ, ed. *Recent results in cancer research. Adjuvant chemotherapy of breast cancer* (Springer Verlag: Heidelberg 1984.)

21 Velez-Garcia E, Carpenter JT, Moore M et al, Post-surgical adjuvant chemotherapy with or without radiotherapy in women with breast cancer and positive axillary nodes: Progress report of a south eastern cancer study group (SEG) trial. In: Salmon SE, ed. *Adjuvant therapy of cancer V.* (Grune and Stratton: Philadelphia 1987.)

22 Hryniuk W, Levine MN, Analysis of dose intensity for adjuvant chemotherapy trials in Stage II breast cancer, *J Clin Oncol* (1986) **4**:1162–70.

23 Cooper RG, Combination chemotherapy in hormone resistant breast cancer, *Proc Am Assoc Cancer Res* (1969) **10**:15 (abstr).

24 Gelman RS, Henderson IC, A re-analysis of dose intensity for adjuvant chemotherapy trials in Stage II breast cancer, *SAKK Bull* (1987) **1**:10–12.

25 Korzun A, Norton L, Perloff M et al, Clinical equivalence despite dosage differences of two schedules of cyclophosphamide, 5-fluorouracil, vincristine and prednisone (CMFVP) for adjuvant therapy of node-positive Stage II breast cancer, *Proc Am Soc Clin Oncol* (1988) **7**:12 (abstr).

26 Howell A, Bush H, George WD et al, Controlled trial of adjuvant chemotherapy with cyclophosphamide, methotrexate and fluorouracil for breast cancer, *Lancet* (1984) **ii**:307–11.

27 Padmanabhan N, Howell A, Rubens RD, Mechanism of action of adjuvant chemotherapy in early breast cancer, *Lancet* (1986) **ii**:411–14.

28 Brincker H, Rose C, Rank F et al, Evidence of a castration-mediated effect of adjuvant cytotoxic chemotherapy in pre-menopausal breast cancer, *J Clin Oncol* (1987) **5**:1771–8.

29 Nissen-Meyer R, Kjellgren K, Malmio K et al, Surgical adjuvant chemotherapy. Results of one short course with cyclophosphamide after mastectomy for breast cancer, *Cancer* (1978) **41**:2088–98.

30 Nissen-Meyer R, The Scandinavian clinical trials. In: Baum M, Kay R, Scheurlen H, eds. *Experienta [Suppl] Clinical Trials in Early Breast Cancer* (1982), **41**.

31 Houghton J, Baum M, Nissen-Meyer R, Is there a role for peri-operative adjuvant therapy in the treatment of early breast cancer?, *Eur J Surg Oncol* (1988) **14**:227–33.

32 CRC Adjuvant Breast Trial Working Party, Cyclophosphamide and tamoxifen as adjuvant therapies in the management of breast cancer, *Br J Cancer* (1988) **57**:604–7.

33 Ludwig Breast Cancer Study Group, Combination adjuvant chemotherapy for node-positive breast cancer. Inadequacy of a single perioperative cycle, *N Engl J Med* (1988) **319**:677–83.

34 Lippman ME, Lichter AS, Edwards BK et al, The impact of primary irradiation treatment of localised breast cancer on the ability to administer systemic adjuvant chemotherapy, *J Clin Oncol* (1984) **2**:21–7.

35 Lippman ME, Edwards BK, Findlay P et al, Influence of definitive radiation therapy for primary breast cancer on ability to deliver adjuvant chemotherapy, *NCI Monogr* (1986) **1**:99–104.

36 Habibollahi F, Fentiman IS, Chaudary MA et al, The influence of radiotherapy on the dose of adjuvant chemotherapy in early breast cancer, *Breast Cancer Res Treat* (1989) **13**:237–41.

37 Ludwig Breast Cancer Study Group, Chemotherapy with or without oöphorectomy in high risk premenopausal patients with operable breast cancer, *J Clin Oncol* (1985) **3**:1059–67.

38 Taylor SG, Kalish LA, Olson JE et al, Adjuvant CMFP versus CMFP plus tamoxifen versus observation alone in postmenopausal node-positive breast cancer patients: three year results of an ECOG study, *J Clin Oncol* (1985) **3**:144–54.

39 Fisher B, Redmond C, Brown A et al, Adjuvant chemotherapy with or without tamoxifen in the treatment of primary breast cancer: 5 year results from the NSABP trial, *J Clin Oncol* (1986) **4**:459–71.

40 Ingle JN, Everson LK, Wieand S et al, Randomised trial of observation versus adjuvant therapy with cyclophosphamide, fluorouracil, prednisone with or without tamoxifen following mastectomy in post-menopausal women with node-positive breast cancer, *J Clin Oncol* (1988) **6**:1388–96.

41 Bianco AR, Gallo C, Marinelli A et al,

Adjuvant therapy with tamoxifen in operable breast cancer. 10 years results of the Naples (GUN) study, *Lancet* (1988) **ii**:1095–9.

42 Taylor GW, Evaluation of ovarian sterilization for breast cancer, *Surg Gynecol Obstet* (1939) **68**:452–6.

43 Cole MD, Suppression of ovarian function in primary breast cancer. In: Forrest APM, Kunkler PB, eds. *Prognostic factors in breast cancer.* (E and S Livingstone: Edinburgh 1968) 146–56.

44 Nissen-Meyer R, Suppression of ovarian function in primary breast cancer. In: Forrest APM, Kunkler PB, eds. *Prognostic factors in breast cancer.* (E & S Livingstone: Edinburgh 1968) 139–45.

45 Nevinny HB, Nevinny D, Rosoff CB et al, Prophylactic oöphorectomy in breast cancer therapy. A preliminary report, *Am J Surg* (1969) **117**:531–5.

46 Ravdin RG, Lewison EF, Slack NH et al, Results of a clinical trial concerning the worth of prophylactic oöphorectomy for breast carcinoma, *Surg Gynecol Obstet* (1970) **131**:1055–64.

47 Bryant AJS, Weir JA, Prophylactic oöphorectomy in operative instances of carcinoma of the breast, *Surg Gynecol Obstet* (1981) **153**:660–4.

48 Tengrup I, Nittby LT, Landberg T, Prophylactic oöphorectomy in the treatment of carcinoma of the breast, *Surg Gynecol Obstet* (1986) **162**:209–14.

49 Meakin JW, Allt WEC, Beale FA et al, Ovarian irradiation and prednisone therapy following surgery and radiotherapy for carcinoma of the breast, *Can Med Assoc J* (1979) **120**:1221–9.

50 Meakin JW, Adjuvant endocrine therapy in premenopausal women with breast cancer, *Reviews in Endocrine Related Cancer* (1987) suppl 20:23–4.

51 Ribeiro G, Swindell R, The Christie Hospital Tamoxifen (Nolvadex) Adjuvant Trial for operable breast cancer—7 year results, *Eur J Cancer Clin Oncol* (1985) **21**:897–900.

52 Fisher B, Brown A, Wolmark N et al, Prolonging tamoxifen therapy for primary breast cancer, *Ann Intern Med* (1987) **106**:649–54.

53 Breast Cancer Trials Committee, Scottish Cancer Trials Office, Adjuvant tamoxifen in the management of operable breast cancer: the Scottish trial, *Lancet* (1987) **ii**:171–5.

54 Jordan VC, Mirecki DM, Gottardis MM, Continuous tamoxifen treatment prevents the appearance of mammary tumours in a model of adjuvant therapy. In: Jones SE, Salmon SE, eds. *Adjuvant therapy of cancer*, IV (Grune and Stratton: New York 1984) 27.

55 Fornander T, Cedermark B, Mattson A et al, Adjuvant tamoxifen in early breast cancer: Occurrence of new primary cancers, *Lancet* (1989) **i**:117–19.

56 Rose C, Thorpe SM, Mouridsen HT et al, Antioestrogen treatment of postmenopausal women with primary high risk breast cancer, *Breast Cancer Res Treat* (1983) **3**:77–84.

57 Nolvadex Adjuvant Trial Organisation, Controlled trial of tamoxifen as single adjuvant agent in management of early breast cancer. Analysis at six years, *Lancet* (1985) **i**:836–40.

58 Nolvadex Adjuvant Trial Organisation, Controlled trial of tamoxifen as a single adjuvant agent in the management of early breast cancer. Analysis at eight years, *Br J Cancer* (1988) **57**:608–11.

59 Singh L, Wilson AJ, Baum M et al, The relationship between histological grade, oestrogen receptor status, events and survival at 8 years in the NATO trial, *Br J Cancer* (1988) **57**:612–14.

60 Rubens RD, Tinson CL, Coleman RF et al, Prednisolone improves the response to primary endocrine treatment for advanced breast cancer, *Br J Cancer* (1988) **58**:626–30.

61 Fisher B, Constantino J, Redmond C et al, A randomised clinical trial evaluating tamoxifen in the treatment of patients with node-negative breast cancer who have oestrogen-receptor-positive tumours, *N Engl J Med* (1989) **320**:479–84.

62 Fisher B, Redmond C, Dimitrou NV et al, A randomised clinical trial evaluating sequential methotrexate and fluorouracil in the treatment of patients with node-negative breast cancer who have oestrogen-receptor-negative tumours, *N Engl J Med* (1989) **320**:473–8.

63 Mansour EG, Gray R, Shatila AH et al, Efficacy of adjuvant chemotherapy in high-risk node-negative breast cancer. An Intergroup Study, *N Engl J Med* (1989) **320**:485–90.

64 Bonadonna G, Valagussa P, Zambetti M et al, Milan adjuvant trials for Stage I–II breast cancer. In: Salmon SE, ed. *Adjuvant therapy for cancer. V* (Grune and Stratton: Orlando 1987) 211–21.

65 Fisher B, Carbone P, Economou SG et al, L-Phenylalanine mustard (L-PAM) in the management of primary breast cancer. A report of early findings, *N Engl J Med* (1975) **292**:117–22.

66 Rubens RD, Knight RK, Fentiman IS et al, A controlled trial of adjuvant chemotherapy for breast cancer using melphalan, *Lancet* (1983) **i**:839–43.

67 Fisher B, Rockette H, Fisher ER et al, Leukaemia in breast cancer patients following adjuvant chemotherapy or postoperative radiation: The NSABP experience, *J Clin Oncol* (1985) **3**:1640–58.

68 Barni S, Lissoni P, Paolorossi F et al, Effects of radical mastectomy on prolactin levels in patients with breast cancer, *Eur J Cancer Clin Oncol* (1987) **23**:1141–5.

69 Wang DY, Hampson S, Kwa HG et al, Serum prolactin levels in women with breast cancer and their relationship to survival, *Eur J Cancer Clin Oncol* (1986) **22**:487–92.

70 Manni A, Wright C, Davis G et al, Promotion by prolactin of the growth of human breast neoplasms cultured in the soft agar clonogenic assay, *Cancer Res* (1986) **46**:1669–77.

71 Fentiman IS, Brame K, Chaudary MA et al, Perioperative bromocriptine adjuvant treatment for operable breast cancer, *Lancet* (1988) **i**:609–10.

72 Danish Breast Cancer Cooperative Group, Increased breast cancer recurrence rate after adjuvant therapy with levamisole, *Lancet* (1980) **ii**:824–7.

73 Kay RG, Mason BH, Stephens EJ et al, Levamisole in primary breast cancer. A controlled study in conjunction with L-phenylalanine mustard, *Cancer* (1983) **51**:1992–7.

74 Lacour J, Lacour F, Spira A et al, Adjuvant treatment with polyadenylic-polyuridylic acid in operable breast cancer: updated results of a randomised trial, *Br Med J* (1984) **288**:589–92.

75 Fentiman IS, Balkwill FS, Cuzick J et al, A trial of human alpha interferon as an adjuvant agent in breast cancer after loco-regional relapse, *Eur J Surg Oncol* (1987) **13**:425–8.

76 Fentiman IS, Matthews PN, Davison OW et al, Survival following local skin recurrence after mastectomy, *Br J Surg* (1985) **92**:14–16.

77 Fentiman IS, Lavelle MA, Kaplan D et al, The significance of supraclavicular fossa node recurrence after radical mastectomy, *Cancer* (1986) **57**:908–10.

78 Fentiman IS, Thomas BS, Balkwill FR et al, Primary hypothyroidism associated with interferon therapy for breast cancer, *Lancet* (1985) **i**:1166.

79 Fentiman IS, Balkwill FR, Thomas BS et al, An autoimmune aetiology for hypothyroidism following interferon therapy for breast cancer, *Eur J Cancer Clin Oncol* (1988) **24**:1299–1303.

CHAPTER 8

PSYCHOLOGICAL STRATEGIES

Nobody is on my side, nobody takes part with me: I am cruelly used, nobody feels for my poor nerves.

Jane Austen

All women with early breast cancer need to make a psychological adjustment to their disease. This is commonly associated with periods of emotional distress and about a quarter develop clinically significant depression or anxiety. Clear, empathetic communication and support from clinicians and nurses can ameliorate distress, and specific psychological and pharmacological interventions are effective in the management of the more severe psychological disturbances.

Various aspects of breast cancer, its treatment and the patient's personal life contribute to the psychological morbidity. These include knowledge of the diagnosis, the unwanted effects of surgery, cytotoxic chemotherapy, endocrine therapy and radiotherapy as well as wider issues of premorbid psychological adjustment and social support. An understanding of the relative importance of these different factors can help surgeons and physicians plan the physical management of a disease for which there are an increasing number of available treatment options. This also allows psychosocial support to be tailored to the specific needs of the individual patient.

Psychosocial consequences of early breast cancer

The influence of early breast cancer on patients' lives has been studied mainly in those treated by mastectomy and has focused on the impact on mood, marital and sexual relationships and work.

Psychological morbidity associated with mastectomy

Recent prospective studies have shown that about a quarter of women undergoing mastectomy develop clinically significant anxiety or depression in the first two years after operation.[1–3] This figure is similar to the prevalence of morbidity reported in patients with other cancers.[4,5] According to Research Diagnostic Criteria[6] used in Dean's study,[3] most of the cases fulfilled the criteria for minor depressive disorder or generalized anxiety disorder. The proportion of cases with a major depressive disorder was no greater than that in a matched random community sample.

Deterioration in sexual relationships has been reported in up to 50 per cent of women undergoing mastectomy in the first 2 years after operation.[1-3] This sexual morbidity has been shown to be significantly associated with psychiatric morbidity.[3] In general, marital relationships are not adversely affected following mastectomy and some actually improve. A deterioration in marital relations has been reported in about 10 per cent of early breast cancer patients and between 6 and 50 per cent report an improvement.[1,3,7]

More than 50 per cent of women are back at work 3 months after mastectomy according to most studies,[1,3,8,9] and over 70 per cent after 1 to 2 years.[1,3]

Significance of loss of the breast

Psychological morbidity associated with loss of the breast itself has been studied by assessing the impact of immediate breast reconstruction on the morbidity associated with mastectomy, and also by comparing the morbidity of mastectomy and breast conservation. A randomized trial of immediate reconstruction after mastectomy versus the option of reconstruction at 1 year demonstrated that immediate reconstruction lowered psychiatric morbidity at 3 months post-mastectomy. At 12 months, however, the psychiatric morbidity had fallen in both groups and the difference was no longer significant.[10] This suggests that breast reconstruction may be effective in lowering *early* psychiatric morbidity following operation.

Contrary to expectation, there is little evidence to suggest breast conservation with radiotherapy reduces the psychiatric morbidity associated with mastectomy. Studies using standardized psychological measures show no difference in postoperative inci-dence of anxiety states and depressive illness amongst women undergoing the two types of treatment.[11-15] Similarly, the loss of sexual interest appears to occur at the same rate in patients undergoing breast conservation and mastectomy. Fallowfield et al, in a retrospective study, reported that over 30 per cent of both the mastectomy and breast-conservation group described loss of libido.[15] Nevertheless, breast conservation does reduce the body-image disturbances associated with mastectomy.[11,13,14] These findings suggest, therefore, that loss of the breast is not the main causal factor in the psychosexual morbidity associated with the diagnosis and management of early breast cancer. The fear and uncertainty associated with the knowledge of having a potentially fatal disease which all patients have in common, regardless of their treatment, may be more important in determining levels of depression and anxiety. Indeed Fallowfield et al suggest that women undergoing a conservation procedure may experience more anxiety related to the possibility of disease recurrence.[15]

Impact of treatment choice

There is preliminary evidence that patients given the choice of treatment between mastectomy and breast conservation experience lower levels of anxiety and depression subsequently than those who are not.[16,17] Offering patients a choice of surgery is not a simple matter however, and there are outstanding problems in presenting options. The authors of these studies stressed the importance of comprehensive pre-operative assessment, giving information and counselling to help women make their choice. Those women who opt for breast conservation seem to have a high degree of concern about their physical appearance and maintenance of a complete body image.[17] Breast conservation is not, however, an automatic choice. A proportion of women offered the choice opt for mastectomy and do so for a number of reasons including fear of recurrence in a conserved breast and desire for rapid treatment for domestic and employment reasons. For these women self-esteem does not seem to be dependent upon maintenance of a complete body image.[17,18]

The choice women make may be determined by their individual priorities in terms of their body image and fear of recurrence. More systematic enquiry is needed to evaluate the process of giving patients an unbiased choice and whether all patients necessarily benefit from the opportunity to choose.

Psychosocial morbidity associated with adjuvant therapy

Adjuvant therapy can increase the psychiatric morbidity associated with breast cancer. Dean found that patients who had adjuvant cytotoxic chemotherapy, radiotherapy or oöphorectomy following mastectomy experienced significantly more psychiatric morbidity at 3 months postoperatively than those treated by mastectomy alone.[3] At 12 months there was no difference in the morbidity between the two groups.

However, no specific association has been shown between adjuvant radiotherapy and this increase in psychiatric morbidity. Two prospective studies found no difference between levels of anxiety and depression in women treated by mastectomy with or without adjuvant radiotherapy.[1,19] Radiotherapy has, nevertheless, been shown to be associated with early social dysfunction and somatic symptoms.

Cytotoxic chemotherapy, on the other hand, does increase postoperative levels of psychiatric morbidity. The extent of physical toxicity associated with adjuvant chemotherapy is well documented. A controlled trial of a five-drug combination (chlorambucil, methotrexate, fluorouracil, vincristine and adriamycin) compared with a single agent (chlorambucil) showed that 42 per cent of the group given the single agent had side-effects sufficient to interfere with their lifestyle, including nausea, vomiting, malaise and alopecia, compared with 79 per cent receiving the five-drug combination.[20] Maguire et al showed that mastectomy and combination adjuvant chemotherapy were associated with significantly more psychiatric morbidity than mastectomy alone or with adjuvant Melphalan and that this morbidity was linked with physical toxicity.[21]

Hughson et al compared psychiatric morbidity following mastectomy in patients with early breast cancer who were randomly allocated to cytotoxic chemotherapy alone, radiotherapy alone or a combination of chemotherapy and radiotherapy.[22] In patients free from recurrence, psychiatric morbidity was the same in the three groups at 1, 3 and 6 months. After 13 months, however, patients who had been allocated chemotherapy had significantly more psychological symptoms, especially depression, than the patients treated with radiotherapy alone. Anticipatory nausea and vomiting increased considerably in the second 6 months of chemotherapy and persisted for up to 1 year. At 18 months and 2 years after the operation, differences in psychiatric morbidity disappeared. This suggests that restricting the duration of courses of cytotoxic chemotherapy would reduce the associated psychiatric morbidity.

Prevention and management of psychosocial problems

Staff/patient communication

Imparting information about cancer to patients is a topic which provokes controversy both within the medical profession and among patients and their families.[23,24] In recent years there has been a shift in emphasis from a paternalistic philosophy of care to one in which the patient is viewed as a health-care consumer with rights to information and access to health professionals. Patient dissatisfaction with information given to them by the doctors has been consistently reported.[25,26] 'Not being told what is wrong' is the most frequent complaint patients make, according to Fletcher.[27] Increasingly, it seems, patients want more information about their cancer, and unnecessary distress could be prevented by improved staff/patient communication.

Simple strategies can be employed to increase the amount of information a cancer patient retains from an interview. These include inviting a close companion to be with the patient during a consultation.[28] Good supplementary information can be provided in the form of information sheets, booklets, posters and audio and video tapes about cancer and its management.[29]

Two recent studies have looked at the benefit of audiotaping consultations between doctors and patients and giving the tapes to the patient.[24,30] First, it was shown that such an intervention was practicable during the routine general surgical and oncology outpatient clinics. Second, patients and their families derived considerable subjective benefit from the opportunity of hearing again the details of their diagnosis and treatment.

Future doctors are also being taught more effective ways of talking to patients about their illness and its treatment. Communication-skills training is being included in the curriculum of some medical schools.[31] Increasingly such courses, funded by cancer charities, are becoming available for trained nurses, doctors and other health professionals.[32] The aim is to improve basic assessment and interviewing skills. Workshops are multidisciplinary and run by experienced tutors, usually a doctor and a nurse. Participants learn how to improve their skills in eliciting

patient concerns and assessing their psychological and social adjustment to their illness. Other communication skills examined include the breaking of bad news, dealing with difficult questions (such as the prognosis of the disease) and handling emotional distress, uncertainty and denial. Teaching techniques involve group discussion, video demonstrations and role-play of interviews with cancer patients.

Follow-up arrangements

Many patients experience considerable distress immediately before and during their follow-up appointments, when fear of detection of disease recurrence is most intense. Such distress can be reduced by ensuring continuity of care, with patients being seen as far as possible by the same clinician at each visit. Improvements in the protracted waiting times and the unfriendly surroundings of many outpatient clinics might also alleviate some of the misery.

Prostheses

A survey of breast prostheses and fitting services on offer in the British National Health Service has revealed the deficiencies and inadequacies of the services that exist in many hospitals.[33] For those women who undergo mastectomy, an adequate prosthesis fitted by a trained, competent fitter is essential to avoid some of the distress which they report as a consequence of their experience of current services.

Patient support groups

Some hospitals organize support groups for cancer patients and their families.[34] The charity Cancerlink provides a directory of self-help groups and information on the training and organization necessary to set up such groups. Regular attenders of support groups report deriving considerable benefit from the information and support they receive. So far, however, there has been little systematic evaluation of their effectiveness for breast-cancer patients.

Detection and evaluation of psychosocial morbidity

Until those patients who develop difficulties adjusting to their disease have been identified and the nature of their problems understood, appropriate psychological support and intervention for them cannot begin.

This is not as straightforward as it would appear and during routine medical care only about 20–25 per cent of cases of clinical anxiety and depression are recognized and referred for appropriate help. Furthermore, in one study of patients undergoing mastectomy none of the 30 per cent of patients who developed sexual problems was recognized and offered help.[35] There are a number of reasons for this disparity between levels of psychological and sexual morbidity and their recognition and referral.

Patients are often reluctant to disclose psychological problems. They do not want to appear inadequate or ungrateful, nor do they want to waste the doctors' and nurses' time on trivial and understandable problems about which they believe nothing can be done. Health professionals, for their part, are reluctant to enquire because they feel they lack the time to do so and the expertise to deal with the distress they may reveal. They may also feel that probing will do more psychological harm than good.

There are also problems in the evaluation of the nature and severity of mood disturbances once they have been recognized. It can be difficult to distinguish between episodes of unhappiness and worry which are normal responses to stress and pathological mood states of depressive illness and anxiety states. The former may be prerequisite to long-term adjustment, but the latter serve no useful purpose, impair quality of survival and merit treatment. It is also difficult to know what significance to ascribe to cases of distress or borderline anxiety and depression. Some will be the prodrome of full-blown psychiatric illnesses, but others are transient disorders which undergo spontaneous remission. These problems are complicated by the fact that mood disorders have physical as well as mental symptoms. Many of these physical symptoms, including lack of energy, sleep disturbance and loss of appetite and weight, can be indistinguishable from the symptoms of metastatic cancer or the side-effects of treatment.

For all these reasons, psychological morbidity amongst breast-cancer patients often goes undetected and consequently untreated. This is an important problem since intervention can be of enormous benefit.

There are three possible ways in which detection may be practicably improved. First, clinicians can be trained in basic psychiatric interview techniques. Alternatively, specialist nurses can be trained to assess systematically patients' psychological, social and physical adjustment to their cancer and its treatment. With the use of standardized assessment interviews, key areas covered should include the patients' understanding and perception of their disease and its treatment and their physical symptoms and functioning. The quality of their relationships with those close to them, in particular their spouse and family, and their domestic, social and occupational circumstances should be elicited. Finally, enquiries about their psychological status focusing on mood and mood-related symptoms are important.[36] A specialist nurse trained to assess and counsel patients with early breast cancer and to monitor their progress and adjustment can raise the detection rate of psychiatric morbidity from 15 to 76 per cent.[37]

The information from a routine standardized psychosocial assessment can contribute to and enhance discussions of patient management on medical and surgical ward rounds. It can also contribute to ward meetings, held specifically to discuss issues of psychosocial management. These may be attended by the nurse specialist who performs the assessments, as well as a ward doctor and nurse, social worker, occupational therapist and physiotherapist.[38]

An alternative approach to improve the detection of psychological morbidity is the use of screening questionnaires which can be administered by untrained personnel. There are a number of existing measures of mood disturbance which can be used, but most contain some somatic symptoms which confound the assessment of psychological and physical morbidity and inflate the rates of psychological disturbance. It is important that somatic symptoms are either excluded or dealt with separately. The Hospital and Anxiety Depression Scale (HADS) has been developed specifically for use amongst physically ill patients and excludes somatic symptoms, concentrating on the psychic manifestations of mood disorder.[39] It is brief and easily completed by patients. It is also quick and easy to score, giving separate values for anxiety and depression. It can be used repeatedly and thus allows monitoring of patients' mood states over time.

The Rotterdam symptom checklist is an alternative self-rating assessment which covers a broader area of adjustment to cancer and its treatment.[40] It assesses not only psychological symptoms, but also activities of daily living, physical toxicity due to treatment and physical symptoms due to disease.

The sensitivity of these instruments is good. Between 80 and 90 per cent of patients with early breast cancer who have clinical anxiety or depression can be correctly identified. However, there are high false-positive rates. Only between one- and two-thirds of high scorers are actual psychiatric cases.[41,42] As with any screening instrument, however, it is better to identify incorrectly as ill an excess of psychologically well women, than to miss those with psychiatric morbidity. Discovering which women actually have a psychiatric illness would, in fact, be a two-stage procedure: screening for psychological distress using a questionnaire and then conducting a psychiatric interview with the high scorers to identify the clinical cases.

Health professionals could be more sensitive to the presence of psychiatric morbidity by being aware of its attendant risk factors. To date these have been shown to include treatment with cytotoxic chemotherapy, pre-operative psychiatric disorder, a previous psychiatric history, lack of social support, in particular lack of opportunity to confide worries and concerns, and pre-existing marital difficulties.[3,22,43] Further study of possible prognostic indicators of psychiatric morbidity and also of sexual morbidity might enable identification of patients at risk of developing psychosexual disturbances who do not necessarily manifest distress or problems at the time of assessment. This might allow early intervention to prevent fully developed psychiatric disorders.

Whichever way it is done, screening for psychological morbidity reveals that a substantial proportion of patients with breast cancer are well adjusted to their illness and its treatment. When assessed they are not distressed, clinically anxious or depressed. They have sufficient personal resources and social support to cope with their situation themselves and do not need specific psychological or social intervention.

Management of distress

Distress or mild psychological disturbance experienced by breast-cancer patients is often transient and closely associated in time and content to some illness-related event, such as news of diagnosis or disease progression. The optimum management of distressed patients has not received much consideration or evaluation. A pragmatic solution is for them to see a nurse specialist who has received a counselling training. She can provide not only practical information about the disease and its management, but also psychotherapeutic support.[38]

Important components of such counselling include explanation of physical and psychological symptoms and challenging false beliefs about cancer. In addition, patients can be encouraged to express their concerns and fears. In this way rational hope can be engendered and any sense of isolation removed. Distressed and bereaved relatives benefit from a similar approach. The recent King's Fund Consensus on the treatment of primary breast cancer stated that 'It is essential that counselling should be available',[44] and clinical experience certainly supports this. To date, study of the benefits of counselling has been methodologically poor and the findings equivocal.[45,46] Systematic evaluation of the impact of counselling and the relative influence of its various components is needed. For counselling to be conducted safely in clinical practice it should be undertaken by those who have received an adequate training. Regular supervision of a counsellor's work is essential to ensure a balanced perspective about what is and is not achievable for a specific patient and to prevent the counsellor becoming emotionally overburdened by her work.[47]

Management of psychiatric morbidity

Patients who have developed more severe psychological disturbances are likely to be-nefit from structured psychotherapy, either alone or in conjunction with psychotropic medication.

Cognitive therapy

A promising approach is provided by cognitive therapy, which aims to bring about improvement in psychological disturbance by altering the underlying maladaptive ways of thinking about cancer.[48] In this context the word 'cognition' is used as if it were synonymous with 'thinking'. In general psychiatric practice, cognitive therapy has been shown to be effective in the management of mild and moderate depressive and anxiety disorders.[49] It has been particularly well developed for the management of cancer-related psychosocial morbidity by Moorey and Greer,[50] and it is being evaluated in a randomized controlled trial.

Cognitive therapy aims to develop coping skills which will enable patients who have become psychologically overwhelmed by the impact of their cancer to deal more effectively with the crisis as well as future crises. In addition, it is designed to reduce anxiety, depression and other psychiatric symptoms and to induce a more positive attitude to the disease and to life in general. This approach promotes in patients a greater sense of personal control over their lives; finally, it focuses on improving communication between the patient and their partner and family.

Cognitive therapy is a relatively brief psychotherapy, usually involving no more than 12 weekly sessions of 1 hour duration each. The therapist is usually a psychologist or a psychiatrist, but may be any health professional trained in the theory and practice of cognitive therapy.

The components of cognitive therapy described by Moorey and Greer include ventilation of feelings, behavioural and cognitive strategies.[50]

Ventilation of feelings

This plays an important part in the management of patients undergoing adjustment reactions to any severe crisis and is usually necessary before a more rational problem-solving approach can be used. Non-directive methods of empathy, listening, reflecting, showing warmth and genuineness facilitate the expression of emotion and are an essential ingredient of cognitive therapy.

Behavioural techniques

Control of symptoms of psychological distress.
An example of this is the management of anxiety using relaxation training or distraction techniques.

Control of environment.
The diagnosis and treatment of cancer often leaves patients feeling a loss of personal control over their body. They may develop a hopeless and helpless response which generalizes this sense of loss of control to other areas of their lives. This may lead in turn to a decrease in activities and a self-perpetuating cycle of decreasing activity and increasing helplessness and hopelessness. Scheduling activities which promote feelings of mastery can help to break that cycle by structuring the day and providing an increased sense of achievement.

Reality testing.
Maladaptive beliefs about cancer and its treatment and the ability to cope with these hurdles can create distress. Patients can be encouraged to treat such beliefs as hypotheses that they then test. Thus for a woman who believes her husband will no longer find her attractive after mastectomy, such a behavioural experiment would involve finding out directly from her husband what he does find attractive about her and his views on the loss of her breast.

Cognitive techniques

Eliciting and challenging negative thoughts.
These are part of the ongoing internal dialogue we all have with ourselves and which has a very strong influence on emotions and moods. A typical negative thought of a patient with cancer who is depressed might be 'Now I have cancer I am a failure and everything has gone wrong'. Such a patient would be encouraged to monitor these thoughts and subsequently to challenge them. This would involve *reality testing*, namely examining the evidence for and against the belief. Evidence for would be, for example, 'clearly, part of my body has failed to function normally'. Evidence against would be 'but that abnormal part has been removed and I have had treatment to try and prevent further problems. In the rest of my life, things are going well. Family life is flourishing: we have just had a good holiday together and my husband and children still love and need me. Work is going well; the boss is keen for me to consider taking on more responsibility.'

Another method of challenging negative thinking is *looking for alternatives*. A patient who feels bleak and hopeless about the future may be encouraged to explore ways in which her life might be changed for the better as a result of the cancer. For example, she may consider spending more time with loved ones, learning to take things easy, planning things which she and her partner have always wanted to do.

Direct confrontation of cancer-related fears is sometimes necessary. This may be appropriate for a patient who is overwhelmingly fearful and preoccupied by thoughts of disease progression. Encouraging them to imagine the possibility of such progression may allow them to realize that, although it may not be easy, there are ways in which they could foresee they would cope with the situation.

Cognitive rehearsal. Problem-solving techniques for dealing with the very real difficulties that distressed cancer patients face can be taught. Once a particular problem has been identified and an adaptive way of dealing with it has been worked out, then rehearsing the strategy within the therapy sessions can be useful. An important example would be preparing to tell family and friends about the diagnosis of a breast cancer.

The following types of psychological problems may benefit from this approach:

Mood disturbances, in particular depression and anxiety.

Body-image problems including difficulty adjusting to loss of the breast, lymphoedema and alopecia. Women describe feelings of being mutilated which can lead to avoidance of looking at or touching their bodies and withdrawing from intimate physical relationships and other social contact.

Dysfunctional coping strategies in response to cancer which cause distress either to the patient or her family, or interfere with management of her disease. Extreme denial and avoidance are important examples. In the presence of an overwhelming threat such as the diagnosis of cancer or disease progression, a common reaction is to believe and act as if nothing has happened. This is often only a transient response. Alternatively, it may only apply to one aspect of the situation; a patient may believe her breast lump is harmless, but be willing to accept a mastectomy 'as a precautionary measure'. Such coping strategies should probably not be

interfered with. However, if a patient's denial or avoidance of her cancer causes her to refuse life-saving treatment, or despite her coping strategies she remains tearful and depressed, then intervention may be indicated. Similarly, prolonged, intense anger or dependence may benefit from treatment.

Marital and sexual problems involving joint therapy with the patient and her partner. Marital therapy usually focuses on issues of communication and adaptation to role changes. In the management of sexual difficulties emphasis is placed on the behavioural aspect of the therapy using Masters and Johnson techniques.[51]

Anticipatory nausea and vomiting associated with cytotoxic chemotherapy can be reduced using behavioural treatments, in particular relaxation techniques and systemic desensitisation.[52,53]

It is important that the psychotherapy is flexible and tailored to the individual needs of the patient. For those presenting in a state of acute and overwhelming crisis the initial objective must be reduction of arousal, resolution of the immediate crisis and restoration to at least the level of functioning that existed before the crisis.[54] For those who have long-standing difficulties coping with the vicissitudes of life and a number of ongoing personal difficulties, a more psychodynamic approach is likely to be of benefit. This involves more detailed consideration of the patient's emotional difficulties in terms of relationships and past life. Such psychodynamic psychotherapy can also be brief and focused on a specific set of issues or problems.[55]

Drug management of depression

Indications for antidepressant medication are listed below. The criteria are that at least five of the following symptoms present during the same 2-week period and represent a change from previous functioning; at least one of the symptoms must be either depressed mood or loss of interest or pleasure.[56]

- Depressed mood
- Marked loss of interest or pleasure in daily activities
- Feelings of worthlessness or excessive and inappropriate guilt
- Significant weight loss or gain when not dieting and in the absence of metastatic disease or treatment with chemotherapy
- Insomnia or hypersomnia, particularly early morning wakening
- Persistent fatigue or loss of energy in the absence of metastatic disease or treatment with chemotherapy or radiotherapy
- Diminished ability to think or concentrate
- Recurrent suicidal ideation
- Psychomotor agitation or retardation
- Diurnal variation of mood, which is worse in the morning

Evidence that the depression is significantly impairing the quality of the patient's life supports the use of antidepressants.

Tricyclic antidepressants have been the standard treatment for depressive illness in general psychiatric practice for 30 years and are the most commonly used antidepressants in patients with cancer. Although they have received little empirical evaluation in depressed cancer patients, existing studies have demonstrated their benefit.[57] To be effective they need to be administered in adequate dosage with good compliance for 6 weeks or more, after which a reduced dose should be continued for a further 4 to 6 months. Ineffective dosage is probably the most important cause of non-response and in clinical practice the development of mild side-effects is a useful determinant of adequate dosage. To ensure good compliance the

rationale for treatment needs to be explained. Patients need to be warned about the development of unpleasant side-effects and the lack of an immediate beneficial response. They often need reassurance that tricyclic antidepressants are not tranquillizers and cannot induce dependence. Easy and immediate access to advice about the drug effects also promotes compliance.

Patients with metastatic disease and those who are receiving cytotoxic chemotherapy appear to have decreased tolerance to the side-effects of tricyclic antidepressants and for this reason they frequently receive their antidepressant medication in the lower end of the therapeutic range. Patients who are both depressed and severely physically ill probably derive less benefit from antidepressants than those who are physically well. However, if the depression is moderate or severe they warrant a trial of drug treatment as it can be beneficial in some cases.

Drug management of anxiety

For severe intractable anxiety states intermittent, flexible dosage regimes of benzodiazepines may be effective. In view of the risk of dependency developing, however, their use should always be restrained and closely supervised. Alternatively, low doses of neuroleptics can be given. When the anxiety is related to a specific situation, for example, administration of chemotherapy then anxiolytic drugs are most beneficial when they are taken directly before and during the stressful event, rather than given on a regular daily basis. Such a pharmacological approach works well when combined with behavioural interventions, particularly anxiety-management techniques, relaxation training and distraction techniques.

Management of psychological consequences of cerebral disorder

Cerebral complications of early breast cancer and its management sometimes have neuropsychiatric manifestations. Such organic reactions may occur in response to cytotoxic chemotherapy, analgesia, steroids, general metabolic disturbance or cerebral metastatic disease.[58] They may benefit from a psychiatric opinion concerning diagnosis or intervention. In particular, the judicious use of psychotropic medication and behavioural strategies may be effective in the management of acute or chronic cerebral disorders.

The role of psychological factors in the prognosis of breast cancer

Recent well-designed studies suggest an association between certain psychological factors and disease outcome in breast cancer. There is accumulating evidence that both mental adjustment to cancer and the experience of stressful life events influence disease prognosis.

The influence of stressful life events on the development of relapse of operable breast cancer has been examined in matched pairs of women in a case-control study.[59] Adverse life events and ongoing difficulties occurring during the postoperative disease-free interval were recorded in 50 women who had developed their first recurrence of early breast cancer, and during equivalent follow-up time in 50 women with operable breast cancer in remission. The cases and controls were matched for the main physical and pathological factors known to be prognostic in breast cancer and sociodemographic variables that influence the frequency of life events and difficulties. A measure of life events and difficulties was used which accurately dated these stressors to ensure that they preceded the clinical onset of

progression of the disease. The measure also attempted to assess the objective threat of life events and difficulties independently of both the subject's emotional reaction and any investigator bias.

Severely threatening adverse life events and ongoing difficulties were shown to be significantly associated with first relapse of breast cancer. Examples include death of a loved one and divorce. Non-severe stressors such as a routine varicose vein operation or a minor road-traffic accident were not found to be associated with relapse.

Two prospective studies have found a relationship between early mental adjustment to cancer and disease outcome. Pettingale et al, in a consecutive series of 57 women with early breast cancer, showed that patients who coped with their disease 3 months postoperatively using attitudes of fighting spirit and denial were more likely to be alive and free from disease after 10 years of follow-up.[60] The patients were similar in terms of some, but not all, of the physical determinants of disease outcome. Hislop et al studied a series of 127 women with early breast cancer and demonstrated an association between extroversion, frequent involvement in social activities and lower levels of anger at the time of diagnosis and survival 4 years later.[61]

The mechanism whereby these psychological factors might affect the prognosis of breast cancer is unknown. Suggested intermediaries include the neuroendocrine and immune systems, which could promote growth of previously dormant or subclinical metastases. Investigation of this is complex and difficult.[62] Modifications in behaviour leading to direct exposure to carcinogens must also be considered as a possible mediating process.

Current evidence concerning the influence of psychological factors on the prognosis of early breast cancer requires corroboration in large prospective studies. The interactions between severe life stress, coping behaviour and social support need to be examined. Improved understanding of the influence of these psychological factors and any interactions between them may have important implications for managing patients, including the refinement of psychological treatments aimed at helping patients with breast cancer adjust to the impact of their disease and cope with the consequences of subsequent severe life stressors.

Providing a comprehensive network of psychosocial care for patients with breast cancer involves the cooperation of a number of health professionals including counsellors, a psychiatrist or a psychologist and social workers. They need to ensure continuity of support by collaborating closely with the medical and nursing staff, as well as liaising with community services including general practitioners and district nurses. Above all, there needs to be a willingness and commitment from the frontline clinicians and nurses to give priority to patients' needs for clear communication and psychological support.

References

1 Morris T, Goodyer HS, White P, Psychological and social adjustment to mastectomy: a two year follow-up study, *Cancer* (1977) **40**:2381–7.

2 Maguire GP, Lee EG, Bevington DJ et al, Psychiatric problems in the first year after mastectomy. *Br Med J* (1978) **1**:963–5.

3 Dean C, Psychiatric morbidity following mastectomy: preoperative predictors and types of illness, *J Psychosom Res* (1987) **31**:385–92.

4 Worden JW, Weisman AD, The fallacy in post-mastectomy depression, *Am J Med Sci* (1977) **273**:169–75.

5 Devlen J, Maguire P, Phillips P et al, Psychological problems associated with diagnosis and treatment of lymphomas. I. A retrospective study. II. A prospective study, *Br Med J* (1987) **295**:953–4, 955–7.

6 Spitzer L, Endicott J, Robins E, Research diagnostic criteria: rationale and reliability. *Arch Gen Psychiatry* (1978) **35**:773–82.

7 Hughes J, Emotional reactions to the diagnosis and treatment of early breast cancer, *J Psychosom Res* (1981) **26**:277–83.

8 Silberfarb PM, Maurer H, Crouthamel CS, Psychosocial aspects of neoplastic disease. I. Functional status of breast cancer: patients during different treatment regimes. *Am J Psychiatry* (1980) **137**:450–5.

9 McArdle CS, Calman KC, Cooper AS et al, The social, emotional and financial implications of adjuvant chemotherapy in breast cancer, *Br J Surg* (1981) **68**:261–4.

10 Dean C, Chetty U, Forrest APM, Effects of immediate breast reconstruction on psychosocial morbidity after mastectomy, *Lancet* (1983) **i**:459–62.

11 Sanger CK, Reznikoff M, A comparison of the psychological effects of breast saving procedures with the modified radical mastectomy, *Cancer* (1981) **48**:2341–6.

12 Schain W, Edwards BK, Gorrell CR et al, Psychosocial and physical outcomes of Stage I breast cancer therapy: mastectomy versus excisional biopsy and irradiation, *Breast Cancer Res Treat* (1983) **3**:377–82.

13 Sternberg MD, Juliano NA, Wise L, Psychological outcome after lumpectomy versus mastectomy in the treatment of breast cancer, *Am J Psychiatry* (1985) **143**:34–9.

14 De Haes JCJM, van Oostrom MA, Welvaart K, The effect of radical and conserving surgery on the quality of life of early breast cancer patients, *Eur J Surg Oncol* (1986) **12**:337–42.

15 Fallowfield LJ, Baum M, Maguire GP, Effects of breast conservation on psychological morbidity associated with the diagnosis and treatment of early breast cancer, *Br Med J* (1986) **293**:1331–4.

16 Morris J, Royle GT, Choice of surgery for early breast cancer: pre and postoperative levels of clinical anxiety and depression in patients and their husbands, *Br J Surg* (1987) **74**:1017–19.

17 Ashcroft JJ, Leinster SJ, Glade PD, Breast cancer—patient choice of treatment: preliminary communication, *J R Soc Med* (1985) **78**:43–6.

18 Wilson RG, Hart A, Dawes PJDK, Mastectomy or conservation: the patient's choice, *Br Med J* (1988) **297**:1167–9.

19 Hughson AVM, Cooper AF, McArdle CS et al, Psychosocial effects of radiotherapy after mastectomy, *Br Med J* (1987) **294**:1515–18.

20 Palmer BV, Walsh GA, McKinna JA et al, Adjuvant chemotherapy for breast cancer: side effects and quality of life, *Br Med J* (1980) **281**:1594–7.

21 Maguire GP, Tait A, Brooke EM et al, Psychiatric morbidity and physical toxicity associated with adjuvant chemotherapy after mastectomy, *Br Med J* (1980) **281**:1179–80.

22 Hughson AVM, Cooper AS, McArdle CS et al, Psychological impact of adjuvant chemotherapy in the first two years after mastectomy, *Br Med J* (1986) **293**:1268–71.

23 Brewin TB, The cancer patient: communication and morale, *Br Med J* (1977) **2**:1623–7.

24 Reynolds PM, Sanson-Fisher RW, Desmond-Poole A et al, Cancer and communication: information-giving in an oncology clinic, *Br Med J* (1981) **282**:1449–51.

25 Stedeford A, Couples facing death—unsatisfactory communication, *Br Med J* (1981) **283**:1098–101.

26 Tuckett D, Williams A, Approaches to the measurement of explanation and information-giving in medical consultations: a review of empirical studies, *Soc Sci Med* (1984) **18**:571–80.

27 Fletcher C, Listening and talking to patients, *Br Med J* (1980) **291**:994–6.

28 Fallowfield LJ, Baum M, Maguire GP, Addressing the psychological needs of the conserva-tively treated breast cancer patient: discussion paper, *J R Soc Med* (1987) **80**:696–700.

29 Ellis DA, Hopkin JM, Leitch AG et al, 'Doctor's orders': a control trial of supplementary written information for patients, *Br Med J* (1979) **i**:456.

30 Hogbin B, Fallowfield LJ, Getting it taped. The 'bad news' consultation with cancer patients, *Br J Hosp Med* **41**:330–3.

31 Rutter DR, Maguire GP, History taking for medical students. II. Evaluation of a training programme, *Lancet* (1976) **i**:558–60.

32 Maguire GP, Faulkner A, Improving the counselling skills of doctors and nurses in cancer care, *Br Med J* (1988) **297**:847–9.

33 Simpson GD, Are you being served? A survey on breast prosthesis and fitting service on offer in the NHS, *Senior Nurse* (1985) **12**:6.

34 Plant H, Richardson J, Stubbs L et al, Evaluation of a support group for cancer patients and their families and friends, *Br J Hosp Med* (1987) **38(4)**:317–22.

35 Maguire P, Communication skills and patient care. In: Matthews A, Steptoe A, eds. *Health care and human behaviour* (Academic Press: London 1984).

36 Tait A, Maguire P, Faulkner A et al, Improving communication skills, *Nursing Times* (1982) **78**:2181–4.

37 Maguire P, Tait A, Brooke M et al, Effect of counselling on the psychiatric morbidity associated with mastectomy, *Br Med J* (1980) **281**:1454–6.

38 Ramirez AJ, Psychosocial care in a clinical oncology unit, *J R Soc Health* (1989) in press.

39 Zigmond AS, Snaith RP, The hospital anxiety and depression scale, *Acta Psychiatr Scand* (1983) **67**:361–70.

40 de Haes JCJM, Pruyn JSA, Knippenberg FCE, Klachtenlijst voor kanker patienten. Eerste ervarngen, *Ned Tijdschariste voor de psychologie* (1987) **38**:403–22.

41 Ibbotson T, Maguire P, Selby P et al, Detection of anxiety and depression in patients with

cancer, Paper presented at the 5th British Psychosocial Oncology Group Annual Conference (1988).

42 Trew M, Maguire P, Further comparison of two instruments to measure quality of life in cancer patients, *Proceedings of the 3rd EORTC workshop on quality of life* (Paris 1982) 111–27.

43 Ramirez AJ, Liaison psychiatry in a breast cancer unit, *J R Soc Med* (1989) **82**:15–17.

44 King's Fund Forum, Consensus Development Conference: Treatment of primary breast cancer, *Br Med J* (1986) **293**:946–7.

45 Watson M, Psychosocial interventions with cancer patients: a review, *Psychol Med* (1983) **13**:839–46.

46 Cunningham A, From neglect to support to coping. The evolution of psychosocial intervention for cancer patients. In: Cooper CL, ed. *Stress and breast cancer* (Wiley: Chichester 1988) 135–54.

47 Fallowfield LJ, Counselling for patients with cancer, *Br Med J* (1988) **297**:727–8.

48 Beck AT, *Cognitive therapy in the emotional disorders* (International Universities Press: New York 1976).

49 Gelder M, Cognitive therapy. In: Granville-Grossman K, ed. *Recent advance in clinic psychiatry*, 5 (Churchill Livingstone: London 1985) 1–21.

50 Moorey S, Greer S, *Psychological therapy for patients with cancer: a new approach* (Heinemann Medical Books: London 1989).

51 Bancroft J, *Human sexuality and its problems* (Churchill Livingstone: Edinburgh 1983).

52 Morrow GR, Morrell C, Behavioural treatment for the anticipatory nausea and vomiting induced by cancer chemotherapy, *N Engl J Med* (1982) **307**(24):1476–80.

53 Redd W, Control of nausea and vomiting in chemotherapy patients. 4. Effective behavioural methods, *Postgrad Med* (1984) **75**(5):105–13.

54 Caplan G, *An approach to community medical health* (Tavistock: London 1961).

55 Rosen B, Brief focal psychotherapy. In: Bloch S, ed. *An introduction to the psychotherapies* (Oxford Medical Publications: Oxford 1985) 65–79.

56 *Diagnostic and statistical manual of mental disorders*, 3rd edn (American Psychiatric Association: Washington DC 1987).

57 Costa D, Mogos I, Toma T, Efficacy and safety of mianserin in the treatment of depression of women with cancer, *Acta Psychiatr Scand* (1985) **72** suppl 320:85–92.

58 Lishman WA, *Organic psychiatry. The psychological consequences of cerebral disorder*, 2nd edn (Blackwell Scientific Publications: Oxford 1987).

59 Ramirez AJ, Craig TKJ, Watson JP et al, Stress and relapse of breast cancer, *Br Med J* (1989) **298**:291–3.

60 Pettingale JW, Morris T, Greer S et al, Mental attitudes to cancer: an additional prognostic factor, *Lancet* (1985) **i**:170.

61 Hislop TG, Waxler NE, Coldman AJ et al, The prognostic significance of psychosocial factors in women with breast cancer, *J Chronic Dis* (1987) **40**:729–35.

62 Cox T, Mackay C, Psychosocial factors and psychophysiological mechanisms in the etiology and development of cancer, *Soc Sci Med* (1982) **16**:381–96.

CHAPTER 9

PREGNANCY AND EXOGENOUS OESTROGENS

Every night and every morn
Some to misery are born.
Every morn and every night
Some are born to sweet delight.
Some are born to sweet delight,
Some are born to endless night.
We are led to believe a lie
When we see not through the eye.

William Blake

Breast carcinoma in pregnancy

Because so few surgeons see cases of breast cancer in pregnancy there is a natural tendency to accept the teaching of the older clinicians who were convinced that like King John, pregnancy carcinoma was a 'bad thing'. Atavistic images of rampant bilateral inflammatory carcinoma arise so that the term induces either radical determination or a fatalistic *laissez faire* attitude. The truth lies somewhere between these two extremes.

Those who have tried to treat inflammatory carcinoma in pregnancy by means of termination, radiotherapy and chemotherapy and have failed to control the disease will have come to the conclusion that this is a fatal condition which cannot be ameliorated by presently available therapies. Others who have been able to control successfully in-

cidental cancers with standard surgical techniques will know that dire generalizations on the prognosis of pregnancy cancer are incorrect.

Irrespective of viewpoint, there is tacit acceptance that the endocrine changes of pregnancy stimulate the growth of breast cancer. The elevation of oestrone, oestradiol and oestradiol concentrations in the blood together with increases in both prolactin and epidermal growth factor would appear to make a potent mitogenic mix so that the incidence of breast cancers should increase during pregnancy and lactation. This is not the case.

Haas, from the German National Cancer Registry, has reported national statistics from 1970–9 for cancers diagnosed during pregnancy.[1] Details of the top three cancers are given in Table 9.1. The commonest is cervical

Table 9.1 Standardized incidence rates of cancers in pregnant women.[1]

	Observed	Expected	O/E	95% CI
Cervix	229	200	1.15	1.01–1.31
Breast	28	78	0.36	0.24–0.52
Ovary	19	36	0.53	0.31–0.82

theoretical consequences of pregnancy being an inhibitor rather than a promoter of malignant expression. In large part these are borne out by the sporadic data derived from patients with pregnancy carcinomas.

cancer which exceeds breast tumours by a factor of 10. Whereas there was an over-representation of cervical cancers there were fewer breast cancers than expected. This approximates to a two-thirds reduction in incidence.

That pregnancy can protect against breast cancer is not a new idea. However, most clinicians have considered this to be a long-term effect and have not envisaged any immediate reduction in incidence. Once this immediate protective effect has been appreciated, the behaviour of cancers which present during pregnancy becomes easier to understand. Rather like cancers in perimenopausal women which present under circumstances of steroid withdrawal, these lesions are innately more aggressive and less responsive to hormonal manipulation since they have emerged from an unfavourable endocrine milieu. Thus the few which evolve will be more aggressive, will more frequently metastasize to axillary nodes and less often respond to endocrine manipulation. The cancers grow despite, not because of, the pregnancy and therefore termination will have either a minimal effect, or alternatively may be deleterious. These would be the

Protective effect of pregnancy

If the growth of pre-existing breast cancers were stimulated by the physiological changes of pregnancy it would be likely that the majority would be found in women undergoing their first pregnancy. This is not so. As Table 9.2 shows, only 9 per cent of women develop the disease during the first pregnancy.[2–4] Approximately half of these cancers occur during the second to fourth pregnancies and one-third in the fifth or later pregnancies. This argues against any direct promotional effect.

When presentation of malignancy is examined within stages of pregnancy there is no evidence of an increase or decrease

Table 9.2 Parity of patients developing carcinoma during pregnancy.

1	2–4	>4	Reference
25	207	51	2
27	117	131	3
7	50	43	4
59 (9%)	374 (57%)	225 (34%)	

Table 9.3 Presentation of breast cancer within trimesters of pregnancy.

1st	2nd	3rd	Reference
28	16	9	2
3	9	13	5
28	20	26	3
21	20	22	6
31	12	27	7
5	4	11	8
116 (38%)	81 (27%)	108 (35%)	

Table 9.4 Effect of termination on prognosis of breast cancer found during pregnancy.

5-year survival (% + 95% CI)		Reference
Termination	No termination	
0	40	5
57	100	9
29	50	10
75	80	11
50	63	3
43	88	4
53	67	6
44 (42–46)	70 (66–74)	

within trimesters. Table 9.3 shows the almost equal distribution of cancers within the three trimesters of pregnancy.[2,3,5–8] This unchanging incidence suggests that the inhibitory effect is an immediate consequence which is maintained throughout the pregnancy.

If the pregnancy exerts a protective effect then this would be lost after termination. This has not been studied in any controlled way, but nevertheless there are some data supporting the protection hypothesis. When the 5-year survival percentages are examined in relation to whether the pregnancy was terminated or allowed to continue, a significantly better prognosis is observed in those who went on to deliver at term. Table 9.4 shows an overall survival of 44 per cent for those whose pregnancies were terminated, compared with 70 per cent for those who did not undergo termination.[3–6,9–11]

In parallel with this, Deemarsky et al have also shown that oöphorectomy is of little value in treatment of pregnancy cancers.[4] For patients with first trimester pregnancies that were aborted, the 5-year survival was 29 per cent for those treated by oöphorectomy and 63 per cent for those whose ovaries were conserved. For second and third trimester cases who had oöphorectomy after normal delivery, or early caesarian section, the 5-year survival was 100 per cent for the oöphorectomy group, and 86 per cent for the non-oöphorectomy group.

This is consistent with the data on oestrogen-receptor measurements in pregnancy carcinoma. Nugent found that 14 out of 19 (71 per cent) of these were oestrogen-receptor negative, further evidence suggesting that those cancers which emerge during pregnancy tend to be of an aggressive, hormone-resistant nature.[12]

That the cancers are more aggressive is witnessed by the rates of axillary-nodal involvement, as shown in Table 9.5.[2,4,5,7] Overall, three-quarters of women with operable pregnancy carcinomas have axillary-nodal involvement, leading to a worsening of prognosis for such cases.

It could be argued that this increased incidence of axillary nodal metastases could be due to delay in diagnosis rather than any innate aggressiveness of pregnancy carcinoma. However, when delay in diagnosis is

Table 9.5 Axillary-nodal metastases in patients with pregnancy carcinoma treated by mastectomy.

N negative	N positive	Reference
13	33	2
30	61	5
22	39	4
14	87	7
79 (26%)	220 (74%)	

examined there does not appear to be any major prolongation in pregnant women.

Montgomery reported on 70 cases of pregnancy cancer and examined the manner of detection both before and after patients had been instructed in breast self-examination (BSE).[13] In the era before BSE, 90 per cent of cancers were detected origin-ally by the patient. After instruction had been given the rate fell slightly to 86 per cent, rather than improved. Delay in diagnosis attributable to the doctor was present in 60 per cent of cases. The major problem is the low index of suspicion among obstetricians since breast cancer will develop in only three women per 100 000 pregnancies.[14] Rose-mond compared survivors with non-survivors and reported a delay of 9 months in the former and 11 months in the latter.[15] It is unlikely that this 2-month difference was a significant contributory factor. Bunker found that 44 per cent of patients had a delay of less than 6 months and suggested that the responsibility for the delay was shared equally by patients and doctors.[5]

This being so, is there evidence of more aggressive tumours being present in pre-gnant women? No large-scale histopatholo-gical comparisons of pregnancy carcinomas and age-matched control cases have been published. Almost all series are small. Tretli et al conducted a case-control study of pregnancy carcinomas and compared tumour grades with controls.[8] Results are shown in Table 9.6. There is a trend towards

Table 9.6 Survival of patients with pregnancy carcinoma.

	5-year survival (%)		10-year survival (%)		Reference
	Stage I	Stage II	Stage I	Stage II	
			35	22	3
	90	50			4
	73	52			6
			62	20	7
AVERAGE	82	51	49	21	

more grade III cancers among the pregnant women, but the numbers are too small to make any definite statement.

Prognosis

When pregnant patients with breast cancer are subdivided on a basis of axillary-nodal histology, their overall survival within stages does not appear to be greater than that of non-pregnant women. Table 9.6 gives 5- and 10-year survival percentages which look very similar to those of the majority of patients with breast cancer.[3,4,6,7]

Three studies have compared directly the survival of pregnant women and age-matched controls.[8,12,16] Peters compared the 5-year survival of 187 pregnant patients with 1992 premenopausal cases and found a reduction in the former group (33 per cent versus 50 per cent).[16] Nugent and O'Connell found no difference in survival, as shown in Table 9.7.[12] In contrast, Tretli et al reported a worse prognosis for pregnant women and stated that the risk of relapse was three times greater than that of non-pregnant cases,

within each stage, although no data have been given concerning within-stage survival.[8]

What this suggests is that the major prognostic determinant in pregnant cases is the axillary-nodal status. Adequate local treatment of Stage I cases can still lead to cure, albeit in a smaller number of women than in the age-matched population.

Treatment of pregnancy carcinoma

If breast cancer is suspected within the first trimester, it is best diagnosed by fine-needle aspiration cytology, needle biopsy or biopsy under local anaesthesia, since a general anaesthetic may damage or destroy the developing fetus. Once the diagnosis has been made, staging needs to be carried out. Bone scanning is probably unnecessary and carries a chance of fetal irradiation, although this can be reduced using low-dose ^{99m}Tc with a urinary catheter in situ, to minimize isotope accumulation within the bladder.[17]

At this stage the treatment possibilities need to be discussed with both the patient and her partner. If they wish the pregnancy to continue the primary treatment suggested should be a modified radical mastectomy. Provided that the axillary nodes are negative, no further therapy will be required. If the nodes are positive the patient should be advised to have adjuvant chemotherapy. Although there may be some oncologists prepared to give cytotoxics to pregnant women, the majority will regard this as a contraindication. In this situation either termination or early delivery should be contemplated, recognizing that extensive nodal involvement will probably mean that the patient will not survive long enough to take care of her child.

If the patient cannot accept mastectomy, the future of the pregnancy has to be

Table 9.7 Comparative 5-year survival of patients with pregnancy cancers and age-matched cancer controls.

Pregnant		Non-pregnant		Reference
Stage I	Stage II	Stage I	Stage II	
100	50	70	48	12
	20		55	8

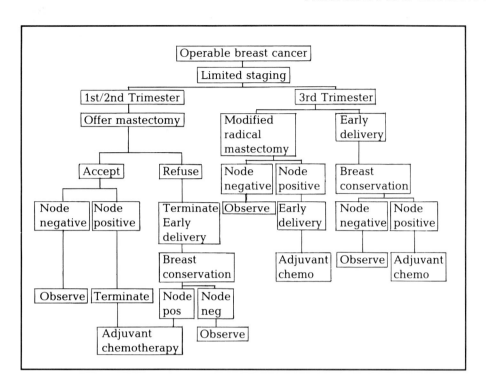

Figure 9.1 Treatment plan for pregnant women with breast cancer.

reconsidered. All effective breast-conserving techniques will include radiotherapy, which cannot be given during pregnancy. Thus the patient will have to be asked to choose between breast conservation and her baby. A suggested treatment plan for pregnant women with breast cancer is given in Figure 9.1. These choices are between standard treatments. Whether it is safe to delay radiotherapy until after delivery in patients opting for breast conservation has yet to be tested.

The two major determinants of treatment are the stage of the pregnancy and the patient's attitude towards breast conservation. Subsequent decisions as to the continuation of the pregnancy will depend upon the axillary-nodal status and the necessity for cytotoxic therapy. Neither termination nor endocrine therapy in the form of oöphorectomy should be considered as routine since these procedures will be unlikely to affect the course of the disease. Realistic estimates of prognosis based on axillary-nodal histology will enable husband and wife to decide whether the pregnancy should continue.

Inflammatory carcinoma

A few may still have a fixed idea that carcinoma in pregnancy is predominantly of the inflammatory type, mimicking an acute infective process and behaving in a very aggressive manner. Such cases are rare and do not occur any more frequently in pregnant rather than non-pregnant women. Lee and Tannenbaum, who were the first to describe inflammatory carcinoma, reported that none of their 28 cases were pregnant.[18] Taylor and Meltzer described a series of 38 women with inflammatory cancers, which comprised 4 per cent of the total group of patients with breast carcinoma.[19] Of these, only two occurred during pregnancy and in one of these the tumour preceded the event.

White, who presented one of the largest combined series of 1413 pregnancy carcinomas, reported that the inflammatory type was responsible for 55 (4 per cent).[14] Similar rarity—1 out of 37 (3 per cent)—was found by Rosemonde.[15] Thus inflammatory carcinoma is no more nor less common during pregnancy in Western women. It is at any time a disease associated with a poor prognosis whose clinical course is only slightly modified by the most aggressive chemotherapy and radiotherapy presently available.

Lactational carcinomas

Many reports of cancer in pregnancy have included patients who developed tumours during the postpartum period (up to 1 year) or while they were lactating. These have been summarized in Table 9.8, which gives the proportions of pregnancy carcinomas diagnosed in lactating women.[2–5,7,8,20] Overall, these comprised 38 per cent of all breast cancers of pregnancy. Since the lactational period (usually up to 1 year) will be greater than the duration of the pregnancy, this

Table 9.8 Breast cancer in lactating women.

L/P*	Node positive (%)	5-year survival (%)	Reference
20/92 (22)	80	14	20
37/150 (25)	–	36	5
80/133 (60)	73	–	2
80/221 (36)	–	36	3
36/100 (36)	–	31	4
43/99 (43)	–	40	7
15/35 (43)	72	33	8
AVERAGE (38)	75	32	

*Percentages in parentheses.
L = Lactating patients.
P = Total patients with pregnancy carcinoma.

proportion suggests that the protective effect of pregnancy continues during the period of lactation, and indeed it is possible that the differentiation of mammary epithelium induced by lactation might result in an increased short-term protection.

The few lactational lesions appear to be as aggressive as other pregnancy cancers. Thus three-quarters of operable cases have axillary nodal metastases. The 5-year survival in these combined series was only 32 per cent, reflecting the aggression of these cancers.

In part this may be the result of delay since small, deeply located cancers will be difficult to detect in the engorged lactating breast. In equivocal cases, and where a galactocoele has been excluded by needle aspiration, it may be necessary to ask the patient to wean rapidly in order that the breast can be reassessed in a non-lactating state. If uncertainty exists the patient should be referred urgently to an experienced surgeon.

Pregnancy subsequent to breast cancer

If pregnancy exerts an inhibitory influence on breast cancer and reduces the incidence of primary tumours it would be likely that it would have a similar effect on micrometastases. Thus pregnancy subsequent to treatment of breast cancer might act in an adjuvant manner. Essentially this is the message that emerges from published work.

Rissanen reported a 5-year survival of 77 per cent in women with breast cancer who subsequently became pregnant, with a 10-year survival of 70 per cent.[11] Holleb and Farrar found a 5-year survival of 38 per cent for Stage II cases and 64 per cent for Stage I patients.

When survival is compared directly between those who do and do not become pregnant subsequently, the former group fare better as shown in Table 9.9, which summarizes the results of Peters and Cooper and Butterfield.[16,21]

Thus should all premenopausal women with breast cancer be advised to become pregnant subsequently? For those who are node-negative this might be to their advantage. For the node-positive group it is more problematic. All will now be offered systemic adjuvant therapy. It is not going to be possible to run a prospective randomized trial comparing the effects of pregnancy and systemic therapy as adjuvants. Careful monitoring of those who elect to become pregnant may yield important data.

Patients with heavy axillary-nodal involvement (greater than 10 nodes) should be actively discouraged from becoming pregnant unless their spouses are prepared single-handedly to raise their issue.

The idea that pregnancy has a beneficial effect both in terms of prevention of breast cancer and as an adjuvant is not new. Twenty years ago, Peters stated 'At the present time there is a common belief that pregnancy has an unfavourable effect on breast cancer in young women. This belief has been responsible for a most aggressive and non-discriminating approach in the management of breast cancer associated with pregnancy.'

We ignore the lessons of history at our patients' peril.

Table 9.9 Survival of patients with breast cancer who subsequently became pregnant compared with cancer controls.

	5-year survival		Reference
	Pregnant	Controls	
Stage I	20/22 (90%)	30/44 (68%)	21
Stage II	1/6 (17%)	4/12 (33%)	
Stage I	(81%)	(70%)	16
Stage II	(76%)	(54%)	

Oral contraception

The last quarter of a century has seen a major shift in both public and private attitudes towards sexual behaviour. One of the major contributory factors in the alteration of heterosexual relationships has been the availability and widespread use of oral contraceptives (OCs). These have had an enormous impact on the independence of women, enabling them to make previously difficult choices between the competing claims of parity and career. However, inside almost every Westerner there is an unreconstructed Calvinist, so that it is assumed that every pleasure incurs a subsequent penalty. This finds expression in those Jeremiahs (male) who unceasingly expound their theories concerning sexual behaviour and the day of payment.

Is there a biological basis for the assertions of the bigots? Does the use of OCs add to or subtract from the total of human happiness? No attempt will be made to answer this latter question. However, the relationship between the use of OCs and risk of breast cancer will be examined in the light of present data which have been derived largely from epidemiological studies using the possibly flawed technique of case-control study.

Problems

There has been an evolution in use of OCs as it has become apparent that inhibition of ovulation can be achieved using progressively lower dosages of oestrogen and that in this way the cardiovascular side-effects can be diminished. Furthermore, a different endocrine approach has been to use progesterone alone, not to stop ovulation but to increase the viscosity of cervical mucus, thereby acting as a biological barrier to sperm penetration.

If OCs mimicked the action of pregnancy it would be expected that a two-thirds reduction in incidence of breast cancer would be observed. Such a measurable effect has not been seen. The question which has remained

open is whether OCs are neutral in respect of breast cancer or whether they do exert a promotional effect, but one which takes some considerable time to manifest. The natural experiment is an impure one. Most individuals do not remain on one particular formulation of OC for many years. Not only do the OCs change but their use may be interspersed with pregnancies which might exert either an antagonistic or possibly a synergistic effect.

Individual recall of OC use may be sketchy. Unlike pregnancy, miscarriage and divorce, use or change of use of OCs does not constitute a major life event and brand names will be forgotten. An ideal experiment would be to study a defined cohort of women, with accurate data on OC use, and prospectively to follow them for a prolonged period (20 years). Such a study would attract little interest from epidemiologists and probably none from grant-giving bodies. As a compromise the case-control study has been used. Because of the accuracy of cancer registration in many countries it has been possible to identify cases fairly easily. Most studies have taken cases aged up to 35 or 40 years. Amongst these cases there will be some with an hereditary predisposition to development of breast cancer, which may or may not be modified by OC use. Others will have endocrine unresponsive breast cancers whose growth may have been totally unrelated to their pre-existing endocrine milieu, with or without exogenous steroids.

Conflict in case-control studies

Oral contraceptives became widely used in parts of the USA in the early 1970s and in Britain in the mid-1970s. The first epidemiological studies gave qualified reassurance that the risk of breast cancer in young women on both sides of the Atlantic was unaffected by use of OCs.[22–4] However, the women of California had been using OCs for the longest period of time, and had a potential 5 years of extra exposure. Pike et al reported that in a study of 163 cases aged less than 32 years, compared with controls, there was a two-fold increase in risk after 6 years of OC usage.[25] However, in a study of 1176 cases and a similar number of controls aged less than 35 years, Vessey et al reported no increase in relative risk with duration of use.[27] This was attributed to differences in availability of controls in California, together with a slightly different age range, and differences in analysis of the data.

Pike extended his work with a case-control study comprising 314 cases aged 37 years or younger, who were compared with neighbourhood-derived controls.[27] His results are summarized in Table 9.10, which shows that when use of OCs before age 25 was examined there was a significant increase in relative risk of breast cancer with duration of exposure, so that after 6 years of use there

was a five-fold increase in risk. This was attributed by Pike to the use of combination OCs containing high dosages of progestogens. This interpretation was criticized,[28] and subsequent work has now shown that increased risk is unrelated to progestogenic potency.[29,30]

One of the largest studies, and therefore one which is able to confirm or refute most accurately the null hypothesis, is that of the Cancer and Steroid Hormone Study Group (CASH study).[30] This comprised 2088 women who had breast cancer diagnosed before the age of 45, and who were compared with 2065 neighbourhood controls, recruited by random-digit dialling after which the individual, if female, was invited to take part. Cases were derived from eight regions within the USA. In 1985, the CASH study reported that there was no increase or decrease in relative risk for OC usage and that this was unaffected by duration of use, or by progestogen potency.

In contrast, Meirik et al reported from a case-control study in Sweden and Norway that there was a two-fold increase in relative risk after 12 years of use.[31] This was unrelated to age at first use, with no evidence of any latent effect.

In 1987, McPherson et al found that there had been a change in the data so that a risk was becoming apparent.[32] The study comprised 1125 women aged 16–64 with proven breast cancer compared with the same number of matched hospital-derived controls. For women aged 45 years or older there was no increase in relative risk for OC users. However, among those under 45 years there was a duration-dependent increase in relative risk, as shown in Table 9.11. This risk persisted after adjustment for age at first full-term birth, age at menarche, menopausal status, family history and prior benign breast disease. Thus there was an adjusted relative risk of 2.6 for women who had taken OCs for more than 4 years before their first full-term pregnancy.

Table 9.10 Relative risk (RR) of breast cancer in relation to oral contraceptive (OC) use and duration before age 25.[27]

OC use (years)	Cases	Controls	RR (95% CI)
0	65	93	1.0
1–2	106	118	1.3 (0.8–2.0)
3–4	79	67	1.7 (1.0–2.7)
5–6	40	29	2.0 (1.1–3.6)
>6	24	7	4.9 (1.9–13.4)

Table 9.11 Relative risk (RR) of breast cancer in relation to oral contraceptive use before full-term pregnancy in women aged less than 45 years.[32]

Duration of use	Unadjusted RR	Adjusted RR
Never	1.0	1.0
1–2 years	1.2	1.0 (0.5–1.9)
3–4 years	2.4	2.0 (1.0–3.8)
> years	3.2	2.6 (1.3–5.6)

Table 9.12 Relative risk of breast cancer in premenopausal women in relation to oral contraceptive use before first full-term pregnancy.[33]

Duration of use	All	Parous	Nulliparous
Women aged 20–44			
Never	1.0	1.0	1.0
<3 years	1.3	1.3	1.2
4–7	1.5	1.3	1.7
8–11	1.4	1.0	1.6
>12 years	2.7	–	2.5
Women aged 45–54			
Never	1.0	1.0	1.0
<3 years	0.7	0.8	0.6
4–7	1.2	1.1	1.2
8–11	0.2	–	0.3
>12 years	0.4	–	0.3

Shortly after this the CASH study reported a similar finding, except that the risk was carried only by the nulliparous.[33] Thus subsequent pregnancy appeared to obliterate any increase in risk. Results are given in Table 9.12, which shows that the nulliparous who had taken OCs for more than 12 years carried an increased risk. This is seen only in those aged 20–44 at the time of diagnosis, but few in the older age group had long exposure to OCs.

Miller et al conducted a study of 407 cases aged less than 45 years, and 424 controls.[34] In this study there was a doubling of relative risk for women who had ever taken OCs, which was found in all categories, and rose to a risk of 4 after 10 years. The controls in this study were hospital-derived who, despite being judged to be suffering from conditions unrelated to OC usage, may not have been representative of the population from whom the cancer cases were derived.

Because of the problem of relatively small numbers in many of the case-control studies, the UK National Case-Control Study Group (UKCCSG) mounted a multicentre study in 11 different areas of Britain.[35] There were 755 cases, each of whom was matched with a control derived from the practice list of her general practitioner. Great care was taken to ascertain accurately the brands of OCs which each individual had used, and to carry out identical interviews for cases and controls. The results are summarized in Table 9.13. There was a highly significant trend of increased risk with increase in duration of OC usage and this was found in both parous and nulliparous women (but greater for the latter group). The effect of OCs was seen both before and after first full-term pregnancy in the parous group.

Thus it appeared that subsequent pregnancy had little effect on risk of breast cancer in young women who had experienced prolonged exposure to the pill. These data could imply that up to 20 per cent of breast cancers in young women might be OC-related. If this were so, there should have been an increase in reported cases, albeit delayed in response to increased sales of OCs. No such increase has been seen.[36] Indeed the incidence rates for young women have remained constant.

Table 9.13 Relative risk of breast cancer in relation to duration of oral contraceptive use and timing of first full-term pregnancy (FFTP).[35]

| Duration of use | All | Parous | | Nulliparous |
		Before FFTP	After FFTP	
Never	1.0	1.0	1.0	1.0
1–4 years	0.95	1.02	1.23	0.98
5–9 years	1.43	1.51	1.4	1.37
>9 years	1.74	1.44	1.97	2.30

Latent period effect

In an attempt to reconcile the discrepant findings, McPherson and Coope have hypothesized that there is a long latent period between first exposure to OCs and clinical manifestation of breast cancers.[37] Thus the studies with the longest follow-up should show a harmful effect in some of these women who have had prolonged usage. Using computer simulation, assuming a relative risk of 3 and a latent period of 20 years, a reasonable fit for the available data was obtained. It was argued that there was a 20-year delay in presentation of breast cancers in survivors of the atomic bombs. However, the two situations are not necessarily similar. The radiation exposure almost certainly had a carcinogenic effect which may have required a long period of subsequent promotion for cancer to manifest. In contrast, it is likely that OCs would act as promoters rather than initiators of pre-existing malignant lesions so that a shorter time-scale might be expected.

In response to this hypothesis, Schlesselman et al re-analysed the CASH data as 4714 cases and 4540 controls and reported that the relative risk remained at unity after up to 14 years of exposure.[38] However, it has still been argued that insufficient time has elapsed for a latency period of 20 years to be discounted.[39]

Effect of formulation of oral contraceptives

Those studies that have shown an increase in risk for women after prolonged OC usage have often attempted to examine the relative roles of the oestrogen and progestogen components. Original claims of an increase in risk with increasing potency of progestogen have now been largely discounted. Indeed, the limited data from the UK study indicated that use of progestogen-only contraception might be associated with a decrease in risk. This is consistent with the known anti-tumour effect of progestogens in advanced breast cancer.

In the first British study to show a deleterious effect, McPherson analysed results of usage of the 30 different brands of OCs which had been prescribed.[39] When these were ranked, the high-dose ethinyl oestradiol containing pills appeared to exert the maximum effect. When multiple logistic analysis was used there was a statistically significant trend for ethinyl oestradiol but no effect for mestranol. This is a little surprising since mestranol is metabolized to ethinyl oestradiol.

In the UK national case-control study, OCs were divided into those containing more than 50 μg oestrogen and those containing 50 μg or less. The relative risk for prolonged usage of the lower dose was only slightly greater than that of controls. In contrast, it was those

165

patients who took the higher dosage who carried the risk.

What advice should be given?

While epidemiologists dispute, patients and their doctors would like some guidelines upon which to decide on whether to use OCs. The case-control studies appear to be showing an increase in relative risk for young women after prolonged usage of OCs. So why are the national incidence figures unchanged for this age group? Stadel has argued that the aggregate effect is zero with only a promotion of cancers in a few patients who would have developed breast cancer even without taking OCs.

To put this into perspective, it has been suggested that, of a cohort of 1000 women aged under 35, 2 would develop breast cancer. The effect of high-oestrogen OCs might increase them to 3 in 1000. If it has taken 20 years to demonstrate a small effect from high-oestrogen pills, it is unlikely that a clinically significant effect will be found for lower-dose oestrogen-containing OCs. It is possible that there will be either no effect or, perhaps because of the progestogen component, there could be a protective effect.

Unlike the cancers which develop during pregnancy, which may be more aggressive, there is no evidence that the prognosis of women who develop breast cancer whilst or after taking OCs is any different from that of those who have never taken the pill.[40-2]

A young woman asking advice should be told that the risks of low-dose oestrogen-containing OCs are very low, and there is little reason why she should not use them. Even those with a family history should not necessarily be discouraged from taking the pill, although maybe they should be encouraged to become pregnant as early as reasonable in order to diminish their chances of breast cancer.

More mature women who require oral contraception should be encouraged to use progestogen-only formulations so that their breast cancer risk may be diminished.

Oral contraceptives have been a major advance in both medical and social terms and it is important that their advantages are not lost by panic reactions. Low-dose oestrogens represent low-risk contraception.

Oestrogen replacement therapy

If the literature relating to oestrogen (hormone) replacement therapy (HRT) and breast cancer is studied after that concerning oral contraceptives and breast cancer, it is difficult to avoid a sense of *déjà vu*. Small, uncontrolled studies originally reported no cause for concern but were followed by larger, better designed studies with longer follow-up which have shown a small but significant increase in relative risk of breast cancer. Just as the potential benefits of HRT on heart and bone have been more accurately quantified, so have the effects on hormone-sensitive tumours of the endometrium and breast. Thus the gains of HRT have to be considered in relation to possible risks. With alterations in formulation it may be possible to arrive at a combination of oestrogen and progestogen which minimizes the risk of not only heart disease and osteoporosis, but also cancers of the breast and endometrium.

For some but not all women the menopausal withdrawal of ovarian hormones represents a physical and psychological assault of an overwhelming nature. Well-recognized symptoms such as vasomotor instability producing hot flushes and palpitation arise from pulsatile discharge of hypothalamic release factors. More severe is the loss of drive and libido, coupled with depression and a sense of worthlessness. This latter is reinforced because the menopause may coincide with a shedding of family responsibility as grown-up children leave home to make their own lives.

The situation is worsened further by the skin changes resulting from oestrogen withdrawal with dryness particularly affecting the vagina and lower urinary tract, leading to dysuria and frequency in the absence of bacterial infections. This latter represents the end-stages of menopausal misery. Hormone replacement therapy acts, in the short term to reverse or prevent the subjective sequelae of oestrogen withdrawal, relieving hot flushes and restoring a sense of well-being.

More easily measured are the effects of HRT on bone and liver metabolism together with indirect reduction in morbidity and mortality from coronary heart disease. It has now been convincingly shown that there is a reduction in these major problems in women who take HRT for 5 years. What is not yet known is the duration of HRT necessary to achieve these effects. Is there an equal trade-off? Is the significant reduction in bone loss equalled by an increase in risk of breast cancer?

Table 9.14 Divergent results of case-control studies of HRT and breast cancer using population- and hospital-derived controls.[43]

Cases	RR, ever used	RR, >5 years	Reference
Population controls			
138	1.1	1.9	44
345	1.4	2.0	45
196	1.4	1.7	46
119	0.7	1.8	47
183	1.1	1.9	48
183	0.6	0.9	49
1960	1.0	1.5	50
1369	1.3	1.6	51
AVERAGE	1.1	1.7	
Hospital controls			
60	1.1	–	52
332	0.9	0.8	53
196	1.4	0.7	46
113	0.6	0.6	54
1610	1.0	1.0	55
161	0.7	0.8	48
AVERAGE	1.0	0.8	

Case-control studies

There is a divergence in the results of case-control studies, some showing an increase in relative risk of breast cancer, others showing a neutral or a protective effect. The situation was clarified by Henderson et al, who showed that studies using population-derived controls almost all demonstrated increases in relative risk, whereas those with hospital-derived controls were negative.[43] Case-control studies of both types are summarized in Table 9.14.[44–55] In the population-based studies there was a slight increase in relative risk (1.1) for those who had ever used HRT, but a significant increase (1.7) among long-term users. This increased relative risk is dependent upon both dosage and duration of HRT.

In contrast, those studies which used hospital-derived controls showed no change in ever users and an apparent reduction after prolonged usage (relative risk 0.8). The only reason for using hospital-derived controls is that this makes case-control studies easier to run, with interviewers working within one location. Such controls are almost certainly unrepresentative of the population from which they derive. They will have had more contact with medical services and are more likely to be prescribed drugs, including HRT. Thus increased usage of HRT within a hospital-derived subset of controls could lead to an apparent reduction in relative risk of cases with which they were compared.

Thus it may be clearly seen that HRT usage carries a significantly increased risk of breast cancer. Is this carried by all women using HRT or are there particular subgroups at increased risk?

Family history, HRT and breast cancer

A consistent effect is seen in almost all the case-control studies that have examined the relationship of family history, HRT usage and breast cancers. With the exception of the data of Kaufman et al,[55] which used hospital-derived controls, all the other studies have shown an increase in risk for users with a family history, as shown in Table 9.15.[45,47–51,53,55] When the relative risk for those with no family history is corrected to unity, the mean relative risk for these studies was 3.1.

This three-fold increase is what would be expected in non-users with a family history. Thus risk is neither amplified nor diminished by HRT usage. However, the combined risk factors would lead to a 4.5–5-fold increase in risk for breast cancer, that is a lifetime risk of approximately 1 in 3, which many might find unacceptable. Thus, women with a first-degree family history of breast cancer need to be advised of the risks that they run if long-term HRT use is contemplated.

Benign breast disease, HRT usage and breast cancer

Because epidemiology is a blunt instrument, the relationship of benign but premalignant histological change has not been examined in respect of HRT use. What has been done is to lump together those who have had a prior benign biopsy of the breast, or alternatively those who have had prior breast symptoms. This 'mish-mash' of uncharacterized conditions is described as benign breast disease. Despite this blurring, a small but consistent elevation of increased risk is seen, as shown in Table 9.16.[44,45,47,48,50,51,53,55] When the relative risk for no prior benign breast disease was converted to unity, the mean relative risk for prior benign breast disease was 1.5.

It is likely that this is not a risk borne by all, but probably by those with florid hyperplasia and atypical change. Combined epidemiological and histological studies will be required to confirm this. Meanwhile, a patient who has had a prior breast biopsy which has not

Table 9.15 Family history (FH), use of HRT and relative risk of breast cancer.

HRT users		Reference
FH+	**FH−**	
1.9	1.0	53
3.9	1.0	45
0.2*	0.9	55
6.0	1.0	47
2.6	1.2	48
1.5	0.9	50
4.5	1.0	49
2.2	1.5	51

*Controls were hospital-derived.

Table 9.16 Prior benign breast disease (BBD), use of HRT and relative risk of breast cancer.

BBD+	BBD−	Reference
5.7	2.1	44
1.6	1.0	53
1.6	1.0	45
1.1	0.7	55
1.5	1.0	47
1.8	1.1	48
1.5	1.2	50
1.0	1.4	51

Obesity, HRT use and breast cancer

Increase in body fat can lead to enhanced oestrogen production in postmenopausal women, as a result of peripheral aromatization of androgens such as androstenedione to form oestrone.[56] Thus, on theoretical grounds, obesity should increase the risk of breast cancer in women receiving HRT. Sherman et al have shown that such an effect does occur.[54] In a study of 113 postmenopausal breast-cancer patients and hospital-derived controls, the relative risk for HRT users was 0.71, which did not differ significantly from unity. When the cases and controls were stratified on a basis of their weight being less than or greater than the median, relative risk for the thinner subjects was 0.41, compared with 1.3 for the fatter women. When entered into a logistic regression model, the interaction term 'relative weight × oestrogen use' emerged as a statistically significant variable. Thus obesity and prolonged use of HRT carry a significant risk of development of breast cancer.

Similar results were reported by Kelsey et al, who found a relative risk of 1.6 for HRT users who weighed more than 125 pounds.[53] However, McDonald did not find any increase in relative risk in heavier women using HRT.[49]

Apart from possible risks of breast cancer, the cardiovascular risks of postmenopausal obesity are such that all such individuals should be actively encouraged to lose weight, possibly holding the carrot of HRT as the prize for those who achieve an appropriate weight.

shown evidence of atypia can be safely advised to take HRT. Those with prior breast symptoms such as mastalgia or cysts can be given HRT but need to be warned that they may continue to have breast pain or may develop subsequent breast cysts.

The woman who as a teenager had a fibroadenoma excised, and who then took OCs for 5 years, can be given HRT. The fibroadenoma puts her at no risk of subsequent malignancy. Whether the 5 years of OC usage will be additive in terms of breast-cancer risk with subsequent HRT usage has yet to be determined. Ross et al have shown a progressive increase in relative risk in relation to accumulated dosage of oestrogen in women with benign breast disease, rising to 5.7 after a dosage of more than 1.5 grams, thereby suggesting that such an interaction might occur.[44]

Hormone replacement therapy in breast-cancer patients

Alteration or suppression of endogenous oestrogen production plays a central role in the management of many patients with both early and advanced breast cancer, either as adjuvant or palliative therapy. Thus there has been a tacit assumption, strongly reinforced by more senior clinicians, that proven breast cancer represents a contraindication for any form of exogenous oestrogen administration.

However, either as a result of planned ovarian ablation or following the natural menopause, many patients will be greatly troubled with menopausal symptoms. Should all these individuals be refused the benefits of HRT? Is it possible to identify a group that are unlikely to be disadvantaged by HRT, thereby suffering acceleration of relapse of breast cancer?

For patients with advanced breast cancer, only under exceptional circumstances will they survive long enough for their menopausal symptoms to be more of a problem than the symptoms arising from their metastatic disease. Thus the need for HRT will not have to be considered.

In those women with early breast cancer treated by either mastectomy or breast conservation, decisions can be based upon their axillary-nodal status and the oestrogen-receptor status (ER) of the primary tumour. A suggested scheme is given in Figure 9.2. For node-negative, ER-negative women who request HRT, this can be given, preferably as a combination of oestrogen and progestogen, and normal follow-up should continue. In the node-negative, receptor-positive cases, HRT is probably best avoided, but if the patient's symptoms do not respond to non-endocrine therapy HRT can be given in combined form

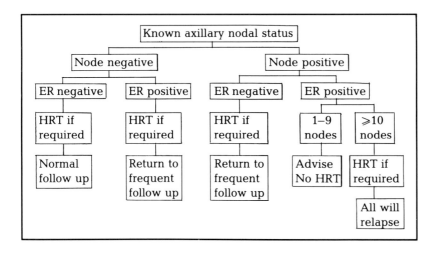

Figure 9.2   Hormone replacement therapy (HRT) in women with early breast cancer.

as the patient will need more frequent follow-up (probably 3-monthly for 2 years). With an approximate 1 per cent annual incidence of contralateral breast cancers it would be likely that an increase in this percentage would be seen among those given HRT. The magnitude cannot be accurately computed but could represent a doubling or more in cumulative risk of contralateral carcinoma. This would mean a 1 in 5 risk after 10 years of follow up.

Node-positive cases are more problematic. It is probable that HRT would have little effect in ER-negative cases, but nevertheless care should be taken when presenting the agent to these patients, who will need close follow up. For ER-positive cases there is a considerable risk that there will be an exacerbation of growth of micrometastases with a decrease in disease-free interval. This has to be weighed against any short-term benefit that the patient may gain in terms of relief of hot flushes and palpitations.

In those with less than ten nodes involved, there is a proportion who may be cured as a result of primary therapy combined with oestrogen suppression or blockade and their survival may be compromised by HRT. Thus this patient group should be advised not to take HRT, or understand the implications if they decide that their menopausal symptoms are unbearable.

For those with ten or more nodes involved, relapse of breast cancer will be an almost inevitable event and all that HRT will achieve will be to shorten the interval before relapse occurs. If the patient's life is being made miserable by menopausal symptoms it may be kinder to prescribe HRT in order that the quality of remaining lifespan is not worsened by these problems.

This is not an area in which dogmatic assertions are useful, and individualization of treatment will be necessary. It is unlikely that such a question could be answered by means of a randomized prospective trial. This particular aspect may be clarified by close monitoring of such cases who elect either to receive or not to be given HRT. Only then can policy decisions be based on data rather than deduction.

References

1 Haas JF, Pregnancy in association with a newly diagnosed cancer: a population-based epidemiologic assessment, *Int J Cancer* (1984) **34**:229–35.

2 Holleb AI, Farrow JH, The relation of carcinoma of the breast and pregnancy in 283 patients, *Surg Gynecol Obstet* (1962) **115**:65–71.

3 Clark RM, Reid J, Carcinoma of the breast in pregnancy and lactation, *Int J Radiat Oncol Biol Phys* (1978) **4**:693–8.

4 Deemarsky LJ, Neishtadt EL, Brea SL, Cancer and pregnancy, *Breast* (1980) **7**:17–21.

5 Bunker ML, Peters MV, Breast cancer associated with pregnancy or lactation, *Am J Obstet Gynecol.* (1963) **85**:312–21.

6 King RM, Welch JS, Martin JK et al, Carcinoma of the breast associated with pregnancy, *Surg Gynecol Obstet* (1985) **160**:228–32.

7 Ribeiro G, Jones DA, Jones M, Carcinoma of the breast associated with pregnancy, *Br J Surg* (1986) **73**:607–9.

8 Tretli S, Kvalheim G, Thoresen S et al, Survival of breast cancer patients diagnosed during pregnancy or lactation, *Br J Cancer* (1988) **58**:382–4.

9 Holman P, Bennett MB, Breast cancer and pregnancy, *S. Afr Med J* (1963) **37**:1236–9.

10 Peete CH, Hunlycutt HC, Cherry MB, Cancer of the breast and pregnancy, *NC Med J* (1966) **27**:514–17.

11 Rissanen PH, Pregnancy following treatment for mammary cancer, *Acta Radiol* (1969) **8**:415–22.

12 Nugent P, O'Connell TX, Breast cancer and pregnancy, *Ann Surg* (1985) **120**:1221–4.

13 Montgomery TC, Detection and disposal of breast cancer in pregnancy, *Am J Obstet Gynecol* (1961) **81**:926–33.

14 White TT, Carcinoma of the breast in the pregnant and the nursing patient, *Am J Obstet Gynecol* (1955) **69**:1277–86.

15 Rosemond GP, Carcinoma of the breast during pregnancy, *Clin Obstet Gynecol* (1963) **6**:994–1001.

16 Peters MV, The effect of pregnancy in breast cancer. In: Forrest APM, Kunkler PB, eds. *Prognostic factors in breast cancer* (Livingstone: Edinburgh 1968.)

17 Baker J, Ali A, Groch MW et al, Bone scanning in pregnant patients with breast carcinoma, *Clin Nucl Med* (1987) **12**:519–24.

18 Lee BJ, Tannenbaum NE, Inflammatory carcinoma of the breast, *Surg Gyncol Obstet* (1924) **39**:580–5.

19 Taylor GW, Meltzer A, Inflammatory carcinoma of the breast, *Am J Cancer* (1938) **33**:33–49.

20 Harrington SW, Carcinoma of the breast. Results of surgical treatment when the carcinoma occurred in the course of pregnancy or lactation and when pregnancy occurred subsequent to operation (1910–1933), *Ann Surg* (1937) **106**:690–700.

21 Cooper DR, Butterfield, J, Pregnancy subsequent to mastectomy for cancer of the breast, *Ann Surg* (1970) **171**:429–33.

22 Paffenbarger RS, Fasal E, Simmons ME et al, Cancer risk as related to use of oral contraceptives during fertile years, *Cancer* (1977) **39**:1887–91.

23 Vessey MP, McPherson K, Doll R, Breast cancer and oral contraceptives: Findings in Oxford Family Planning Association Contraceptive Study, *Br Med J* (1981) **282**:2093–4.

24 Royal College of General Practitioners, Breast cancer and oral contraceptives: Findings in Royal College of General Practitioners Study, *Br Med J* (1981) **282**:2089–93.

25 Pike MC, Henderson BE, Casagrande JJ et al, Oral contraceptive use and early abortion as risk factors for breast cancer in young women, *Br J Cancer* (1981) **43**:72–6.

26 Vessey MP, McPherson K, Yeates D et al, Oral contraceptive use and abortion before first term pregnancy in relation to breast cancer risk, *Br J Cancer* (1982) **45**:327–31.

27 Pike MC, Henderson BE, Krailo MD et al, Breast cancer in young women and use of oral contraceptives: Possible modifying effects of formulation and age at use, *Lancet* (1983) **ii**:926–9.

28 Swyer GIM, Progestagen 'potency' and breast cancer, *Lancet* (1983) **ii**:1416.

29 McPherson K, Neil A, Vessey MP et al, Oral contraceptives and breast cancer, *Lancet* (1983) **ii**:1414–15.

30 Stadel BV, Rubin GL, Webster LA, Oral contraceptives and breast cancer in young women, *Lancet* (1985) **ii**:970–3.

31 Meirik O, Lund E, Adami H-O et al, Oral contraceptive use and breast cancer in young women, *Lancet* (1986) **ii**:650–3.

32 McPherson K, Vessey MP, Neil A et al, Early oral contraceptive use and breast cancer: Results of another case-control study, *Br J Cancer* (1987) **56**:653–60.

33 Stadel S, Schlesselman JJ et al, Oral contraceptives and premenopausal breast cancer in nulliparous women, *Contraception* (1988) **38**:287–99.

34 Miller DR, Rosenberg L, Kaufman DW et al, Breast cancer before age 45 and oral contraceptive use: New findings, *Am J Epidemiol* (1989) **129**:269–80.

35 UK National Case-Control Study Group, Oral contraceptive use and breast cancer risk in young women, *Lancet* (1989) **i**:973–82.

36 Caygill CPJ, Hill MJ, Oral contraceptives and breast cancer, *Lancet* (1989) **i**:125–8.

37 McPherson K, Cooper PA, Early oral contraceptive use and breast cancer risk, *Lancet* (1986) **ii**:685–6.

38 Schlesselman JJ, Stadel BV, Murray P et al, Breast cancer in relation to early use of oral contraceptives. No evidence of a latent effect, *JAMA* (1988) **259**:1828–33.

39 McPherson K, Latent effect of oral contraceptives on breast cancer, *JAMA* (1988) **260**:1240–1.

40 Matthews PN, Millis RR, Hayward JL, Breast cancer in women who have taken contraceptive steroids, *Br Med J* (1981) **282**:274–6.

41 Rosner D, Lane WW, Brett RP, Influence of oral contraceptives on the prognosis of breast cancer in young women, *Cancer* (1985) **55**:1556–62.

42 Millard FC, Bliss JM, Chilvers CED et al, Oral contraceptives and survival in breast cancer, *Br J Cancer* (1987) **56**:377–8.

43 Henderson BE, Ross R, Bernstein L, Estrogens as a cause of human cancer: The Richard and Hilda Rosenthal Foundation Award Lecture, *Cancer Res* (1988) **48**:246–53.

44 Ross RK, Paganini-Hill A, Gerkins VR et al, A case control study of menopausal estrogen therapy and breast cancer, *JAMA* (1980) **243**:1635–9.

45 Hoover R, Glass A, Finkle WD et al, Conjugated estrogen use and breast cancer risk in women, *J Natl Cancer Inst* (1981) **67**:815–20.

46 Huika BS, Chambliss LE, Deubner DC, Breast cancer and oestrogen replacement therapy, *Am J Obstet Gynecol* (1982) **143**:638–44.

47 Hiatt RA, Bawol R, Friedman GD et al, Exogenous estrogen and breast cancer after bilateral oöphorectomy, *Cancer* (1984) **54**:139–44.

48 Nomura AMY, Kolonel LN, Hirohata T et al, The association of replacement estrogens with breast cancer, *Int J Cancer* (1986) **37**:49–53.

49 McDonald JA, Weiss NS, Daling JR et al, Menopausal estrogen use and the risk of breast cancer, *Breast Cancer Res Treat* (1986) **7**:193–9.

50 Brinton LA, Hoover R, Fraumeni JF, Menopausal oestrogens and breast cancer risk: an expanded case-control study, *Br J Cancer* (1986) **54**:825–32.

51 Wingo PA, Layde PM, Lee NC et al, The risk of breast cancer in postmenopausal women who have used oestrogen replacement therapy, *JAMA* (1987) **257**:209–15.

52 Jick H, Walker AM, Watkins R et al, Replacement estrogens and breast cancer, *Am J Epidemiol* (1980) **112**:586–94.

53 Kelsey JL, Fischer DB, Holford TR et al, Exogenous estrogens and other factors in the epidemiology of breast cancer, *J Natl Cancer Inst* (1981) **67**:327–33.

54 Sherman B, Wallace R, Bean J, Estrogen use and breast cancer. Interactions with body mass, *Cancer* (1983) **51**:1527–31.

55 Kaufman DW, Miller DR, Rosenberg L et al, Non-contraceptive oestrogen use and the risk of breast cancer, *JAMA* (1984) **252**:63–7.

56 Grodin J, Siiteri P, MacDonald P, Source of estrogen production in postmenopausal women, *J Clin Endocrinol Metab* (1973) **56**:207–14.

CHAPTER 10

NON-INFILTRATING CARCINOMA

It was not suddenly bred,
It will not swifly abate
Through the chill years ahead
When time shall count from the date

Rudyard Kipling

There is a tendency to consider the evolution of cancer in Darwinian terms. According to this model there is a slow progression with altered normal cells dividing and becoming hyperplastic, and giving rise to atypical daughter cells which gradually evolve into in situ cancer and ultimately manifest as infiltrating carcinoma. From this viewpoint the fossil record is incomplete. Although the pathologist may report the presence of a variety of precursors of malignancy in tissue surrounding invasive carcinoma, it is not uncommon for a cancer to be present in isolation with no evidence of a non-infiltrating component in its environs, and no clue as to the nature of the progenitors of the disease.

Because of the propensity of invasive breast carcinoma to metastasize at an apparently early clinical stage, this provides a compelling reason to try and identify malignancy before the basement membrane has been breached. However, can this be achieved? Can the natural history of breast cancer, in population terms, be influenced by treatment of pre-invasive lesions? Will aggressive treatment save lives, or merely add morbidity to a group who might never have suffered from clinical breast cancer? These are some of the questions that must be addressed when studying the relationship of in situ carcinoma to infiltrating breast cancer. In addition, is there sufficient information available in order to formulate appropriate interventional strategies for those women who, either as a result of symptoms, or alternatively as a consequence of screening, are found to have non-invasive breast lesions?

Many workers have tended to treat lobular and ductal variants of in situ carcinoma as subtypes which are broadly similar. However, this is not borne out by a close examination of the biological behaviour of LCIS and DCIS. The conditions may have different aetiologies: they certainly have divergent behaviour, and this has important implications for treatment. The extended period during which change occurs from non-infiltrating to invasive breast carcinoma means that both the inadequacies of under-treatment and the morbidity of overtreatment may be missed in the passage of time. Despite this, and possibly because of the success of breast-conserving treatments for early invasive disease, the role of mastectomy in the management of in situ breast cancer is being questioned with increasing frequency.

Lobular carcinoma in situ (LCIS)

Histology

This self-effacing lesion is often diagnosed only after the most meticulous histological examination of biopsy specimens. It had largely eluded the attention of pathologists until the description by Foote and Stewart in 1941:[1]

'Microscopically the process shows the following characters: there is a sudden and abrupt alteration in lobular cytology. A group of normal lobules is interrupted by the presence of a lobule or group of lobules in which the cells are large. They are perhaps twice the size of those in normal lobules and their nuclei are in proportion. The nuclei tend to be clear, the cytoplasm is apt to be opaque. The compact orderly arrangement of the epithelium gives place to a decided looseness, a loss of cohesion.

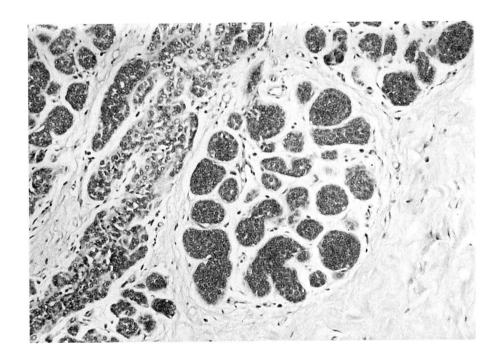

Figure 10.1   Lobular carcinoma in situ.

Cells are progressively displaced towards the lumina in a disorderly fashion eventually obliterating the space. Mitoses are rare. The cells lose polarity, varying in shape, while maintaining surprisingly uniform size'.

An example of LCIS is shown in Figure 10.1, which indicates the excellence of the original description by Foote and Stewart. They also described spread of the cells into the terminal lobular duct which they dubbed 'Pagetoid' spread. Foote and Stewart were convinced that the process was always present in several lobules and they were not prepared to make the histological diagnosis unless more than three lobules were involved. This quantitative rather than qualitative approach to diagnosis was subsequently challenged by Wheeler and Enterline, who argued that no relationship had been demonstrated between prognosis and the number of lobules involved.[2] Nevertheless, it is at the earliest detectable stage that there may be diagnostic problems for the pathologist trying to differentiate between LCIS and atypical lobular hyperplasia, which is shown in Figure 10.2.

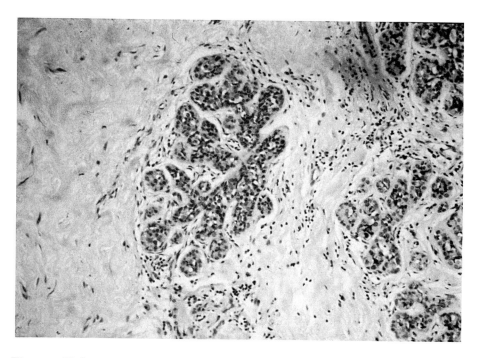

Figure 10.2   Atypical lobular hyperplasia.

Clinical aspects

The epithelial cells within the lobules do not form tumours, nor excite any inflammatory reaction. They do not cause nipple discharge and do not undergo necrosis with subsequent calcification, so that the lesion is usually undetectable mammographically. All these factors conspire to mask the presence of LCIS, which is almost always an unexpected histological finding. After it had been named lobular carcinoma in situ by Foote and Stewart, this induced a predictable reaction among surgeons who treated the lesion by mastectomy. These largely unnecessary operations have at least served to highlight the histopathological characteristics and distribution of LCIS within mastectomy specimens.

The pathological findings are listed in Table 10.1, which shows the incidence of residual LCIS, presence of infiltrating carcinoma and axillary lymph node involvement in mastectomy specimens following a biopsy diagnosis of LCIS.[3-8] In addition, the incidence of LCIS in contralateral breast biopsies is given. A consistent pattern emerges. Contralateral LCIS is detectable in 30 per cent of biopsies, whether mirror-image or random biopsy is performed. Residual or multifocal LCIS is present in the ipsilateral breast in up to 70 per cent of cases. Foci of occult invasion are a rare event and axillary lymph nodes are almost never involved with metastases from a coexisting infiltrating lesion. Follow-up of cases treated in these studies showed that none had developed recurrence of cancer.

Taken together, these findings suggest that although mastectomy may prevent ipsilateral problems, it represents overtreatment with regards to the axilla, and also to the breast since 30 per cent of cases showed no residual disease. Although there is a high incidence (30 per cent) of contralateral LCIS, the significance of this is unclear.

Clues to the incidence of LCIS in the population have been obtained from autopsy

Table 10.1 Mastectomy findings after biopsy showing LCIS.

	No	Contralateral LCIS present	Contralateral biopsy	Residual LCIS	Invasion	Axillary metastases	Reference
	26	6	18	27	0	0	3
	13	2	5	13	0	0	4
	28	6	15	21	0	?	5
	118	?	?	79	0	0	6
	24	1	?	14	0	0	7
	49	27	44	31	3	1	8
TOTAL	258	42 (30)	82 (71)	185 (72)	3 (1)	1 (0.4)	

*Percentages in parentheses.

material. Alpers and Wellings found no cases of LCIS in 185 random autopsies, but discovered LCIS in eight breasts from 59 women with clinically apparent primary carcinomas.[9] None of these were in women aged 15–39, two were 40–49, four were 50–59 and one was 60–69. In the contralateral breasts of 44 women with known breast primaries, LCIS was present in six (14 per cent), four aged 39–49 and two aged 50–59. Nielsen et al studied 110 medico-legal autopsy cases of women aged 20–54 years and found LCIS alone in four (4 per cent) and LCIS with DCIS in one (1 per cent).[10] In a similar study, but using hospital-derived autopsy cases, LCIS was present in eight out of 83 (10 per cent) and LCIS with DCIS in three (4 per cent).[11]

These studies do suggest that LCIS can be present in an asymptomatic form in women particularly between the ages of 30 and 50 years. Haagensen has suggested that LCIS should be renamed lobular neoplasia.[12] Although this may deliver reassurance to the patient and possibly persuade the surgeon to eschew mastectomy, it still fails to define whether this is a truly pre-malignant lesion or merely an epiphenomenon of breast cancer.

LCIS and invasive breast cancer

With the gradual realization that mastectomy represented overtreatment there was a trend towards a more conservative approach, treating such patients by excision followed by close observation, and this is now the standard treatment for LCIS. In addition, because of the difficulty of sampling histological specimens, subsequent more extensive reviews have shown LCIS to be present in approximately 3 per cent of biopsies originally reported as benign.[12–14]

These cases have provided an opportunity to study the progress of patients bearing LCIS but not subjected to mastectomy. The five long-term follow-up studies of such patients are summarized in Table 10.2, which

Table 10.2 Ipsilateral invasive carcinoma after biopsy of LCIS.

No	Mean follow-up (years)	5 years (%)	10 years (%)	15 years (%)	20 years (%)	Reference
50	19.5	8	15	27	35	15
25	17.5	0	0	4	4	16
47	15	9	11	13	17	17
211	14	3	7	10	18	12
99	24	–	–	–	19	18
MEAN (%)		5	8	14	19	

Table 10.3 Contralateral invasive carcinoma after biopsy of LCIS.

	5 years (%)	10 years (%)	15 years (%)	20 years (%)	References
	4	11	16	25	15
	0	7	12	12	16
	0	4	6	9	17
	6	7	9	15	12
	–	–	–	16	18
AVERAGE	3	7	11	15	

gives the risk of development of ipsilateral invasive breast cancer after up to 20 years of follow-up.[12,15–18]

With the exception of the smallest study,[16] all the others are in broad agreement. Mean percentages for developing ipsilateral cancers are 5 per cent at 5 years, 8 per cent at 10 years, 14 per cent at 15 years and 19 per cent after 20 years. The carcinomas evolving in such patients were a mixture of both infiltrating lobular and infiltrating ductal carcinomas.[18]

From the same studies, the proportions of patients developing contralateral breast carcinoma are given in Table 10.3, and here the results are all remarkably similar. The mean percentages developing contralateral breast cancer were 3 per cent at 5 years, 7 per cent at 10 years, 11 per cent at 15 years and 15 per cent at 20 years. Thus over 30 per cent of patients with LCIS will develop either an ipsilateral or a contralateral infiltrating carcinoma after 20 years of follow-up. The mean

age at diagnosis of LCIS in these studies was 45 years, so that assuming a female life expectancy of 80 years, this represents an average of 35 years of risk with a likelihood of infiltrating breast carcinoma possibly rising to 50–60 per cent. From these studies the ratio of ipsilateral to contralateral carcinomas would be 1.6 : 1. If considered in this way, lobular carcinoma is one of the most powerful risk factors for the subsequent development of breast cancer. However, LCIS is not necessarily the precursor lesion of infiltrating lobular carcinoma. The development of infiltrating ductal carcinomas after LCIS suggests the lesion is tumour-associated rather than tumourigenic. Thus extensive local treatment is an inappropriate management for LCIS.

Endocrine function and LCIS

It has been reported that between 67 and 85 per cent of women with LCIS are premenopausal.[3,5,7,19,20] This propensity of the premenopausal does suggest that the withdrawal of steroid hormones at the menopause may induce the regression of LCIS lesions and possibly prevent development of infiltrating carcinoma. The relatively rare finding of LCIS in the postmenopausal might be due either to higher levels of endogenous or exogenous steroids, or alternatively the emergence of a cell population capable of autocrine stimulation. This has implications for both acceleration and also prevention of progression of LCIS to infiltrating carcinoma.

First, it is possible that the use of oral contraception or hormone replacement therapy might promote such progression. To date there is no compelling evidence of such an event occurring. Nevertheless, when patients with proven LCIS request contraceptive advice, if it is decided to prescribe contraceptive steroids such a patient will require very close follow-up. Similarly, although hormone replacement therapy is not absolutely con-traindicated, nevertheless great caution needs to be exercised and such cases are probably best followed in a breast clinic.

A more exciting possibility is the chance to reduce the risk of subsequent development of infiltrating carcinoma. There are various theoretical approaches including the use of progestogens, anti-oestrogens or ovarian ablation either by irradiation or medically with an LHRH agonist. The anti-oestrogen tamoxifen is a promising candidate for a prevention trial since it would not only block endogenous oestrogen,[21] but also might inhibit autocrine growth factors such as transforming growth factor alpha.[22]

Against this there are theoretical risks of oestrogen blockade, including bone de-mineralization and also alteration in serum lipids and lipoproteins leading to an in-creased risk of osteoporosis and ischaemic heart disease, both degenerative conditions being known to be associated with meno-pausal oestrogen deprivation and both being preventable by exogenous oestrogens. However, these fears have arisen from an incomplete understanding of the action of tamoxifen, which is not a pure oestrogen antagonist but actually possesses oestrogen agonist activity. Thus, the administration of tamoxifen leads to a slight alteration in lipoprotein profiles consistent with oestroge-nic effect which certainly does not appear likely to increase the risk of coronary heart disease.[23,24] Tamoxifen has been given to premenopausal women without malignancy, but who were suffering from cyclical mastal-gia. For this indication it is a very effective agent with an acceptable profile of side-effects including menstrual irregularity, hot flushes and occasional nausea.[25] These side-effects can be further reduced when the dosage is changed from 20 mg to 10 mg daily.[26] Follow-up of such cases who have taken tamoxifen for up to 12 months has shown no change in bone mineral density measured by dual photon absorptiometry

after up to 3 years following completion of tamoxifen treatment.[27] Furthermore, no changes in calcium, phosphate, alkaline phosphatase or osteocalcin were found either during or after such treatment.

Nevertheless, the oestrogen agonist effects may carry other risks. Studies of rats given high dosages of tamoxifen have shown the development of both cataracts and hepa-tocellular carcinoma, both of which may occur in rodent models after high dosages of oestrogen. To date, no cases of hepatocellu-lar carcinoma have been reported in women taking tamoxifen and it has been argued, without contradiction, that the risk of tamox-ifen is minimal and is not a contraindication to its use for prevention.[28] Certainly consid-ering individuals with LCIS where the life-time risk of invasive cancer may be up to 70 per cent, this is of a different order of magnitude to the risks of treatment. Another possible risk of tamoxifen therapy would be the promotion of endometrial carcinoma and an association has been suggested.[29] Never-theless, this risk, if any, remains very small in relation to the more major risk of, and mortality from, invasive breast cancer.

For these reasons a trial has been set up by the EORTC Breast Cancer Cooperative Group to examine the role of tamoxifen in the prevention of infiltrating carcinoma in women with LCIS.[30] Eligible cases include women with no previous history of carcinoma who are found to have LCIS on a biopsy, without evidence of DCIS or of invasive disease. No further surgery is performed and patients are randomized to observation or to receive tamoxifen, 20 mg once daily, for 5 years. The major obstruction to the successful conduct of such a trial as this is logistic. The incidence of LCIS at any institution will usually be directly proportional to its work-load, that is the number of biopsies being performed. Even the largest centres may only see two or three cases of LCIS every year and it is of course difficult for a variety of clinicians to remember to put such rare cases into a multicentre study. National screening programmes will have little influence on the pick-up rate of LCIS. Nevertheless, if such a trial can be completed this should provide very interesting evidence as to whether there is a preventative role for tamoxifen in women with LCIS.

Ductal carcinoma in situ (DCIS)

Whereas the link between LCIS and infiltrating carcinoma is somewhat tenuous, a closer relationship between ductal carcinoma in situ and infiltrating ductal cancer can be postulated. Unlike LCIS, where the diagnosis may be a surprise to both clinician and pathologist, DCIS may produce symptoms and certainly may be strongly suspected on clinical and radiological grounds before definite histological diagnosis has been obtained. Whereas the absolute incidence of LCIS is related to the number of biopsies being performed, the numbers of cases of DCIS diagnosed will increase as more mammograms are performed, either for symptomatic patients or as part of screening programmes. The rarity of LCIS means that few have a great deal of experience and therefore dogmatic statements on management are rare. In contrast, DCIS has been treated by most surgeons, who will therefore hold strong views as to the respective merits of mastectomy and breast conservation, together with the role of radiotherapy in the treatment of DCIS. However, is there sufficient evidence to shed light upon the problem and allow definitive pronouncements on the management of DCIS?

Histological subtypes

The threshold for acceptance of histological evidence of DCIS will vary from pathologist

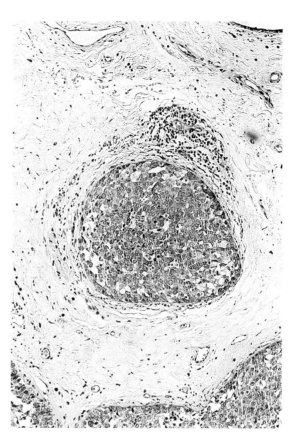

Figure 10.3   Solid DCIS × 125 magnification.

to pathologist and probably in 10 per cent of cases no pathological consensus can be obtained. Thus it is somewhat subjective as to whether certain lesions are called atypical ductal hyperplasia or possibly clinging or low-papillary DCIS. Most pathologists recognize six subtypes of DCIS: solid, cribriform, comedo, clinging, papillary and low papillary, with frequent mixtures of these patterns (Figures 10.3–10.6). In terms of likely tumour

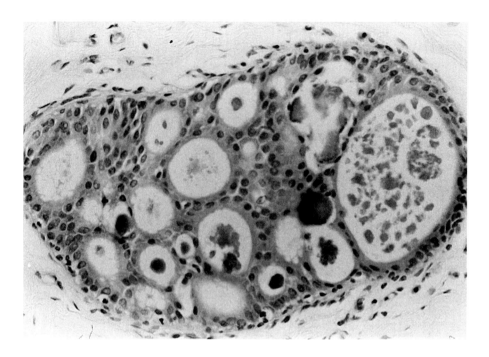

Figure 10.4   Cribriform DCIS × 125 magnification.

burden, the least would be the low papillary and clinging and the most the solid and comedo types, although in the latter many of the intraductal cells are necrotic.

Clinical features

The clinical features at presentation of women with DCIS in eight series are given in Table 10.4.[31–8] Where the average age has been given this has been remarkably consistent, being 52 years, an average of 7 years

later than that of published series of LCIS cases. Gump distinguished between patients with microscopic DCIS (average age 50 years) and gross DCIS (average age 57 years), giving some indication of the protracted time-scale of progression from histological to clinical disease in patients with DCIS.[38]

The commonest symptom among patients was a lump, reported by approximately 60 per cent. A nipple discharge was the presenting symptom in 10 per cent. When specified, the discharge was either blood-stained or contained haemoglobin on testing in 75 per

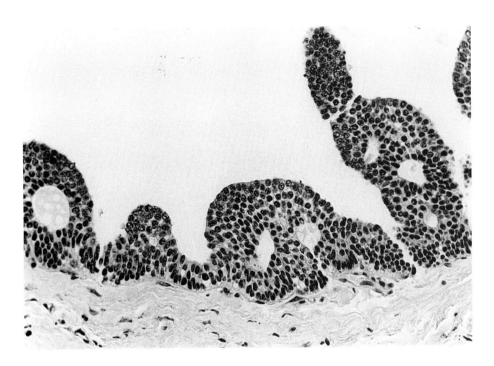

Figure 10.5   Papillary DCIS × 125 magnification.

cent of cases.[32,34] A combination of both nipple discharge and palpable lump was reported in 8 per cent of cases. Not all series have included patients whose original presentation was with Paget's disease of the nipple, but this accounts for approximately 5 per cent of cases of DCIS. Nowadays in breast clinics approximately 20 per cent of patients with DCIS will be diagnosed on a basis of mammographic abnormality, without any abnormal physical signs being present. Review of mammograms of patients with DCIS shows the presence of microcalcification in approximately 50 per cent. Not all

patients with breast symptoms and DCIS necessarily have a lump or discharge as a direct result of the premalignancy. For some the lump is due to fibrocystic disease or the nipple discharge due to a duct papilloma or duct ectasia. Nevertheless, the majority do have symptoms directly attributable to DCIS.

Analysis of the British Breast Group's data showed no difference in overall survival of patients who originally presented with a lump or discharge and those who had mammographic abnormalities (unpublished work). This might be the result of the treatment, which was predominantly mastec-

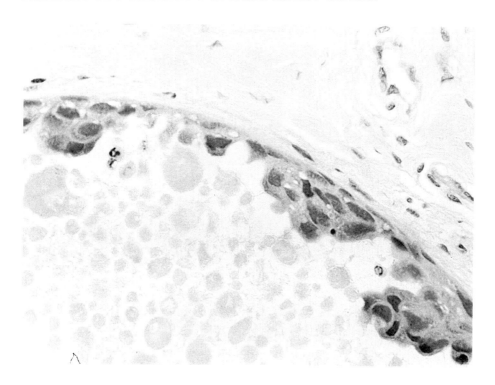

Figure 10.6   Clinging DCIS × 500 magnification.

Table 10.4 Clinical features of patients with DCIS.

	No	Age	Lump	Discharge	Paget's	Asymptomatic	X-ray	Reference
	36	0	20	9	0	7	0	31
	40	0	34	1	0	1	4	32
	55	53	44	11	0	0	0	33
	53	51	38	11	0	0	4	34
	101	52	54	15	11	0	21	35
	70	52	49	3	13	0	5	36
	100	52	40	0	1	0	59	37
	70	mg 57/50	48	0	4	3	15	38
TOTAL	525	52	327 (62%)	50 (10%)	29 (5%)	11 (2%)	108 (20%)	

m = Microscopic disease.
g = Gross disease.

Table 10.5 Histological findings after mastectomy for DCIS.

No	No residual	Residual	Multifocal	Invasion	Axillary metastases	Reference
38	5	25	–	7	4	8
50	16	20	10	3	0	39
53	25	–	17	11	1	40
47	23	–	18	6	0	34
82	30	20	19	13	0	35
45	15	28	–	2	1	36
52	–	–	9	1	1	41
49	11	38	27	–	0	37
61	27	10	24	3	1	38
Mean (%)	36	43	31	11	2	

tomy, and the relative shortness of follow-up. Nevertheless, it is suggestive that mammographically detected DCIS is not different from symptomatic DCIS with regard to its behaviour and prognosis.

Mastectomy findings

Until very recently the majority of patients with DCIS were treated by either total or radical mastectomy. From the study of such cases the pattern of DCIS, its association with infiltrating carcinoma and the incidence of axillary-nodal metastases together with outcome can be evaluated. The results from nine series are summarized in Table 10.5.[8,34–41] This indicates the frequency of residual DCIS at the original biopsy site, present in up to 78 per cent of cases (average 43 per cent). A multifocal DCIS was present in up to 55 per cent (average 31 per cent) and a co-existing

unsuspected infiltrating carcinoma was present in 11 per cent (range 2–18 per cent) and this was usually associated with multifocal DCIS. Axillary-nodal metastases were only very rarely present (2 per cent). Such metastases were present either when the pathologist found a co-existing infiltrating carcinoma or alternatively in the absence of any apparent invasive disease. This underlines the difficulty involved in accurately sampling breast tissue from a patient with DCIS. It does provide clear evidence of the redundancy of axillary dissection in the treatment of staging of patients with biopsy-proven DCIS.

Electron microscopic examination of DCIS material will often provide evidence of damage to, or microinvasion through, the basement membrane but this has not so far been shown to be of value in the routine prognostic evaluation of tissue from such cases.[42] These results do provide evidence that a biopsy alone would leave residual disease in over half of patients and would miss an invasive carcinoma in 10 per cent. A wider excision might detect the majority of adjacent infiltrating carcinomas. If histological confirmation was obtained that the wider excision specimen had completely cleared DCIS, then multifocal disease would still be left behind in up to 30 per cent of patients. Although a total or radical mastectomy would achieve almost 100 per cent local control of breast cancer, the mortality rate following such a procedure for DCIS is 1–3 per cent as a result of co-existing metastatic infiltrating carcinoma.

women-years represents an annual percentage of less than 0.01 per cent, as compared with 0.08 per cent for patients with infiltrating carcinoma and 1–2 per cent for those with LCIS. Thus there would appear to be no justification for mirror-image biopsy of the contralateral breast of a patient with DCIS. The difference in annual incidence compared with infiltrating carcinoma is possibly a reflection of the diminished risk of progression of DCIS to infiltrating lesions and is more circumstantial evidence supporting DCIS as an actual precursor lesion in the involved breast rather than a marker of malignant chance.

Bilaterality of DCIS

The risk of development of infiltrating carcinoma in the contralateral breast after a histological diagnosis of DCIS appears to be of a very low order. The four studies which have either examined this question or given data allowing its examination are shown in Table 10.6.[8,35,36,43] The only two cases of contralateral infiltrating carcinoma per 2344

Follow-up of biopsied DCIS

Several studies have followed patients for DCIS where the original diagnosis was missed by the pathologist or alternatively the patient or surgeon was reluctant for a mastectomy to be performed. The follow-up studies are summarized in Table 10.7.[33,44–8] Under these circumstances, which probably

Table 10.6 Development of contralateral infiltrating carcinoma after DCIS.

No	Mean follow-up	Women years	DCIS	Infiltrating carcinoma	Reference
38	6.2	235	0	0	8
101	5	505	2	0	35
70	8	560	1	2	36
116	9	1044	0	0	43
325		2344	3	2	

Table 10.7 Development of ipsilateral infiltrating carcinoma after biopsy of DCIS.

No	Follow-up (years)	Infiltrating carcinoma	Reference
25	4	5	44
11	10	2	48
4	4	0	33
10	10	7	45
15	18	10	46
25	15	7	47
TOTAL 90		31 (34%)	

Table 10.8 Development of ipsilateral infiltrating carcinoma after wide excision of DCIS.

No	Follow-up (years)	Infiltrating (carcinoma)	Reference
11	10	2	49
20	4	3	40
22	3	5	50
TOTAL 53		10 (19%)	

embrace some of the earliest forms of DCIS, there is an overall 50 per cent incidence of infiltrating carcinoma developing within the original breast with a minimal risk on the contralateral side. Other series have followed patients in whom a wide excision of the area was performed, although in the majority of these studies there is no information as to whether the area of DCIS was completely excised.[40,49,50]

Despite this inadequacy, Table 10.8 shows that more extensive surgery does reduce the risk of development of infiltrating carcinoma within the affected breast with an average overall incidence of infiltrating carcinoma of 19 per cent. In addition, a wider excision will uncover an infiltrating carcinoma, missed by the original biopsy in 5–10 per cent of patients.

Although this is an improvement it still suggests that uncontrolled surgery, that is surgery with inadequate pathological information as to the completeness of excision, will lead to an unacceptably high rate of progression to infiltrating carcinoma. This, therefore, provides an argument in favour of more extensive surgery. However, it is paradoxical that mastectomy should be regarded as the treatment of choice for precursor of infiltrating carcinoma whereas invasive early breast cancer can be treated by proven safe breast-conservation techniques. With increasing patient awareness of alternative techniques to mastectomy there will be more frequent requests for breast conservation in DCIS, particularly screen-detected. Surgical techniques, however, almost always rely on radiotherapy to supplant less extensive surgery in patients with infiltrating carcinoma. Is this a reasonable approach for patients with DCIS?

Radio-sensitivity of DCIS

Almost all trials of treatment of early breast cancer have excluded patients with DCIS. However, within two trials, subsequent histological review of biopsy material has shown that some cases originally deemed to have infiltrating carcinoma (as a result sometimes of frozen section) were found to have pure DCIS. In the Guy's wide excision trial there were six cases treated by wide excision followed by external radiotherapy (38 cGy to the breast and 30 cGy to the axilla).[51] None of these cases has developed local or systemic relapse of breast carcinoma, although of course it is not possible to determine whether the successful outcome was the result of surgery or radiotherapy. This result does suggest that therapeutic doses of radiation may inhibit progression of DCIS and certainly does not accelerate the process.

In the NSABP trial B-06, which compared total mastectomy and axillary clearance with partial mastectomy and axillary clearance, with or without radiation, there were found to be 78 out of 2072 (3.8 per cent) patients who had DCIS without evidence of invasion.[50] In all cases except one, the original biopsy showed complete excision of the lesion. Of the 51 patients treated by partial mastectomy, 29 received postoperative radiation (50 cGy) and 22 were not given any further local treatment. Seven patients developed local relapse, although this was an infiltrating carcinoma in only four and DCIS in three. Of the relapses 5/22 (23 per cent) were in the non-irradiated group and 2/29 (7 per cent) in the irradiated group. With a

mean follow-up of 39 months, definite conclusions cannot be drawn, but there is a suggestion of a benefit for patients treated with radiotherapy.

The results of those studies in which external radiotherapy was given as part of the treatment of DCIS are shown in Table 10.9.[37,52-4] On average, only 5 per cent of such cases developed subsequent infiltrating carcinoma, which again suggests a benefit from external radiotherapy.

However, against these encouraging findings there have been doubts expressed, particularly in relation to DCIS and risk of recurrence of infiltrating carcinoma after breast conservation.[55] Several studies have suggested that the extent of DCIS within the original biopsy specimen, together with tumour grade and lymphatic permeation, may be an important determinant of risk of relapse. However, the extent of DCIS and differentiation of infiltrating carcinoma may be a reflection of both aggressiveness and tumour burden, which may differ under circumstances where infiltration has developed rather than at a pre-invasive state. This question must be regarded as unanswered at present.

Two multicentre controlled trials of treatment for DCIS are under way, one run by the NSABP and the other by the EORTC. The broad outline of both trials is similar and both seek to answer the question 'Does radiotherapy alter the natural history after apparent complete excision of DCIS?'. Eligible cases are women who have had a pathologically confirmed complete excision of DCIS with no evidence of invasion. Patients are randomized to observation alone or alternatively to receive external radiotherapy to the breast (50 cGy) without treatment of the axilla and without a boost to the primary excision site. It is hoped that these trials will be able to answer the role of radiotherapy in the management of localized DCIS. However, at present no trial is under way to examine the role of radiotherapy in the treatment of more

Table 10.9 Development of infiltrating carcinoma after breast irradiation of patients with DCIS.

	No	Follow-up (years)	Infiltrating carcinoma	Reference
	42	3	3	52
	7	4	2	53
	29	3	2	50
	54	4	1	54
	51	2	1	37
TOTAL	183		9 (5%)	

extensive DCIS, either histologically or radiographically. These may comprise up to 50 per cent of cases with DCIS. At the present time total mastectomy is regarded by most surgeons as the most appropriate treatment for proven multifocal DCIS.

Prognostic factors in DCIS

It would be very useful to identify those patients with DCIS who are most at risk of developing infiltrating carcinoma. A variety of techniques has been employed with this objective. First the cell type of DCIS may give an indication of risk. Vijver et al used two monoclonal antibodies for the immunohistochemical detection of *neu* proto-oncogene expression in a variety of formalin-fixed breast-cancer biopsies.[56] The *neu* oncogene (synonymous with c-erb B2) has extensive homology with the receptor for epidermal growth factor (EGF-R) and is a putative marker of poor prognosis. *Neu* oncogene overexpression was detected in all the 19 comedo-type DCIS lesions. All of these contained large cells. In contrast, no overexpression of oncogene was seen in the small DCIS cases (papillary and cribriform). Thus it is possible that the comedo (large cell) variants are more at risk of progression to infiltration, but this still remains an open question. The extent of DCIS within the original biopsy has been claimed to predict the likelihood of multifocal disease and risk of infiltrating carcinoma,[41] but others have not found this to be the case.[57] Measurement of ploidy in the DCIS cells has been suggested as a predictor of risk of subsequent infiltrating carcinoma. Carpenter et al reported that 4 out of 13 (31 per cent) lesions from patients with atypical hyperplasia were aneuploid, compared with 4/12 (33 per cent) of those with DCIS and 23/26 (88 per cent)

from cases with DCIS and associated infiltrating carcinoma.[57] It was postulated that aneuploidy might predict for progression to infiltrating carcinoma. However, Erhardt and Aver found aneuploidy in 6/9 (67 per cent) of cases of DCIS and 7/9 (78 per cent) of infiltrating lesions, casting some doubt on the association between ploidy and progression.[58]

Nielsen et al carried out short-term culture of cells from DCIS and invasive carcinomas, performed chromosome banding and found different ploidy levels without any consistent chromosome abnormalities.[59] The most frequent ploidy levels were hypodiploid/hypotriploid in invasive cancer and hyperdiploid/hypertriploid in DCIS.

De Potter et al measured the Feulgen DNA content of cells from atypical hyperplasia and DCIS and were unable to distinguish between the two conditions.[60] However, mitotic activity was significantly increased in DCIS alone or in association with infiltrating carcinoma.

The thymidine-labelling index (TLI) was measured in 61 in situ carcinomas by Meyer, who found that the TLI was significantly lower in cribriform and papillary DCIS than in comedo DCIS (1.8 versus 5.2 per cent). Solid DCIS was intermediate with a mean TLI of 3.3 per cent.[61] Because of the rarity of DCIS lesions it has not been possible to conduct a multivariate analysis to examine the relative predictive values of type of DCIS, TLI, ploidy and extent of DCIS in determination of risk progression to infiltrating lesions.

References

1 Foote FW, Stewart FW, Lobular carcinoma in situ. A rare form of mammary cancer, *Am J Pathol* (1941) **17**:491–6.

2 Wheeler JE, Enterline HT, Lobular carcinoma of the breast in situ and infiltrating, *Pathol Annu* (1976) **11**:161–8.

3 Newman W, In situ lobular carcinoma of the breast: report of 26 women with 32 cancers, *Ann Surg* (1963) **157**:591–9.

4 Benfield JR, Jacobson M, Warner NE, In situ lobular carcinoma of the breast, *Arch Surg* (1965) **91**:130–5.

5 Lewison EF, Finney GC, Lobular carcinoma in situ of the breast, *Surg Gynecol Obstet* (1968) **126**:1280–6.

6 Farrow JH, Clinical considerations and treatment of in situ lobular breast cancer, *AJR* (1968) **102**:652–6.

7 Dall'Olmo CA, Ponka JL, Horn RC et al, Lobular carcinoma of the breast in situ. Are we too radical in its treatment, *Arch Surg* (1975) **110**:537–42.

8 Carter D, Smith RRL, Carcinoma in situ of the breast, *Cancer* (1977) **40**:1189–93.

9 Alpers CE, Wellings SR, The prevalence of carcinoma in situ in normal and cancer-associated breasts, *Hum Pathol* (1985) **16**:796–807.

10 Nielsen M, Thomsen JL, Primdahl S et al, Breast cancer and atypia among young and middle-aged women: a study of 110 medico-legal autopsies, *Br J Cancer* (1987) **56**:814–19.

11 Nielsen M, Jensen J, Andersen J, Precancerous and cancerous breast lesions during lifetime and at autopsy, *Cancer* (1984) **54**:612–15.

12 Haagensen CD, Lane N, Lattes R et al, Lobular neoplasia (so-called lobular carcinoma in situ) of the breast, *Cancer* (1978) **42**:737–69.

13 Gaton E, Czernobilsky B, Lobular carcinoma in situ of the breast, *Isr J Med Sci* (1974) **10**:1106–11.

14 Harvey DG, Fechner RE, Atypical lobular and papillary lesions of the breast: a follow-up study of 30 cases, *South Med J* (1978) **71**:361–4.

15 McDivitt RW, Hutter RVP, Foote FW et al, In situ lobular carcinoma. A prospective follow-up study indicating cumulative patient risks, *JAMA* (1967) **201**:82–6.

16 Wheeler JE, Enterline HT, Roseman JM et al, Lobular carcinoma in situ of the breast. Long-term follow-up, *Cancer* (1974) **34**:554–63.

17 Andersen JA, Lobular carcinoma in situ: a long-term follow-up in 52 cases, *Acta Pathol Microbiol Scand* (1974) **82**:519–33.

18 Rosen PP, Kosloff C, Lieberman PH et al, Lobular carcinoma in situ of the breast, *Am J Surg Pathol* (1978) **2**:225–51.

19 Rosen PP, Senie RT, Farr GH et al, Epidemiology of breast carcinoma: age, menstrual status and exogenous hormone usage in patients with lobular carcinoma in situ, *Surgery* (1979) **85**:219–24.

20 Rosner D, Bedwani RN, Vana J et al, Non-invasive breast carcinoma. Results of a national survey by the American College of Surgeons, *Ann Surg* (1980) **192**:139–47.

21 Jordan VC, Anti-oestrogenic and anti-tumour properties of tamoxifen in laboratory animals, *Cancer Treat Rep* (1976) **60**:1409–19.

22 Lippman ME, Dickson RB, Bates S et al, Autocrine and paracrine growth regulation of human breast cancer, *Breast Cancer Res Treat* (1986) **7**:59–70.

23 Rossner S, Wallgren A, Serum lipoproteins and proteins after breast cancer surgery and effects of tamoxifen. *Atherosclerosis* (1984) **52**:339–46.

24 Caleffi M, Fentiman IS, Clark GM et al, The effect of tamoxifen on oestrogen binding, lipid and lipoprotein concentration and blood clotting parameters in premenopausal women with breast pain, *J Endocrinol* (1988) **119**:335–9.

25 Fentiman IS, Caleffi M, Brame K et al, Double-blind controlled trial of tamoxifen therapy for mastalgia, *Lancet* (1986) **1**:287–8.

26 Fentiman IS, Caleffi M, Hamed H et al, Dosage and duration of tamoxifen treatment for mastalgia: a controlled trial, *Br J Surg* (1988) **75**:845–6.

27 Fentiman IS, Caleffi M, Rodin A et al, Bone mineral content of women receiving tamoxifen for mastalgia, *Br J Cancer* (1989) **60**:262–4.

28 Fentiman IS, Powles TJ, Tamoxifen and benign breast problems, *Lancet* (1987) **2**:1070–2.

29 Hardell L, Tamoxifen as risk factor for carcinoma of corpus uteri, *Lancet* 1988) **ii**:563.

30 Fentiman IS, Surgery in the management of early breast cancer: a review, *Eur J Cancer Clin Oncol* (1988) **24**:73–6.

31 Gillis DA, Dockerty MB, Claggett OT, Pre-invasive intraductal carcinoma of the breast, *Surg Gynecol Obstet* (1960) **110**:555–62.

32 Brown PW, Silverman J, Owens E et al, Intraductal 'non-infiltrating' carcinoma of the breast, *Arch Surg* (1976) **111**:1063–7.

33 Ashikari R, Huvos AG, Snyder RE, Prospective study of non-infiltrating carcinoma of the breast, *Cancer* (1977) **39**:435–9.

34 Von Rueden DG, Wilson RE, Intraductal carcinoma of the breast, *Surg Gynecol Obstet* (1984) **158**:105–11.

35 Fentiman IS, Fagg N, Millis RR et al, In situ ductal carcinoma of the breast: implications of disease pattern and treatment, *Eur J Surg Oncol* (1986) **12**:261–6.

36 Peterse JL, Gelderman WAH, Van Dongen JA et al, Ductal carcinoma in situ of the breast: a clinicopathological analysis of 70 cases, *Ned. Tijdschr. Geneeskd* (1986) **130**:308–10.

37 Silverstein MJ, Rosser RJ, Giersan ED et al, Axillary lymph node dissection for intraductal breast carcinoma—is it indicated? *Cancer* (1987) **59**:1819–24.

38 Gump FE, Jicha DL, Ozzello L, Ductal carcinoma in situ (DCIS): a revised concept, *Surgery* (1987) **102**:790–5.

39 Rosen PP, Senie R, Schottenfeld D et al, Non-invasive breast carcinoma. Frequency of unsuspected invasion and implications for treatment, *Ann Surg* (1979) **18**:377–82.

40 Lagios MD, Westdahl PR, Margolin FR et al, Duct carcinoma in situ, *Cancer* (1982) **50**:1309–14.

41 Schuh ME, Nemoto T, Penetrante B et al, Intraductal carcinoma. Analysis of presentation, pathologic findings and outcome of disease, *Arch Surg* (1986) **121**:1303–7.

42 Ozzello L, The behaviour of basement membrane in intraductal carcinoma of the breast, *Am J Pathol* (1959) **35**:887–99.

43 Webber BL, Heise H, Neifeld JP et al, Risk of subsequent contralateral breast carcinoma in a population of patients with in situ breast carcinoma, *Cancer* (1981) **47**:2928–37.

44 Farrow JH, Current conception. The detection and treatment of early breast carcinomas, *Cancer* (1970) **25**:468–77.

45 Betsill WL, Rosen PP, Lieberman PH et al, Intraductal carcinoma. Long-term follow-up after treatment by biopsy alone, *JAMA* (1978) **239**:1863–6.

46 Rosen PP, Braun DW, Kinne DF, The clinical significance of pre-invasive breast carcinoma, *Cancer* (1980) **46**:919–25.

47 Page DL, Dupont WD, Roger LW et al, Intraductal carcinoma of the breast: follow-up after biopsy only, *Cancer* (1982) **49**:751–8.

48 Carter D, Orr SL, Merino MJ, Intracystic papillary carcinoma of the breast. After mastectomy, radiotherapy or excisional biopsy alone, *Cancer* (1983) **52**:14–19.

49 Millis RR, Thynne GSJ, In situ intraduct carcinoma of the breast: a long-term follow-up study, *Br J Surg* (1975) **62**:957–62.

50 Fisher ER, Sass R, Fisher B et al, Pathologic findings from the National Surgical Adjuvant Breast Project (Protocol 6). 1. Intraductal carcinoma (DCIS), *Cancer* (1986) **57**:197–208.

51 Atkins HJB, Hayward JL, Klugman DJ et al, Treatment of early breast cancer: a report after ten years of a clinical trial, *Br Med J* (1972) **2**:423–9.

52 Goodman RC, Danoff BF, Recht A et al, Intraductal carcinoma of the breast: results of

treatment with excisional biopsy and irradiation, *Int J Radiat Oncol Biol Phys* (1984) **10** suppl 2:121.

53 Morgan DAL, Hinton CP, Blamey RW, Management of intraduct carcinoma, *Lancet* (1984) i:1082.

54 Zafrani B, Fourquet A, Vilcoq JR et al, Conservative management of intraductal breast carcinoma with tumourectomy and radiation therapy, *Cancer* (1986) **57**:1299–1301.

55 Recht A, Connolly JL, Schnitt SJ et al, The effect of young age on tumour recurrence in the treated breast after conservative surgery and radiotherapy, *Int J Radiat Oncol Biol Phys* (1988) **14**:3–10.

56 Van de Vijver MJ, Peterse JL, Mooi WJ et al, Neu-protein overexpression in breast cancer. Association with comedo-type ductal carcinoma in situ and limited prognostic value in Stage II breast cancer, *N Engl J Med* (1988) **319**:1239–45.

57 Carpenter R, Gibbs N, Matthews J et al, Importance of cellular DNA content in premalignant breast disease and pre-invasive carcinoma of the female breast, *Br J Surg* (1987) **74**:905–6.

58 Erhardt K, Aver GU, Mammary carcinoma. Comparison of nuclear DNA content from in situ and infiltrative components, *Analyt Quant Cytol Histol* (1987) **9**:263–7.

59 Nielsen KV, Andersen JA, Blichert-Toft M, Chromosome changes of in situ carcinomas in the female breast, *Eur J Surg Oncol* (1987) **13**:225–9.

60 De Potter CR, Praet MM, Slavin RE et al, Feulgen DNA content and mitotic activity in proliferative breast disease. A comparison with ductal carcinoma in situ, *Histopathology* (1987) 1307–19.

61 Meyer MS, Cell kinetics of histologic variants of in situ breast carcinoma, *Breast Cancer* (1986) **7**:171–80.

CHAPTER 11

BREAST CANCER IN THE ELDERLY

What is the worst of foes that wait on age?

Lord Byron

For many women, their final years of life, instead of being the acme of their achievements, are lived out in an increasing misery of widowhood, financial deprivation and loneliness. Those unlucky enough to develop breast cancer may fare even worse because of a regrettable tendency to undertreat the disease in the elderly, partly from a misunderstanding of the biology of breast cancer in older women, and also because of groundless fear that operative treatment carries a high mortality rate. The reluctance of surgeons to operate on the elderly has been reinforced by the emergence of non-toxic endocrine therapies and there has been an almost gadarene stampede away from mastectomy in the elderly. Only very recently has any information been available from controlled trials of treatment for early breast cancer in older women, and much of the data is apparently contradictory.

The expression 'atrophic scirrhous carcinoma' is deeply rooted in the consciousness of many clinicians, and yet this belief that breast cancer runs a more indolent course in older women is totally at variance with the information available. An attempt will be made to destroy this mythical creature, and to construct an appropriate framework for management of what will be an increasing part of our clinical workload. Breast cancer is

an unforgiving foe if a less than mortal blow is delivered as a first strike. Inadequate treatment on dubious grounds of frailty will usually not be disguised by the premature death of the patient from concurrent illness.

It is arguable whether the age of 70 years should be taken as the threshold for patients being regarded as elderly. Publications on breast cancer in the elderly have variously used thresholds of between 65 and 80 years. For most trials of treatment in early breast cancer, women over 70 years have been excluded. The average life expectancy of a 70-year-old Western woman is approximately 15 years. Thus the majority of 70-year-old women are non-fragile patients with a low risk of operative mortality. As a result of an improvement in dietary habits, and provided that smoking rates can be reduced, it is to be expected that both the proportion and absolute numbers of the elderly will increase by the end of this century.

The annual incidence of breast cancer in Britain is 24 000.[1] Of these, 8000 patients are over the age of 70 years. Thus, so defined the elderly represent one-third of the total cases of breast cancer and this proportion is likely to increase. It is not possible at present to predict what effects screening will have on this population, since women over the age of 65 will not be routinely offered screening in

Britain. Eventually, as a byproduct of screening, some slow-growing variants will have been detected and possibly screened individuals will be more breast aware. Unless there is a knock-on effect from screening younger women, the reduction in population mortality will be less than that which is predicted, because of breast cancers in unscreened elderly women.

Stage at presentation

It is commonly believed that elderly women tend to delay in presenting with breast cancer so they have higher stage tumours when first seen. Approximately one-quarter of patients aged over 75 with breast cancer will present with Stage III or Stage IV disease. Representative series are summarized in Table 11.1.[2–5] The largest of the series was that from the Cancer Registry of Norway, which presented data on a total of 31 594 women of all ages. Of those women aged less than 75, 49 per cent had Stage I lesions (51 per cent in those over 75), 37 per cent were Stage II (21 per cent in those over 75), 5 per cent Stage III (11 per cent in those over 75) and 6 per cent Stage IV (11 per cent in the elderly) and 3 per cent were of unknown stage (6 per cent in the elderly). Thus, although there was a trend towards more advanced cancers in the elderly, in clinical terms this did not amount to a significant effect.

Nevertheless, this does reflect a delay in presentation which has been confirmed by the studies summarized in Table 11.2.[6–8] This shows that 36 per cent of women aged over 70 years delayed for more than 6 months, compared with only 26 per cent of younger women.

The reasons for this delay are manifold. A few patients will be unaware of any problem as a result of either dementia or depression. Others who are caring for sick husbands may not wish to report their problem because they fear that there will be no one to take their place as nurse/housekeeper for their ailing

Table 11.1 TNM stage at presentation in the elderly.

No of cases	I	II	III	IV	Total	Reference
>80	23 (31)	15 (20)	18 (24)	19 (25)	75	2
>80	73 (52)	25 (18)	8 (6)	35 (24)	141	3
>80	39 (25)	77 (49)	24 (15)	16 (10)	156	4
>75	2907 (53)	1221 (22)	686 (12)	698 (13)	5512	5
	3042 (52)	1338 (23)	736 (12)	768 (13)	5884	

Figures in parentheses are percentages.

Table 11.2 Age and delay at presentation.

<70		70+		Reference
<6 months (%)	6 months + (%)	<6 months (%)	6 months + (%)	
72	28	58	42	6
72	28	65	35	7
78	22	71	29	8
74	26	64	36	

spouse. Having delayed for some time, they then become concerned that their own doctor will be angry with them if they admit to having put off their consultation. Other reasons may include an ignorance of those breast symptoms that do require assessment. It is to be hoped that as a result of increased public awareness of the importance of early diagnosis, together with participation in screening and adoption of regular breast self-examination this ignorance may diminish. However, the message has not yet been heard and accepted. There are still those with the fatalistic approach that nothing can be done and who therefore do not consult a doctor because they feel wrongly that no patient is ever cured of breast cancer. Such attitudes are frequently expressed by elderly women who had not considered that it was worthwhile to have any treatment. This is a situation where the family doctor can reinforce the value of early diagnosis and use the opportunity of an examination of a patient with chest symptoms to perform additionally a breast examination, together with some basic health information about the need to report painless breast lumps.

Tumour aggressiveness in the elderly

The aggressive nature of any cancer may be measured in a variety of ways, including tumour type and histological grade. A better index is the extent of lymph node invasion and the most direct is the effect on relapse-free and overall survival of the patient. Those studies that have compared the histology of breast cancer in younger and older women are shown in Table 11.3, which confirms that the majority of infiltrating carcinomas in the elderly are of the ductal and lobular types and that the percentages in older women are very similar to those in younger cases.[8-10]

Rosen et al graded infiltrating ductal carcinoma pathologically in women aged under 35 and over 75.[9] Of the younger women, 4 per cent had grade I lesions, 42 per cent grade II and 54 per cent grade III. In the elderly group, 5 per cent were grade I, 55 per cent grade II and 39 per cent grade III. Thus, although fewer of the elderly had poorer differentiated lesions, this does not represent a major shift in the elderly towards less aggressive tumours.

Table 11.3 Comparative histology of infiltrating carcinomas in elderly and younger women.

Age	Ductal	Medullary	Lobular	Papillary	Reference
<65	1896 (74)	115 (5)	291 (11)	40 (2)	8
>65	468 (76)	14 (2)	44 (7)	20 (3)	
<35	122 (76)	17 (10)	4 (2)		9
>75	130 (77)	2 (1)	19 (11)		
<75	961 (69)	40 (3)	96 (7)		10
>75	290 (71)	4 (1)	20 (5)		

Percentages in parentheses.

Table 11.4 Axillary nodal involvement in operable breast cancer in the elderly.

No of cases	Nodal involvement	Reference
>70	133/242 (55)	6
>75	29/44 (66)	11
>65	43/92 (47)	12
>75	33/58 (57)	13
>70	22/56 (39)	14
>75	566/1299 (44)	15
>75	85/163 (52)	16
>80	54/116 (47)	4
	965/2070 (47)	

Percentages in parentheses.

Table 11.5 Five-year survival after mastectomy.

No of cases	Localized (%)		Regional (%)		Reference
	Crude	Adjusted	Crude	Adjusted	
<65	82	85	49	51	8
>65	71	90	43	55	
<70	73	79	50	55	17
>70	64	89	58	80	

When tumour aggression is measured by invasive potential, that is axillary nodal involvement, combined studies show that 47 per cent of the elderly have histopathological evidence of nodal metastases. Table 11.4 is a summary of series reporting nodal involvement.[4,6,11–16] A survey of the American College of Surgeons[15] comprised a total of 24 136 patients and among patients under 75 years treated by mastectomy, 47 per cent had pathologically involved axillary nodes compared with 44 per cent of those aged 75 years or more. This again argues against any significant reduction in the aggressiveness of breast cancers in the elderly.

As measured by overall survival, the crude 5-year rates do show impaired survival in elderly women. However, when deaths from other causes are allowed for, the rates are then very similar, as is shown in Table 11.5.[8,17] Thus, adequate treatment achieves good local control and comparable survival from breast cancer among older and young women.

However, older women are more often undertreated by minimal surgery or by simple mastectomy without nodal irradiation.[18,19] This latter operation represents suboptimal treatment with regard to the axilla. Table 11.6 shows the significantly increased local relapse rate in women treated by simple mastectomy compared with those who had a modified radical mastectomy.[2,3] There is also a reduction in the overall survival at 5 years in those treated by total mastectomy, as shown in Table 11.7.[2,6,12,13,17] Of course this may not be the direct result of treatment since these patients were not entered into randomized trials. Selection of the more frail patients for simple mastectomy may have biased the results. From the patient's viewpoint, the functional difference between a total mastectomy and a modified radical mastectomy is minimal, and yet the latter will achieve better local control. Viewed objectively, with regard to operative mortality after different types of mastectomy,

Table 11.6 Local relapse-free survival at 5 years in women treated by simple mastectomy and modified radical mastectomy.

Simple (%)	Modified radical (%)	Reference
52	100	2
41	83	3

Table 11.7 Overall survival at 5 years.

Simple (%)	Modified (%)	Radical (%)	Reference
	60		6
		79	12
	85	88	13
33	44	53	17
24	85		2
———	———	———	
29	69	73	

Table 11.8 Operative mortality after mastectomy in the elderly.

No of cases	Radical	Modified radical	Simple	Reference
>70	5/148	0/94	–	6
>75	2/75	–	–	11
>80	–	–	1/7	20
>65	0/92	–	–	12
>65	1/339	0/75	–	8
>75	–	0/58	0/40	13
>70	1/56	–	–	14
>65	–	1/52	–	21
>70	0/53	0/44	0/33	17
>75	–	0/13	0/21	2
	———	———	———	
	9/763 (1.2%)	1/336 (0.3%)	1/101 (1%)	

Table 11.8 shows the very low rates after radical mastectomy (1.2 per cent), modified radical (0.3 per cent) and simple mastectomy (1 per cent)[2,6,8,11–14,17,20,21] There is little justification for the continued use of simple mastectomy in the management of elderly patients unless the procedure is performed as a salvage operation in order to free the patient of a troublesome ulcerating chest-wall lesion.

Can mastectomy be avoided in the elderly?

Although a modified radical mastectomy can yield good local control in elderly patients, together with information on the nodal status which might be used to determine the need for adjuvant therapy, there is still a reluctance on the part of many surgeons and patients to take part in such procedures. In contrast, there is a belief among aggressive surgeons that the elderly are not bothered by vanity, self-esteem and sexual needs. Not only is this untrue, but also many elderly women are very loath to undergo changes in their body image and many offered mastectomy as treatment will ask for alternative breast-preserving therapy. Less aggressive surgeons who are worried about operative mortality may undertreat patients because of their fear of prolonged general anaesthesia.

Proven techniques of breast conservation all include an axillary clearance and external radiotherapy. The radiation component (46–50 Gy) means that the patient has daily treatments for 5–6 weeks. The travelling to and from hospital, possibly using public transport, represents a heavy burden for an elderly woman and thus the patient may require admission during treatment. Partly because this blocks beds, most centres do not recommend radiation as first-line treatment in older patients. Nevertheless, it has been reported by Toonkel et al that radiotherapy can be successfully delivered with good local control and overall survival similar to that following modified radical mastectomy.[22]

By changing dose fractionation and possibly giving interstitial rather than external irradiation, it may be possible to truncate treatment, and this could be of major benefit for older women with breast cancer. Such an approach is, however, experimental and no evidence is presently available to support such changes. Because of the limited availability of radiotherapy resources and surgical reluctance to operate on frail patients, there has evolved a tendency to treat the elderly with first-line systemic treatment and this usually takes the form of hormonal therapy. Originally, oestrogens were used as treatment, but because of the toxicity of this therapy stilboestrol and ethinyloestradiol were discarded when the agent tamoxifen became widely available.

Tamoxifen and the elderly

Because of its low subjective and objective toxicity, together with the opportunity for once-daily oral administration, tamoxifen has become the most widely prescribed endocrine treatment for patients with breast cancer. In particular, the drug has been widely used as first-line treatment instead of surgery in the elderly with early disease. Can this approach be justified? What are the penalties for not using some form of surgery?

Because of a reluctance to subject the elderly to a general anaesthetic for a biopsy, several groups have made the diagnosis of malignancy by cytology, trucut needle biopsy or on mammographic grounds alone. With dosages of 30–40 mg daily, patients have been treated without excision of the primary tumour. The results of four uncontrolled

Table 11.9 Uncontrolled studies of tamoxifen treatment for elderly women with operable breast cancer.

No of cases	Age	Dosage	Immediate failure		Late failure		Reference
			SD	PD	PR	CR	
67	>75	20 bd	17 (25)	18 (27)	1/14	2/18	23
27	>65	20 bd	2 (7)	5 (19)	2/5	0/15	24
160	>70	20 bd	38 (46)	27 (17)	7/49	21/46	25
100	>60	10 tds	22 (22)	10 (10)	2/29	10/39	26
354			79 (22)	60 (17)	12 (3)	33 (9)	

Percentages in parentheses.
SD = Static disease.
PD = Progressive disease.
PR = Partial remission.
CR = Complete remission.

studies are shown in Table 11.9.[23–26] The responses have been separated into immediate failure, where disease progression or static disease was reported on first treatment, and subsequent failure, where a patient who had complete or partial remission then developed recurrent disease. Static disease was reported in an average of 22 per cent of cases and progressive disease in 17 per cent. Thus approximately one-third of patients failed to respond to tamoxifen, although late response may be achieved up to 2 years after starting treatment.[25] Although static disease may be regarded by the clinician as a form of disease control, the patient may perceive this as a failure to eradicate the cancer that she had been told was present in her breast. It is not known whether apparently static disease will provide an opportunity for hormone–independent cells to metastasise from the primary tumour site.

During the period of follow up in these studies, a further 12 per cent of patients relapsed within the breast. Of those who originally had a partial response, 25 per cent relapsed compared with 27 per cent of those going into complete remission. These similar rates suggest that what is regarded as a partial response, that is a 50 per cent reduction in tumour size, originally conceived as a measurement as response in advanced breast cancer,[26] may truly be a complete response in early breast cancer. The presence of a residual mass may be the result of the fibrotic reaction engendered by the original cancer, rather than the presence of active malignancy.

Overall, among patients treated by tamoxifen alone, 49 per cent were reported to remain in remission, but it is likely that this percentage would diminish with time, as a result of the tumouristatic rather than tumouricidal action of tamoxifen.[27] Indeed, the study with the longest follow up, which also contained the largest number of patients, reported that only 42 per cent of patients were disease free.[25] The majority of patients who relapse will require either salvage surgery or radiotherapy at a time when they will be both older and weaker. There is now some evidence that local relapse after tamoxifen is associated with subsequent increase in mortality, and this, together with the reduced rate of local control with tamoxifen, does argue for caution in its uncontrolled use in the elderly. In particular, when a response has been achieved the agent should not be stopped but should be continued on a lifetime basis.

Randomized trials of tamoxifen in the elderly

Two prospective randomized trials have recently been published, both of which have compared tamoxifen and surgery in elderly women with potentially operable breast cancer.[28,29] The conclusions drawn by the authors of the two papers are contradictory, one claiming tamoxifen to be the equal of surgery, the other stating that the drug is inferior to surgical treatment. Can these conflicting conclusions be reconciled? Yes. Not only do these two studies raise methodological issues, but they also highlight the problems of relapse after suboptimal surgery. These trials will be discussed and the results compared with those derived from an ongoing randomized trial at Guy's Hospital, which now forms part of EORTC trial 10850.

The first trial was conducted at St George's Hospital, London, and the aim was to compare surgical treatment with the use of tamoxifen alone, in as broad a group of elderly patients as possible with operable

breast cancer, T_1 to T_4. Eligible cases were aged 70 years or more and all had to be deemed fit for surgery. During the accrual period, 222 elderly patients were seen in the clinic, but only 116 were entered into the study. Reasons for ineligibility were refusal (22), prior treatment (21), inoperable disease (15), serious intercurrent illness (21), psychiatric illness (11), second malignancy (10), intercurrent disease (8) and other reasons (8). Thus, taking out the 15 locally-advanced cases, the study population comprised 116 out of 199 (58 per cent) of the 'operable' elderly group.

The trial plan and results are shown in Figure 11.1. There was a close balance in the proportions of T_1,T_2 cases (early) and T_3,T_4 cases (advanced) in both treatment arms. However, the surgical management was not standardized. Total mastectomy was used for 18 per cent of early cases and 67 per cent of advanced cases. Wide excision alone was performed for 82 per cent of early cases and 33 per cent of advanced patients.

Results were reported after a median follow up of 3 years. For patients with early disease treated by wide excision, 35 per cent had relapsed locally, a similar percentage to that reported in the non-irradiated segmental mastectomy group in the NSABP trial B6.[30] Interestingly, only 17 per cent of patients with T_3,T_4 lesions relapsed locally after wide excision, although of course this procedure would have necessarily removed much more tissue in patients with larger tumours.

Patients treated by total mastectomy showed a high local relapse rate of 29 per cent in early and 75 per cent in advanced cases. The tamoxifen-treated group responded in a very similar way to patients described in the previously reported uncontrolled studies. Thus, 47 per cent relapsed in the St George's trial, compared with 52 per cent of those in the pilot studies.

With similar rates of relapse-free and overall survival, the authors stated that tamoxifen was equivalent to surgery. A

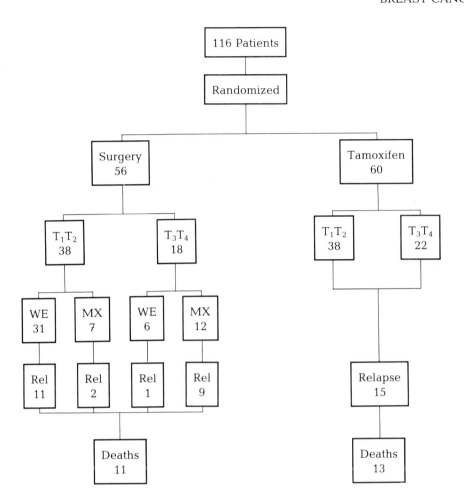

Figure 11.1   Results of St George's hospital trial which compared surgery with tamoxifen for women aged over 70 years with operable breast cancer.

sceptical observer might conclude that suboptimal surgery is as unsuccessful as tamoxifen in achieving local control in the elderly. The study underlines the point that wide excision alone is inadequate treatment of T_1, T_2 lesions and that total mastectomy alone does not achieve local control in the majority of patients with advanced cancers. Thus, different surgical approaches may be necessary to achieve good local control in the elderly. The study demonstrated a similar response rate in those patients given 20 mg once daily to that reported in the literature for women given 20 mg twice daily. This does have important economic consequences if life-long tamoxifen administration, to what will be a substantial proportion of the population, is being considered.

In the second control trial, in Nottingham, results were reported after a median follow up of 2 years. Eligible patients were aged over 70 with operable tumours measuring less than 5 cm in diameter. The histological diagnosis was made by trucut biopsy and 68 were randomized to tamoxifen alone (20 mg twice daily) and 67 were treated by mastectomy. The details of the trial design and outcome are presented in Figure 11.2. At surgery, a wedge mastectomy was performed, that is the breast was drawn away from the chest wall and excised around its base. This was therefore a much speedier procedure than a total mastectomy, although it did leave behind some breast tissue. Only symptomatic axillary lymph nodes were excised. Thus, the treatment given in each of the two arms was standardized.

Possibly as a result of the brevity of general

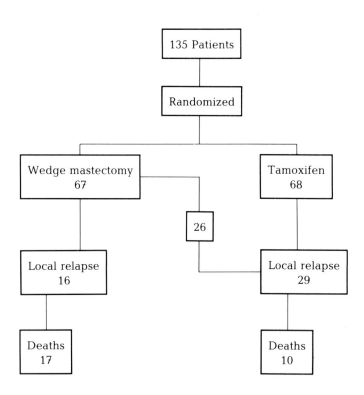

Figure 11.2   Results of Nottingham trial which compared wedge mastectomy with tamoxifen for women aged over 70 years with operable breast cancer.

anaesthesia for wedge mastectomy there were no operative deaths. However, the immediate saving of several minutes of operation time and possibly some lives led to a fairly high rate of local relapse (24 per cent) with 11 per cent of patients dying of metastatic disease. Again, the response rate in the tamoxifen-treated group was consistent with the literature and 43 per cent relapsed after a shorter follow up than in the St George's trial.

The authors concluded that wedge mastectomy achieved significantly better local control than tamoxifen alone. What neither trial attempted was to compare a modified radical mastectomy with the use of tamoxifen.

In the design of the Guy's trial, several interconnected factors were taken into account. First, what is the standard treatment in this age group? Unfortunately, there is no standard, and individual surgeons may recommend either total or radical mastectomy. However, from the literature it did emerge that optimal local control was achieved by modified radical mastectomy. This carries a lower operative mortality than a Halsted procedure, since conservation of pectoralis major may be important for those patients with chronic respiratory disease in whom this functions as a secondary muscle of respiration. Removal of the axillary contents results in an almost negligible rate of local relapse, which was again an important consideration.

For the tamoxifen-treated group it was of great interest to know whether receptor status predicted for risk of relapse. At the time when the trial started immunocytochemical methods of receptor measurement were not available. Therefore it was necessary to obtain sufficient tissue for the dextran charcoal assay. Another question related to whether the tumour type and grade bore any relation to the risk of relapse and again this needed a sample of tissue larger than that which could be derived from a trucut needle biopsy. It was hypothesized that the patient might be less worried if the primary tumour

was excised and also that this might lead to an improvement in local control if combined with tamoxifen. The decision whether to prescribe 20 mg or 40 mg tamoxifen daily was difficult, but there appeared little evidence to support the use of a higher dosage. Thus, the study was designed as a randomized comparison of modified radical mastectomy against tumourectomy and tamoxifen 20 mg once daily for life, or until the development of relapse. Eligible patients had operable breast cancer with no evidence of metastatic disease and all were aged 70 years or more. Patients had to be fit enough to withstand a general anaesthetic, in either procedure, and had to be capable of complying with the instruction to take tamoxifen on a prolonged daily basis.

A total of 124 patients were entered into the trial, of which three were withdrawn because staging investigations showed the presence of metastases. Of the 123 eligible cases, 60 were randomized to modified radical mastectomy and 63 to treatment by tumourectomy and tamoxifen.

The study outline and results after a median follow up of 4 years are shown in Figure 11.3. Within the tamoxifen-treated group there have been 16 (25 per cent) relapses within the breast. Nevertheless, a higher rate of local control (75 per cent) is achieved when tumourectomy is performed before starting the tamoxifen rather than leaving the cancer intact. Only one patient who relapsed on tamoxifen had inoperable disease and therefore needed treatment by radiotherapy.

Of much greater concern is the overall survival. So far there have been two deaths (one postoperative) among those treated by mastectomy, and neither of these were associated with relapse. However, there have been 10 deaths (seven from breast cancer) in the group treated by tumourectomy and tamoxifen. This difference is now statistically significant. Thus tumourectomy and tamoxifen emerges as a substandard treatment.

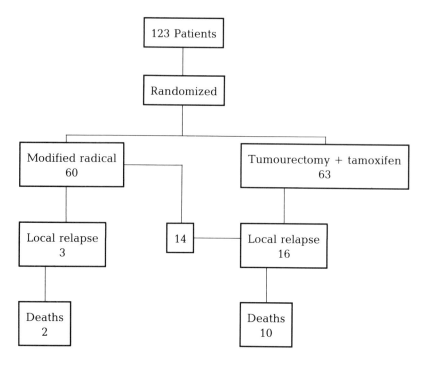

Figure 11.3   Results of Guy's Hospital trial which compared modified radical mastectomy with tumourectomy and tamoxifen for women aged over 70 years with operable breast cancer.

If these results are confirmed by other trials in progress, a reconsideration of primary treatment for the elderly will be required.

If modified radical mastectomy is to be replaced, then an attempt should be made to improve local control. The desire to keep elderly patients out of hospital, and in particular out of anaesthetic rooms, may not serve their best interests. A local or wide excision together with tamoxifen may gain many months and possibly years, which may therefore achieve local control in those patients refusing mastectomy. It is of course possible that high-dose implant treatment may achieve local control in the elderly without recourse to mastectomy and this is an

important reason for studying such an approach. A determined attempt to achieve local control when an elderly patients presents with breast cancer will minimize the chances of such a patient returning later with local relapse. Indeed, her loss of faith over the failure of the primary treatment to achieve control may be responsible for her delay in reporting the recurrence, which may then not be amenable to local treatment or to non-toxic systemic therapies.

For the elderly, the unacceptability of mastectomy and the inadequacy of tamoxifen could be circumvented by use of high-dose implants provided that they can be shown to achieve good long-term control.

References

1 Office of Population Censuses and Surveys, *Cancer statistics registrations*, Series MBI No 12 (1980) 6–7.

2 Chryssos AE, Bondi RP, Breast cancer in women over the age of 80, *Breast* (1984) **10**:13–15.

3 Robins RE, Lee D, Carcinoma of the breast in women 80 years of age and older: still a lethal disease, *Am J Surg (1985)* **149**:606–9.

4 Davis SJ, Karrer FW, Moor BJ et al, Characteristics of breast cancer in women over 80 years of age, *Am J Surg* (1985) **150**:655–8.

5 Host H, Age as a prognostic factor in breast cancer, *Cancer* (1986) **57**:2217–21.

6 Berg JW, Robbins GF, Modified mastectomy for older, poor risk patients, *Surg Gynecol Obstet* (1961) **113**:631–4.

7 Devitt JE, The influence of age on the behaviour of carcinoma of the breast, *Can Med Assoc J* (1970) **103**:923–6.

8 Schottenfeld D, Robbins GF, Breast cancer in elderly women, *Geriatrics* (1971) **26**:121–32.

9 Rosen PP, Lesser ML, Kinne DW, Breast carcinoma at the extremes of age: a comparison of patients younger than 35 years and older than 75 years, *J Surg Oncol* (1985) **28**:90–6.

10 Allen C, Cox EB, Manton KG et al, Breast cancer in the elderly. Current patterns of care, *J Am Geriatr Soc* (1986) **34**:637–42.

11 Kraft RO, Block GE, Mammary carcinoma in the aged patient, *Ann Surg* (1962) **156**:981–5.

12 Papadrianos E, Cooley E, Haagensen CD, Mammary carcinoma in old age, *Ann Surg* (1965) **161**:189–94.

13 Cortese AF, Cornell GN, Radical mastectomy in the aged female, *J Am Geriatr Soc* (1975) **23**:337–42.

14 Kesseler HJ, Seton JZ, The treatment of operable breast cancer in the elderly female, *Am J Surg* (1978) **135**:664–6.

15 Nemoto T, Vang J, Bedwani RN et al, Management and survival of female breast cancer. Results of a National survey by the American College of Surgeons, *Cancer* (1980) **45**:2917–24.

16 Schaefer G, Rosen PP, Lesser ML et al, Breast carcinoma in elderly women: pathology, prognosis and survival, *Pathol Annu* (1984) **19** (1):195–219.

17 Herbsman H, Feldman J, Seldera J et al, Survival following breast cancer in the eldery, *Cancer* (1981) **47**:2358–63.

18 Greenfield S, Blanco DM, Elashoff RM et al, Patterns of care related to age of breast cancer patients, *JAMA* (1987) **257**:2766–70.

19 Chu J, Diehr P, Feigl P et al, The effect of age on the care of women with breast cancer in the community hospitals, *J Gerontol* (1987) **42**:185–90.

20 Leis HP, Mersheimer WL, Varadi J et al, Breast cancer in the ninth and tenth decades, *J Am Geriatr Soc* (1964) **12**:527–37.

21 Hunt KE, Fry DE, Bland KI, Breast carcinoma in the elderly patient: an assessment of operative risk, morbidity and mortality, *Am J Surg* (1980) **140**:339–42.

22 Toonkel LM, Fix L, Jacobson LH et al, Management of elderly patients with primary breast cancer, *Int J Radiat Oncol Biol Phys* (1988) **14**:677–81.

23 Preece PE, Wood RAB, Mackie CR et al, Tamoxifen as initial sole treatment of localised breast cancer in elderly women: a pilot study, *Br Med J* (1982) **284**:869–70.

24 Helleberg A, Lundgren B, Norin T et al, Treatment of early localised breast cancer in elderly patients by tamoxifen, *Br J Radiol* (1982) **55**:511–13.

25 Bradbeer JW, Treatment of primary breast cancer in the elderly with 'Nolvadex' alone, *Reviews in Endocrine Related Cancer* (1985) **Suppl 17**:77–80.

26 Allan SG, Rodger A, Smyth JF et al, Tamoxifen as primary treatment of breast cancer in elderly or frail patients: a practical management, *Br Med J* (1985) **290**:358.

27 Hayward JL, Carbone PP, Heuson JC et al, Assessment of response to therapy in advanced breast cancer: a project of the programme of clinical oncology of the International Union Against Cancer, *Cancer* (1977) **39**:1289–94.

28 Gazet J-C, Markopoulos C, Ford HT et al, Prospective randomised trial of tamoxifen versus surgery in elderly patients with breast cancer, *Lancet* (1988) **i**:679–81.

29 Robertson JFR, Todd JH, Ellis IO et al, Comparison of mastectomy with tamoxifen for treating elderly patients with operable breast cancer, *Br Med J* (1988) **297**:511–14.

30 Fisher B, Bauer M, Margolese R et al, Five year results of a randomised clinical trial comparing total mastectomy and segmental mastectomy with or without radiation in the treatment of breast cancer, *N Engl J Med* (1985) **312**:665–73.

31 Furr BJA, Jordan VC, The pharmacology and clinical uses of tamoxifen. *Pharmacol Ther* (1984) **25**:127–205.

CHAPTER 12

MALE BREAST CANCER

One man among a thousand have I found.

Ecclesiastes

Ask any medical student what they know about male breast cancer and the likely answer will be that this rarity represents 1 per cent of all mammary malignancies. Even the most experienced clinicians have seen only a few cases so that the available literature abounds with small series.

In 1889, Mr Roger Williams, who was then a surgical registrar at the Middlesex Hospital in London, reported a series of 100 cases.[1] His description began as follows

'In most treatises on diseases of the breast this subject is dismissed in a few lines. Considering the large amount of material available, such a state of things is extremely unsatisfactory. That fuller information about cancer of the male breast is desirable, both on its own account and because of the value of such knowledge as a factor in the solution of many problems relating to cancerous disease in general, I have not the slightest doubt.'

Plus ça change, plus c'est la même chose.

Those series which have included more than 100 cases of male breast cancer are summarized in Table 12.1.[2–7] The mean duration of symptoms was 18 months, suggesting that males delay consulting a doctor

with breast symptoms, either because they are unaware of the possibility of developing breast malignancy, or alternatively because they are embarrassed by the nature of the problem. Mean age at diagnosis was 60 years, as compared with 53 for females. Interestingly, the laterality of tumour is similar in both sexes with a right/left ratio of 1/1.1. This asymmetry is difficult to explain, and in females has been frivolously related to handedness of partners. It is possible that during intra-uterine development the differential development of the myocardium might lead to an increase in the left mammary anlage, thereby increasing the number of potential target cells.

Endocrinology

The hundred-fold increase in risk for females strongly suggests the involvement of ovarian steroid hormones in the development of malignancy. However, this is likely to be promotional rather than directly carcinogenic. Both sexes are equally exposed to environmental carcinogens, such as natural radiation and water- and food-borne mutagens. Thus in males, conditions tending

Table 12.1 Summary data from large series of male breast-cancer cases.

No of cases	Symptom duration (months)	R/L	Bil	Mean age (years)	Reference
342	29	163/170	3	53	2
205	23	99/106	3	57	3
146	9	63/82	1	52	4
257	21	120/136	0	65	5
135	9	68/67	0	69	6
138	18	68/69	1	61	7
AVERAGE	18	1/1.1	0.7%	60	

R = Right.
L = Left.

to reduce androgen synthesis or to increase oestrogen production will then lead to an overexpression of the malignant phenotype.

This would be suggested from endocrine studies of male breast cancer. The combination of castration and exogenous steroids has been shown to lead to breast cancer in trans-sexual men taking oestrogens,[8,9] and in patients with prostatic carcinoma prescribed oestrogen.[10,11] Another group of men over-represented among those with breast cancer are individuals who have Klinefelter's syndrome (XXY), in which affected individuals have gonadal hypoplasia, aspermia, gynaecomastia and elevated urinary gonadotrophins. In a combined series of 187 male breast-cancer cases, eight individuals were found to be chromatin positive.[12–14] This represented a frequency of 33 cases of Klinefelter's per 1000 cases of breast cancer. In the population, the incidence of Klinefelter's is 1.9 per 1000 new-born males, so that the XXY genotype results in a 16-fold increase in risk.

Another source of hyperoestrogenization is the failure of hepatic degradation, which may be a consequence of bilharzia. This is postulated to be the cause of the observed high incidence of male breast cancer in Egypt.[15]

Other investigators have sought to determine whether an underlying endocrine abnormality is present in the majority of males with breast cancer and, as with similar studies on females, the results have been contradictory. It is generally found, when cases of Klinefelter's are excluded, that no differences in serum testosterone levels exist between cases and controls, as shown in the studies summarized in Table 12.2.[16–19] Both Calabresi[16] and Nirmul[18] reported higher levels of oestradiol in the sera of cases. The group studied by Nirmul were predominantly black South Africans and the elevated levels of oestradiol in both cases and controls may have been partly dietary in origin. More important than the total level of oestradiol is the biologically-available fraction. Nirmul

Table 12.2 Case-control studies of serum testosterone and oestradiol in male breast cancer.

Mean testosterone (nmol/l)		Mean oestradiol (pmol/l)		Reference
Cases	Controls	Cases	Controls	
17	15	71	37	16
23	17	95	67	17
18	12	223	101	18
17	17	103	94	19

Table 12.3 Case-control studies of urinary oestrogen excretion in male breast cancer.

E_1		E_2		E_3		References
Cases	Controls	Cases	Controls	Cases	Controls	
7.3	3.0	2.6	1.6	8.8	3.5	20
6.9	3.0	6.4	2.7	7.9	3.4	21
6.4	6.9	3.8	3.9	12.9	13.8	19

E_1 = oestrone; E_2 = oestradiol; E_3 = oestriol.
Values are given in μg per 24 hours.

found this to be elevated, but no differences were found by Casagrande.[19]

Similarly confusing data emerge from studies of urinary oestrogen excretion, shown in Table 12.3. Dao reported increased excretion of all urinary oestrogens (E_1, E_2, E_3) in men with breast cancer.[20] Everson studied a group of men with familial breast cancer and found increased excretion of oestrogens,[21] but Casagrande found no differences between cases and controls.[19]

Olsson measured prolactin levels in 15 male patients and found hyperprolactinaemia in five.[22] To determine whether this was a consequence or a contributory factor, a case-control study was mounted, using data derived from the Swedish Southern Health Centre Area Registry.[23] When men with breast cancer were compared with others suffering from either lung cancer or non-Hodgkins lymphoma (NHL), a history of prior head injury, with concussion, was reported more frequently by those men with breast cancer. Since hyperprolactinaemia was an occasional sequel of closed head injury,[24] Olsson postulated that prolonged exposure to elevated levels of prolactin by promotion of growth of mammary epithelium might lead to an increased risk of breast cancer in males.[23] As supportive evidence, Olsson found an increase in relative risk for individuals taking prolactin-elevating drugs.

Gynaecomastia

Gynaecomastia is commonly assumed to be associated with, or a forerunner of, male breast cancer. However, it is difficult to implicate such a common condition. Nydick examined boys aged 10–16 years attending Scout Summer Camp and found evidence of gynaecomastia in 39 per cent, which rose to a peak of 65 per cent in those aged 14.[25] In an

autopsy study of 447 cases from an age group more comparable with those developing breast cancer, there was gross breast enlargement in only four (1 per cent).[26] However, histological examination showed evidence of gynaecomastia in 40 per cent. This was of type I (florid) in 38 (21 per cent) and type II (quiescent) in 140 (79 per cent). Nuttall examined men aged between 17 and 58 and reported an increasing incidence of gynaecomastia with age, so that 47 per cent of men aged over 44 displayed breast enlargement.[27]

Those series which have given incidence rates of gynaecomastia in men with breast cancer are summarized in Table 12.4.[4–7,28–30] Overall, gynaecomastia was present in 7 per cent, although this may represent an overestimate since for some cases the presentation of the malignancy will have been in the form of breast swelling. Scheike carried out a histological evaluation of mastectomy specimens of 79 cases and found evidence of gynaecomastia in 21 (27 per cent).[5] Of these, six (29 per cent) were type I and 15 (71 per

Table 12.4 The incidence of gynaecomastia in male breast cancer cases.

Breast-cancer cases	Gynaecomastia	Percentage	Reference
100	0	0	4
265	10	4	5
87	12	14	28
138	0	0	7
135	9	7	6
39	4	10	29
52	13	25	30
		MEAN 7	

cent) were type II, which is very similar to the incidence reported by Williams in her autopsy study.[26]

Thus gynaecomastia cannot be regarded as a premalignant state, and men with breast enlargement do not require more intensive follow up as they are not a high-risk group.

Familial breast cancer

Among women with breast cancer, Lynch et al suggested that 5 per cent may have an hereditary disease.[31] It is probable that the group with an inherited susceptibility form an even smaller proportion of males with breast cancer. Series giving a history of a female relative with breast cancer are shown in Table 12.5.[5,31–4] Overall, only 3 per cent of cases gave such a history. A history of a male relative with the disease is even rarer, being reported by less than 1 per cent.[7,5,35] Nevertheless, rare cases of families with more than one affected male have been recorded involving brothers,[21,36] father/son[37] and uncle/nephew.[38] These represent a clinically insignificant yet aetiologically important aspect of the male disease. Thus genetic studies of such families may lead to the identification of the chromosomal abnormality responsible for not only familial but also sporadic male breast cancer.

Epidemiology

Epidemiological studies of male breast cancer have provided enticing glimpses of some of the predisposing factors for the disease. However, rather as with the epidemiology on the female disease, the studies have yielded more questions than answers.

International variations

As has been mentioned, the highest incidence of male breast cancer is found in Egypt, but this is probably the result of schistosomiasis, rather than any national genetic or dietary susceptibility. Schottenfeld et al have given international mortality figures for male breast cancer and these are shown in Table 12.6.[35] In most countries there is an inverse relationship between death rates of men with the disease and female/male death ratio. Thus the countries with the lowest incidence rates of male breast cancer also have a smaller proportion of male cases in the total numbers of breast cancers. Finland has the highest female/male ratio and the lowest male rate per million. The highest rate was among American

Table 12.5 Family history of breast cancer in female relatives of male breast cancer cases.

No of cases	Family history	Percentage	Reference
32	1	3	32
28	3	11	33
265	5	2	5
32	1	3	34
	MEAN	3	

Table 12.6 Annual death rates from male breast cancer per million population.

Country	Male deaths per million	Ratio of female/male breast cancer deaths
Finland	0.4	293
Sweden	1.5	126
W. Germany	2.1	72
Canada	2.2	100
Denmark	2.3	105
England/Wales	2.5	93
USA (whites)	2.5	87
France	3.4	41
USA (blacks)	3.5	55
Japan	0.7	56

negroes. Japan is an exception. The rate in males is low, but so is the female/male ratio at 56/1.

Occupation

McLaughlin analysed data from the Swedish Cancer Environment Registry to examine occupational risks for male breast cancer.[39] The highest relative risk (7.6) was found among men working in the soap and perfume industries. Journalists, editors and mental health attendants carried a six-fold increase in risk. Newspaper printers had a four-fold risk. Other occupations with a significantly increased risk included iron and steel workers, brewers, gardeners and business administrators. It is difficult to discern a unifying risk factor among these disparate jobs. All involve some exposure to potentially toxic chemicals, albeit only in the form of printer's ink.

Other factors

Schottenfeld et al compared male breast-cancer patients with those having gynaecomastia and others suffering from carcinoma of the colon.[35] The breast-cancer cases reported prior orchitis or orchidectomy with increased frequency. In addition, they more frequently gave a family history of male breast cancer and prior breast irradiation. Of the breast-cancer cases, 22 per cent had one or more of these characteristics compared with 8 per cent of the gynaecomastia cases and only 2 per cent of colon-cancer patients.

In a case-control study, Casagrande et al examined a wide variety of endocrine factors. These included fertility, obesity, smoking, alcohol consumption, prior breast irradiation and family history of breast cancer. None of these emerged as being significant risk factors except obesity. Those individuals who had weighed in excess of 80 kg at age 30 had a doubled risk of male breast cancer.

Clinical features

Taking the clinical features of patients in the larger series, the commonest presenting symptom was a painless lump, as shown in Table 12.7.[4,5,17,28,40] Of the lumps, only 5 per cent were painful.[17,28] The second commonest presenting symptom was nipple

Table 12.7 Presenting features of male breast cancer.

Lump	Nipple retraction	Ulcer	Nipple discharge	Paget's	Other	Nil	Reference
105	4	7	8	5	3	–	4
182	10	17	11	2	28	5	5
158	7	20	7	–	5	3	17
43	19	16	7	–	2	3	28
38	28	7	14	–	12		40
526	68	67	47	7	50	11	
(68%)	(9%)	(9%)	(6%)	(1%)	(6%)	(1%)	

retraction (9 per cent), with or without a palpable mass being present. Almost equally common was ulceration, which was separate from the nipple in approximately 50 per cent of cases.

Paget's disease of the nipple is a rare presenting feature of breast cancer. The literature was reviewed by Satiani et al[41] and Johnson et al.[42] Of the 24 reported patients, the average age was 60 years (no different from other cases of male breast cancer). Axillary nodal metastases were present in 58 per cent and therefore Satiani suggested that such cases carried a worse prognosis and argued that any suspicious nipple changes in the male should be biopsied.

Other presenting features included pain in 10 per cent of Scheike's series,[5] and very occasionally diffuse erythema or hardening. Axillary nodal enlargement, without a clinically detectable cancer, was present in nine (1 per cent) of reported cases. It was exceeding-ly rare for the breast carcinoma to be picked up by routine clinical examination.

Histopathology

Four large studies have reported the histo-pathological diagnoses in patients with male breast cancer and the results of these are given in Table 12.8. Findings are remarkably consistent. The majority (87 per cent) of male cancers are of the infiltrating ductal type, and only occasionally of infiltrating papillary or medullary types.[43] Not surprisingly, since the male breast does not contain lobules, none of these series reported cases of infiltrating lobular carcinoma. However, small-cell car-cinomas of the male breast have been recorded,[44,45] and in one of these there was lobular proliferation of terminal ducts.[44]

213

Table 12.8 Histological types of male breast cancer.

Type	Reference				Total (%)
	4	5	43	7	
Infiltrating ductal	96	157	67	113	443 (87)
Infiltrating papilloma	5	5	4	9	23 (5)
Mucoid	–	5	1	–	6 (1)
Medullary	2	4	–	14	20 (4)
Tubular	–	–	1	–	1
Lobular	–	–	–	–	0
DCIS	7	5	4	–	16 (3)

Table 12.9 Oestrogen receptor (ER) positivity in male breast cancer.

ER+	ER–	Reference
3	1	46
5	1	47
14	0	48
10	2	49
12	1	50
16	1	51
7	1	52
15	8	53
82 (85%)	15 (15%)	

Table 12.10 TNM stage at presentation of male breast cancer.

I	II	III	IV	Reference
4	2	4	11	33
89	28	107	29	5
76	38	55	41	17
55	37	33	14	7
26	36	25	17	54
9	15	6	2	34
259 (34%)	156 (21%)	230 (30%)	114 (15%)	

Non-infiltrating cancers form a very small proportion (3 per cent) of male breast carcinomas.

Oestrogen receptors

No large series exist of oestrogen receptor (ER) assays in male breast cancer. Several small studies have been combined in Table 12.9, which shows that overall, 85 per cent of male breast cancers were ER positive.[46–53] This is a higher proportion than would be expected in an unselected female series. In part, this may be because there is less endogenous oestradiol to block the receptor, but it may also reflect the better response to endocrine therapy that may be expected in males with breast cancer.

Stage at presentation

Representative series which have given TNM stages for all males presenting with breast cancer are shown in Table 12.10.[5,7,17,33,34,54] This shows that many males have advanced breast cancer in Stages III/IV. Thus if all males are compared with females, there will appear to be a worse prognosis overall for men. However, this effect disappears when results of comparable stages of disease are examined.

Treatment and outcome

The absence of clinical trials or even of consistent treatment policies makes for difficulty in interpretation of published results. Because of small numbers, patients with disparate stages treated in different ways have often been combined. The 5-year results for men treated by total mastectomy and radical mastectomy, with or without postoperative radiotherapy, are summarized in Table 12.11.[5–7,28,29,32,33] Firm conclusions cannot be drawn from this type of data, but they suggest that 5-year survival is better after radical rather than total mastectomy. However, frailer patients may have been selected for total mastectomy and then subsequently died from non-malignant causes.

Some authorities have suggested that postoperative radiotherapy should be an intrinsic part of the management of male breast cancer, but these data do not show any clear survival advantage.[55] This needs testing.

Both adjuvant tamoxifen and cytotoxic chemotherapy have been given to males with breast cancer.[56] Although likely to be of benefit, no survival advantage can be claimed since no trials have been conducted.

The future

To some extent, improvements in the treatment of female breast cancer will help with the management of male disease. Thus, for patients with advanced disease, orchidectomy has been replaced by tamoxifen as first-line therapy. Tamoxifen will probably prove to be of value in an adjuvant role for male breast cancer. Advances in breast conservation will have little impact on the male disease where anatomical and cultural factors make the psychological effect of mastectomy less devastating. In addition, the

Table 12.11 Five-year overall survival (percentage) after different primary treatments for male breast cancer.

TM		TM + RT		RM		RM + RT		Reference
I	*II*	*I*	*II*	*I*	*II*	*I*	*II*	
				83	13			32
				100	64			33
63		58		67		82		5
						77	38	28
71	36			77	33			7
				91	63			6
				88	55			29
67	36	58	–	85	38	80	38	

TM = total mastectomy; RT = radiotherapy; M = radical mastectomy.
I = Stage I; II = Stage II.

relative sizes of tumour and organ with the inevitable subareolar location will make criteria for safe conservation difficult to establish.

It will be more important to define the role of skin-flap irradiation after mastectomy and to determine whether survival can be prolonged by adjuvant tamoxifen. Thus an easy national study would be a factorial design trial with males being allocated to one of four treatment schedules: radical mastectomy (RM), RM plus skin-flap irradiation (RM + RT), RM plus tamoxifen and RM + RT plus tamoxifen.

In Britain there are approximately 300 new cases of male breast cancer every year. It is likely that half might agree to take part in a trial so that, over a 3-year period, over 400 cases could be accrued with 100 in each treatment arm. This type of approach would be an important step towards the rationalization of treatment for the male disease. The most important requirement would be the acceptance by surgeons of the concept of national trials for rare tumours. As a secondary matter, funding for the central collection and collation of data would be needed. Is it really going to be necessary for us to wait for the death of a famous and influential man before this aspect of breast cancer becomes seriously studied by clinical trial?

References

1 Williams WR, Cancer of the male breast, based on the records of one hundred cases; with remarks, *Lancet* (1889) **ii**:261–3.

2 Wainwright JM, Carcinoma of the male breast, *Arch Surg* (1927) **14**:836–60

3 Sachs MD, Carcinoma of the male breast, *Radiology* (1941) **37**:458–67.

4 Treves N, Holleb AJ, Cancer of the male breast. A report of 146 cases, *Cancer* (1955) **8**:1239–50.

5 Scheike O, Male breast cancer, *Acta Pathol Microbiol Scand* (1975) suppl **251**:1–33.

6 Carlsson G, Hafstrom L, Jonsson P, Male breast cancer, *Clin Oncol* (1981) **7**:149–55.

7 Ramantanis G, Besbeas S, Garas JG, Breast cancer in the male: a report of 138 cases, *World J Surg* (1980) **4**:621–4.

8 Symmers WStC, Carcinoma of breast in transsexual individuals after surgical and hormonal interference with the primary and secondary sex characteristics, *Br Med J* (1968) **2**:83–5.

9 Pritchard TJ, Pankowsky DA, Crone JP et al, Breast cancer in a male-to-female transsexual. A case report, *JAMA* (1988) **259**:2278–80.

10 McClure JA, Higgins JC, Bilateral carcinomas of male breast after oestrogen therapy, *JAMA* (1951) **146**:7–9.

11 Schlappack OK, Braun O, Maier U, Report of two cases of male breast cancer after prolonged estrogen treatment for prostatic carcinoma, *Cancer Detect Prev* (1986) **9**:319–27.

12 Jackson AW, Muldal S, Ockey CH et al, Carcinoma of male breast in association with Klinefelter's Syndrome, *Br Med J* (1965) **i**:223–5.

13 Nadel M, Koss LG, Klinefelter's syndrome and male breast cancer, *Lancet* (1967) **ii**:366.

14 Harnden DG, Maclean N, Langlands AO, Carcinoma of the breast and Klinefelter's syndrome, *J Med Genet* (1971) **8**:460–1.

15 El-Gazayerli MM, Abdel-Aziz AS, On bilharziasis and male breast cancer in Egypt: preliminary report and review of the literature, *Br J Cancer* (1963) **17**:566–71.

16 Calabresi E, De Giuli A, Becciolini P et al, Plasma oestrogens and androgens in male breast cancer, *J Steroid Biochem* (1976) **7**:605–9.

17 Ribeiro GG, Phillips HU, Skinner LG, Serum oestradiol-17β, testosterone, luteinising hormone and follicle-stimulating hormone in

males with breast cancer, *Br J Cancer* (1980) **41**:474–7.

18 Nirmul D, Pegoraro RJ, Jialal I et al, The sex hormone profile of male patients with breast cancer, *Br J Cancer* (1982) **48**:423–7.

19 Casagrande JT, Hanisch R, Pike MC et al, A case-control study of male breast cancer, *Cancer Res* (1988) **48**:1326–30.

20 Dao TL, Morreal C, Nemato T, Urinary oestrogen excretion in men with breast cancer, *N Engl J Med* (1973) **289**:138–40.

21 Everson RB, Li FP, Frameni JF et al, Familial male breast cancer, *Lancet* (1976) **i**:9–12.

22 Olsson H, Alm P, Aspegren K et al, Increased plasma prolactin levels in a group of men with breast cancer, *Proceedings of the European Congress on Clinical Oncology and Cancer Nursing, Stockholm* (1985) 249.

23 Olsson H, Ranstam J, Head trauma and exposure to prolactin-elevating drugs as risk factors for male breast cancer, *J Natl Cancer Inst* (1988) **80**:679–83.

24 Matsuura H, Nakazawa S, Wakabayashi C, Thyrotropin-releasing hormone provocative release on prolactin and thyrotopin in acute head injury, *Neurosurgery* (1987) **16**:791–5.

25 Nydick M, Bustos J, Dale JH et al, Gynaeco-mastia in adolescent boys, *JAMA* (1961) **178**:449–54.

26 Williams MJ, Gynaecomastia. Its incidence recognition and host characterisation in 447 autopsy cases, *Am J Med* (1963) **34**:103–17.

27 Nuttal FQ, Gynaecomastia as a physical finding in normal men, *J Clin Endocrinol Metab* (1979) **48**:338–40.

28 Yap HY, Tashima CK, Blumenschein GR et al, Male breast cancer. A natural history study, *Cancer* (1979) **44**:748–54.

29 Axelsson J, Andersson A, Cancer of the male breast, *World J Surg* (1983) **7**:281–7.

30 Mabuchi K, Bross DS, Kessler II, Risk factors for male breast cancer, *J Natl Cancer Inst* (1985) **74**:371–5.

31 Lynch HT, Albano WT, Danes BS et al, Genetic predisposition to breast cancer, *Cancer* (1984) **53**:612–22.

32 Crichlow RW, Kaplan EL, Kearney WJ, Male mammary cancer. An analysis of 32 cases, *Ann Surg* (1972) **175**:489–94.

33 Donegan WL, Perez-Mesa CM, Carcinoma of the male breast, *Arch Surg* (1973) **106**:273–9.

34 Lefor AR, Numann PJ, Carcinoma of the breast in men, *NY State J Med* (1988) **88**:293–6.

35 Schottenfeld D, Lilienfeld AM, Diamond H, Some observations on the epidemiology of breast cancer among males, *Am J Public Health* (1963) **53**:810–97.

36 Marger O, Urdaneta N, Fischer JJ, Breast cancer in brothers. Case reports and a review of 30 cases of male breast cancer, *Cancer* (1975) **36**:458–60.

37 Schwartz RM, Newell RB, Hauch JF et al, A study of familial male breast carcinoma and a second report, *Cancer* (1980) **46**:2697–701.

38 Kozak FK, Hall JG, Baird PA, Familial breast cancer in males. A case report and review of the literature, *Cancer* (1986) **58**:2736–9.

39 McLaughlin JK, Malker HSR, Blot WJ et al, Occupational risks for male breast cancer in Sweden, *Br J Ind Med* (1988) **45**:275–6.

40 Erlichman C, Murphy KC, Elhakim T, Male breast cancer: a 13-year review of 89 patients, *J Clin Oncol* (1984) **2**:903–9.

41 Satiani B, Powell RW, Mathews WH, Paget's disease of the male breast, *Arch Surg* (1977) **112**:587–92.

42 Johnson TJ, Tomek CS, Patterson KB et al, Paget's disease of the male breast, *Nebr Med J* (1987) **72**:10–13.

43 Heller KS, Rosen PP, Schottenfeld D et al, Male breast cancer: a clinicopathologic study of 97 cases, *Ann Surg* (1978) **188**:60–5.

44 Giffler RF, Kay S, Small-cell carcinoma of the male mammary gland. A tumour resembling infiltrating lobular carcinoma, *Am J Clin Pathol* (1976) **66**:715–22.

45 Yogore MG, Sahgal S, Small cell carcinoma of the male breast. Report of a case, *Cancer* (1977) **39**:1748–51.

46 Duffy MJ, Duffy GJ, Multiple steroid receptors in male breast carcinomas, *Clin Chim Acta* (1978) **85**:211–14.

47 Gupta N, Cohen JL, Rosenbaum C et al, Estrogen receptors in male breast cancer, *Cancer* (1980) **46**:1781–4.

48 Ruff SJ, Bauer JE, Keenan EJ et al, Hormone receptors in male breast carcinoma, *J Surg Oncol* (1981) **18**:55–9.

49 Friedman MA, Hoffman PG, Dandolos EM et al, Estrogen receptors in male breast cancer: clinical and pathological correlations, *Cancer* (1981) **47**:134–7.

50 Pegoraro RJ, Nirmul D, Joubert SM, Cytoplasmic and nuclear estrogen and progesterone receptors in male breast cancer, *Cancer Res* (1982) **42**:4812–14.

51 Mercer RJ, Bryan RM, Bennett RC, Hormone receptors in male breast cancer, *Aust NZ J Surg* (1984) **54**:215–18.

52 Pacheco MM, Oshima CF, Lopes MP et al, Steroid hormone receptors in male breast diseases, *Anticancer Res* (1986) **6**:1013–18.

53 Bezwoda WR, Hesdorffer C, Dansey R et al, Breast cancer in men. Clinical features, hormone receptor status and response to therapy, *Cancer* (1987) **60**:1337–40.

54 van Geel AN, van Slooten EA, Mavrunac M et al, A retrospective study of male breast cancer in Holland, *Br J Surg* (1985) **72**:724–7.

55 Robison R, Montague ED, Treatment results in males with breast cancer, *Cancer* (1982) **49**:403–6.

56 Bagley CS, Wesley MN, Young RC et al, Adjuvant chemotherapy in males with cancer of the breast, *Am J Clin Oncol (CCT)* (1987) **10**:55–60.

CHAPTER 13

RARER PROBLEMS

They are ill discoverers that think there is no
land when they can see nothing but sea.

Francis Bacon

Paget's disease of the nipple

'I believe it has not yet been published that
certain chronic affections of the skin of the
nipple and areola are very often succeeded
by the formation of scirrhous cancer in the
mammary gland. I have seen about 15
cases in which this has happened and the
events were in all of them so similar that
one description may suffice.'

Thus wrote Sir James Paget in 1874.[1] He was
both right and wrong – right in his elegant
description of the disease, but wrong because the lesion had been described previously by Velpeau.[2] Nevertheless, thereafter this rarity has been called Paget's disease.
In 1889 Crocker described the first case of
extra-mammary Paget's disease affecting the
perineal skin.[3]

Paget postulated that the chronic inflammatory process on the nipple might lead on
to the development of an underlying cancer,
since he had seen patients with chronic
balanitis who subsequently progressed to
penile carcinoma. A variety of histogenetic
theories have been propounded, but the
recent use of monoclonal antibody markers
has enabled the determination of the source

of Paget cells within the epidermis. As this
question has been answered, so other uncer-
tainties have arisen. Should the treatment of
Paget's disease of the nipple be by mastectomy, or is there a role for conservative
treatment?

Clinical presentation

Paget described the disease as an eruption
beginning on the nipple and areola with an
intensely red-raw surface which was finely
granular, as if the epidermis had been
removed. It looked like either an acute
diffuse eczema or psoriasis and was associated with a copious clear exudate together
with tingling, itching or burning, but with no
disturbance of general health (Figure 13.1).
The changes that Paget described preceded
the development of a palpable lump in the
breast. However, most large series have
included patients with palpable lumps in
whom the nipple changes of Paget's were
apparent either clinically or sometimes on
histological examination of the mastectomy
specimen.[4–11] These are summarized in
Table 13.1. In just over half the cases a

Table 13.1 Presentation of Paget's disease.

Nipple erosion	Nipple erosion + lump	Histological finding	Reference
2	16	5	4
56	67	14	5
13	13		6
21	32		7
96	113		8
68	49	42	9
19	31		10
24	11		11
299 (47%)	332 (53%)		

Table 13.2 Associated symptoms in patients with Paget's disease of nipple.

Eczema	Bleeding/ discharge	Pain	Itch	Erythema	Inversion	Reference
23	10	10	8			7
17	13	7		5	3	10
	15	9		10	1	11

palpable lump was present. In the three series which included histologically rather than clinically diagnosed Paget's, this comprised 21 per cent of the total cases.[4,5,9]

The other symptoms associated with Paget's disease were, in order of frequency, bleeding/discharge, erythema/dermatitis, pain, itching and nipple inversion. Series giving this information are shown in Table 13.2.[7,10,11]

In the absence of a palpable breast lump, the major clinical dilemma lies not so much in missing early cases, but in the dismissal of the nipple eruption as being part of the patient's known eczema or psoriasis. In an individual who gives a history of skin disease and in whom Paget-like changes are present on the nipple or areola, a short course of topical steroid will clear the lesion if it is eczematous in origin. If, at review after 2 weeks of topical therapy, the lesion has not resolved, a biopsy should be performed under local anaesthesia, to establish a histological diagnosis.

Histogenesis

The histological appearance of Paget's disease of the nipple was originally described by Darier.[12] The pathognomic feature is the presence within the epidermis of large clear (ballooned) cells, as shown in Figure 13.2. A variety of theories have been advanced by pathologists to try and explain the nature and origin of Paget cells. This illustrates the capacity of classical histology to generate hypotheses and its inability to refute or confirm them. Morphology is not enough. Only after the advent of immunohistochemistry has it been possible to assign a lineage to Paget cells.

Darier believed that the cells were epidermal in origin and resulted from dyskeratosis.[12] Orr and Parish examined specimens of Paget's disease from Indian patients, and concluded that the Paget cells were only one feature amid general disorganization of the epidermis.[13] Because the numbers of Paget cells were similar in both early and advanced

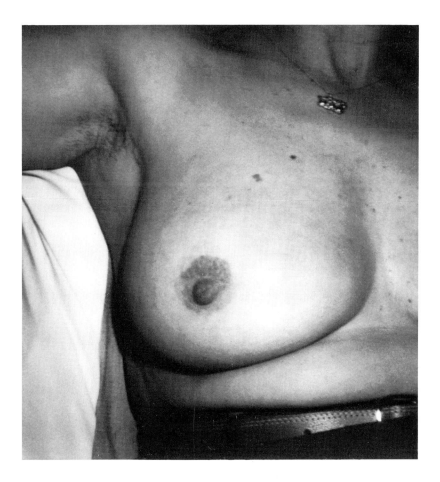

Figure 13.1   Paget's disease of the nipple.

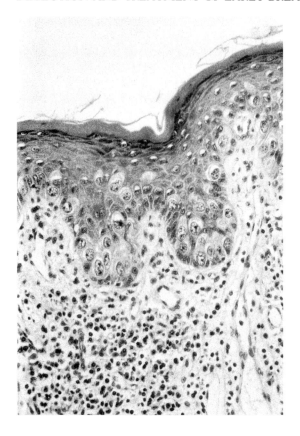

Figure 13.2   Microscopical appearance of Paget's disease of the nipple.

cases, and because the cells did not invade the dermis and were surrounded by dendritic melanoblasts, it was postulated that the cells were non-malignant degenerated melanocytes. Cheatle and Cutler suggested that the cells were premalignant and epidermally derived,[14] but Willis regarded them as malignant cells which had arisen within the nipple skin.[15]

The other group of theories regarded Paget cells as being derived from breast ductal epithelium which had migrated. Muir found an almost universal association of Paget's disease with intraductal carcinoma and postulated that intra-epithelial invasion occurred so that cylinders comprising intraductal carcinoma spread along the ducts in centripetal fashion, eventually passing the epidermocuboidal junction and spreading within the epidermis.[16] Inglis had a similar theory, except that he believed that the process started at the epidermo-cuboidal junction and spread centrifugally so that the intraductal carcinoma arose from the Paget cells rather than vice versa.[17]

With the use of transmission electron microscopy, Sagebiel was able to study the ultrastructure of Paget cells.[18] The cells were

Table 13.3 Immunohistochemical characterization of cells in Paget's disease of nipple.[11]

Cytokeratin	Mab	Breast		Paget's cells	Nipple epidermis	
		Basal	Luminal		Basal	Suprabasal
8	LE41	−	+	+	−	−
	TROMA1	−	+	+	−	−
18	LE61	−	+	+	−	−
	MO8	−	+	+	−	−
19	LP2K	−	+	+	−	−
	BA16	−	+	+	−	−
	BA17	−	+	+	−	−
20	RKSE60	−	−	−	−	+

easily identified and had cytoplasm which was less dense than that of the surrounding cells. Numerous cytoplasmic organelles were present, including smooth and rough endoplasmic reticulum, lysosome bodies and free ribosomes. Multiple irregular mitochondria were present, together with prominent Golgi membranes. Both microvilli and intracellular canaliculi were seen and plasma membranes were united by desmosomes. These findings were consistent with a mammary-gland origin. Despite the occasional presence of melanin, these cells were not degenerate melanocytes because of the presence of desmosomes which are not found in melanocytes.

Immunohistochemistry

Bussolati and Pinch used a polyclonal antibody raised against human casein as part of an immunoperoxidase technique to examine formalin-fixed specimens of both mammary and extra-mammary Paget's disease.[19] This stained positively both normal duct epithelium and intraductal carcinoma. In addition, the Paget cells were strongly stained, together with epidermal cells which were indistinguishable morphologically from normal keratinocytes. Casein was also apparently detected in both sebaceous and apocrine

glands within the skin, which casts some doubt on the specificity of the antibody.

Nadji et al used a polyclonal antiserum to carcino-embryonic antigen (CEA).[20] This stained all Paget cells, ductal carcinoma cells and both eccrine and apocrine gland secretions. Neither keratinocytes nor melanocytes were stained and it was therefore suggested that Paget cells were derived from glandular epithelium. Vanstapel et al used both monoclonal and polyclonal antisera to CEA and monoclonal antibodies raised against milk fat globule (HMFG).[21] The cases of mammary Paget's were positive with anti-HMFG and negative with monoclonal anti-CEA. Two cases with anal Paget's showed positively with anti-CEA and weak staining with anti-HMFG. The other cases of extra-mammary Paget's were negative for CEA and positive for HMFG. This suggests a different origin for some extra-mammary Paget's cells.

A panel of monoclonal antibodies raised against specific cytokeratins was used in a study from Guy's in which 13 cases of mammary Paget's were examined.[11] The outline results are given in Table 13.3. This shows that cytokeratins 8, 18 and 19 were expressed in breast epithelial cells and Paget cells. They were not present in myoepithelial cells nor in basal or suprabasal cells of the epidermis. Keratin 20 was found in suprabasal epidermal cells, but in one of the other cell

Table 13.4 Milk-fat-globule membrane glycoproteins in mammary and extra-mammary Paget's disease.[23]

MFGM-gp	Breast		Skin			Paget's	
	Duct	Lobule	Epidermis	Apocrine	Eccrine	Mammary	Extra-mammary
70	+	+	−	+	−	+	+
155	−	+	−	−	−	+	−

types. This strongly suggests a breast ductal lineage for Paget cells, with no similarity between the cytokeratins of Paget cells and epidermal cells.

Support for the derivation of Paget cells from breast ductal epithelium was provided by the study of Ordonez et al.[22] A monoclonal antibody had been raised against 40, 45 and 52 kd cytokeratins. This was used in an immunoperoxidase method and found to stain breast epithelium, Paget cells, apocrine and eccrine glands, but not keratinocytes. Similar staining patterns were obtained using a monoclonal antibody recognizing 54 kd keratin. Ordonez et al concluded that mammary Paget's derived from underlying malignancy but that extra-mammary Paget's might arise from intra-epithelial glandular cells.

Imam et al examined mammary and extra-mammary Paget's disease using two monoclonal antibodies raised against separate glycoproteins present within milk-fat-globule membrane (MFGM-gp 70 and MFGM-gp 155).[23] The distribution of these glycoproteins is given in Table 13.4. These data suggest a different origin for the two types of Paget's disease. Although the Paget cells are morphologically indistinguishable,

it is likely that the Paget cells on the nipple are derived from intraduct breast carcinoma, whereas those of extra-mammary disease may arise from apocrine glands. Very rarely, Paget's disease of the nipple might be similarly derived from malignant apocrine cells, and mammary Paget's disease without any evidence of breast cancer has been reported.[24]

Prognosis

Three inter-related factors are the major determinants of outcome in patients with Paget's disease. One is determined clinically and that is the presence or absence of an associated breast lump. The other two are pathological variables: the presence or absence of infiltration and the status of the axillary lymph nodes.

As shown in Table 13.1, approximately 50 per cent of cases have both Paget's disease and a breast lump. When survival is examined in relation to this finding, a significant difference emerges as is demonstrated in Table 13.5.[5-9] At 5 years the mean survival

Table 13.5 Prognosis of Paget's disease in relation to the presence or absence of a breast lump.

5-year survival (%)		10-year survival (%)		Reference
Lump	No lump	Lump	No lump	
0	83	0	73	6
43	70			5
41	94			7
		56	81	9
43	42	38	87	8
—	—	—	—	
32	85	31	81	

is 32 per cent for those with lumps but 85 per cent where no lump is palpable. Interestingly, over the next 5 years little change occurs, with an overall survival of 31 per cent for those with lumps and 81 per cent for patients with Paget's disease without a lump. Thus the majority of patients who have had adequate treatment for Paget's (modified

radical mastectomy) and who are relapse-free at 5 years will continue in this state for the next 5 years and probably for the rest of their life.

Of the lumps associated with Paget's disease, 94 per cent are due to infiltrating carcinoma.[7,8] In the absence of a lump only 30 per cent of cases will prove to have an underlying infiltrating carcinoma, the others having ductal carcinoma in situ (DCIS). For patients who have DCIS and Paget's disease, 5-year survival rates of 94–100 per cent have been reported.[5,7,8]

True DCIS does not infiltrate and therefore cannot spread to axillary lymph nodes. Results have usually been reported, not in relation to underlying pathology, but in terms of the presence or absence of a lump and the presence or absence of axillary nodal metastases in the mastectomy specimens. These are summarized in Table 13.6, which shows that only 9 per cent of patients without lumps have nodal metastases compared with 64 per cent of those in whom a lump is present. [4,6–9,11,25,26]

When survival is examined in relation to axillary nodal involvement the prognosis is, not surprisingly, greatly improved when the axillary nodes are negative. Both 5- and 10-year survival percentages are shown in Table 13.7. Maier et al reported that premenopausal node-positive patients with

Table 13.6 Axillary nodal metastases in relation to presence of a breast lump in Paget's disease.

No mass		Mass		Reference
No of cases	*Node positive*	*No of cases*	*Node positive*	
11	1	12	8	25
5	0	16	11	4
8	0	12	8	26
13	0	13	10	6
16	0	18	9	7
96	13	113	74	8
56	3	38	25	9
24	3	11	5	11
229	20 (9%)	233	150 (64%)	

Table 13.7 Survival of patients with Paget's disease in relation to axillary nodal status.

	5-year survival (%)		10-year survival (%)		Reference
	Node negative	*Node positive*	*Node negative*	*Node positive*	
Premenopausal	55	0			5
Postmenopausal	96	33			
			79	20	9
	88	25	83	22	8
			44	10	10

Paget's had a dire prognosis, with none surviving 5 years.[5] Paone and Baker found that amongst patients with Paget's and infiltrating carcinoma, 10 per cent of those with nodal involvement survived 10 years compared with 44 per cent of the node-negative group.[10]

Breast conservation in Paget's disease

The major trials of breast conservation have excluded patients with Paget's disease of the nipple. The rarity of the condition has precluded the running of single-centre controlled trials. Nevertheless, there is some evidence that Paget's disease may be treatable by radiotherapy. At the Institute Curie in Paris a series of 20 patients with Paget's but no associated lump were given external radiotherapy.[27] The diagnosis was confirmed by incision biopsy of the nipple and only three patients had excision of the nipple and/or areola. Cases were treated with a ^{60}Co unit giving a median dose of 57 Gy to the breast and 72 Gy to the nipple/areola. After a median follow up of 7.5 years, none of the patients had died of breast cancer. There had been three relapses, all in the form of Paget's disease. All three were treated by mastectomy and none showed evidence of either infiltrating or non-infiltrating cancer on pathological examination.

This does therefore support the safety of breast conservation for patients with Paget's but without a lump. Nevertheless, the standard treatment is still a modified radical mastectomy. An alternative approach would be to excise the nipple/areola and reconstruct with a free labial graft, with or without the use of postoperative radiotherapy. Some patients might accept nipple excision without reconstruction. The role of radiotherapy under these circumstances needs to be defined and this could only be answered by an international cooperative trial.

Modified radical mastectomy remains the treatment for patients with a breast lump and Paget's disease, provided that the tumour is operable. However, a reasonable case could be made for breast conservation when the tumour is less than 4 cm in diameter, provided that an axillary clearance is performed and that the tumour is excised. Booster doses of radiation would be required for both tumour site and nipple. Proponents of minimal treatment for Paget's disease need to present their evidence for the safety of lesser procedures.

Bilateral breast cancer

The myths

Associated with diagnosis of bilateral breast cancer, various myths have evolved, in part because of a misunderstanding of the pathobiology of the disease, but also because of mis-classification, together with the publication of data derived from too few patients followed for too short a period of time.

Some still believe that bilateral breast cancer, either synchronous or metachronous, is invariably a manifestation of metastatic disease and therefore associated with a poor prognosis. Others assume that bilaterality is the almost exclusive behavioural characteristic of infiltrating lobular carcinoma, just because non-infiltrating lobular carcinoma is associated with an almost equal propensity for development of subsequent infiltrating carcinoma in the ipsilateral or contralateral breast.

Because of the risks of subsequent or synchronous bilateral disease, extensive contralateral biopsy has been used routinely in some centres and bilateral mastectomy has been advocated by others as treatment. This has been reinforced because some have assumed that because radiation is known to induce bilateral breast cancers, breast-conservation treatment including radiotherapy will lead to an increased risk of new primary tumours in both the treated and non-treated breast.

The realities

A synchronous tumour is a carcinoma diagnosed in the contralateral breast within 6 months of presentation of an ipsilateral lesion. In seven large series, comprising over 40 000 patients with primary breast cancer, 230 (0.6 per cent) had synchronous breast cancers.[28-34] Not surprisingly, the lowest rate (0.3 per cent) was recorded in a series from Japan.[31]

A metachronous breast cancer is one which develops in the contralateral breast (or another quadrant of the same breast) more than 6 months after diagnosis of the first primary tumour. Differentiation of such a tumour from a metastasis is in part by exclusion.

A confident histological diagnosis of a metachronous second primary can be made when the two tumours differ in type or grade. This is strengthened by the finding of in situ disease around the putative second primary tumour. In such cases there will be no evidence of other metastatic disease. When the contralateral tumour resembles the primary, has a rounded gross appearance, is situated in the medial half of the breast and has no non-infiltrating component, a metastasis is much more likely. These are rare and occur in less than 0.3 per cent of patients with primary breast cancers.

Metachronous second primaries occur at a rate of 1 per cent for every year of follow up in patients with primary breast cancer.[28] Thus after 20 years, approximately 20 per cent of patients would have developed contralateral primaries. Such statistics have been calculated for women treated by mastectomy, with only one breast at risk. A likely doubling in incidence would be seen for women treated by breast conservation with twice the number of breast epithelial cells which could undergo malignant transformation. When risk is computed in relation to women who have not had a prior breast carcinoma, the relative risk is 3.0 and this remains constant for every year of follow up.

These findings underline the essential nature of annual mammography in the follow up of patients with breast cancer. Expensive screening for metastatic disease is a waste of time, but the early detection of a new primary may save patients' lives. In addition, the use of mammography in the preoperative evaluation of patients with early breast cancer has led to an increase in diagnosis of synchronous primary tumours, which can be as high as 5 per cent.[35-7]

Contralateral breast biopsy

The concept and practice of aggressive surgical treatment for prophylaxis of contralateral breast carcinoma arose in New York. For women deemed to be at high risk, Leis et al carried out prophylactic contralateral simple mastectomies on 83 patients and malignancy was found in 15 (17 per cent).[38] However, of these cancers the majority were non-infiltrating, only 6 per cent had invasive carcinoma.

Rather than carry out an immediate ablative procedure, Urban et al biopsied the contralateral breast in 954 patients with proven malignancy, and found cancer in 12.5 per cent.[39] The patients were divided into three groups. In the first group cancer was suspected, in the second there was an area of nodularity or calcification and in the third

Table 13.8 Results of contralateral breast biopsy.[39]

		No of cases	Infiltrating carcinoma	In situ carcinoma
Group 1	Suspected carcinoma	28	20 (71)	2 (7)
Group 2	Equivocal	625	30 (5)	44 (7)
Group 3	Normal	301	5 (2)	18 (6)
	TOTAL	954	55 (6)	64 (7)

Percentages in parentheses.

Table 13.9 Contralateral carcinoma risk in relation to histology of primary tumour.

Invasive ductal	Invasive lobular	DCIS	LCIS	Reference
30/418 (7)	2/24 (8)			40
44/934 (5)	4/110 (4)	8/83 (10)	6/36 (17)	33

Percentages in parentheses.

group no abnormality was present, either clinically or radiologically.

The results for each group are shown in Table 13.8. Overall, 6 per cent of the biopsies resulted in a diagnosis of infiltrating carcinoma. Over half the patients with malignancy had in situ disease, and not all of them would have progressed to infiltrating carcinoma. Thus over 90 per cent of the biopsies were unnecessary and for this reason the technique has largely fallen into disuse.

There are some who still perform mirror-image biopsies for certain histological subtypes of breast cancer, namely patients with lobular carcinoma in situ or infiltrating lobular carcinoma. Is a biopsy justified under these circumstances?

Histological subtypes and bilaterality

The literature on histological subtypes and bilaterality is replete with assertions, but often lacking in assessable data. Many authors have not distinguished between infiltrating and non-infiltrating carcinomas, particularly of the lobular type. This makes for difficulties in interpretation. No patient has yet died of lobular carcinoma in situ, although many have suffered as a result of unnecessary surgery. Studies which have examined the risk of contralateral carcinoma in relation to defined histological subtypes are shown in Table 13.9.[33,40] This confirms that LCIS is frequently a bilateral condition and that no particular histological feature is associated with risk of contralateral infiltrating carcinoma.

It has been claimed that bilateral breast cancer is a systemic disease affecting all quadrants.[41] Such an hypothesis is an oversimplification, but multicentricity of carcinoma is certainly associated with bilaterality. This has been studied at the Memorial Sloan-Kettering Cancer Centre in a series of 880 patients with invasive breast carcinoma.[42] Multicentricity was defined as the presence of carcinoma in more than one quadrant. There were 71 patients with synchronous carcinoma, of whom 18 per cent had multifocal infiltrating carcinoma and 20 per cent had unilateral in situ. Among those who had contralateral mastectomies without evidence of malignancy, multicentric infiltration and in situ carcinoma were present in the ipsilateral breast of 13 per cent. A similar increase in both multicentric infiltration and in situ carcinoma was seen in the first breast of those who developed metachronous tumours.

Bilaterality was reported to be more common in those patients with infiltrating carcinoma and LCIS in surrounding tissue. However, the histological breakdown of the second primaries was not given so that some may have been LCIS rather than infiltrating carcinoma.

Family history and bilaterality

Anderson reported in 1972 that a premenopausal woman who had a first-degree relative with bilateral breast carcinomas which developed before the age of 50 carried an eight-fold increase in relative risk of breast cancer.[43] These data were derived from analysis of cancer families, and several reports have described clusters of familial bilateral breast carcinoma.[44-7] Others have linked Peutz-Jeghers Syndrome (peri-oral

pigmentation and jejunal polyposis) with bilateral breast carcinoma.[48,49] However, such cases inherited in a Mendelian dominant manner are very rare. Population and case-control studies examining familial breast cancer and bilaterality have yielded more equivocal results.

Sakamoto et al compared 92 Japanese patients who had bilateral breast cancer with 490 women with unilateral disease.[50] A first-degree family history was reported by 12 per cent of the bilateral group compared with only 1 per cent of those with unilateral disease. A Swedish study compared 1330 breast-cancer patients with a similar number of population-derived controls.[51] A first-degree family history was reported by 149 cases and 90 controls. The relative risk for breast cancer was 1.7 for those with unilateral family history and 2.2 for those with bilateral family history, the difference being non-significant. Bilateral breast carcinoma developed in 6 per cent of patients with a family history and 5 per cent of those without this risk factor.

Chaudary et al examined the family histories of 54 women with bilateral disease and compared these with 208 patients with unilateral disease.[52] A first-degree family history was reported by 28 per cent of those with bilateral cancers compared with 13 per cent for those with unilateral disease. As part of the Cancer and Steroid Hormone (CASH) study, Sattin conducted a case-control study comprising 4735 women with breast cancer and 4688 population-derived controls.[53] Although family history of breast cancer carried a significant increase in relative risk, this was greater for those who had a mother or sister with unilateral disease, as shown in Table 13.10.

Divergent results were found in a case-control study from California, conducted by Ottman.[54] The study group comprised 82 women with bilateral breast cancer, 213 with unilateral disease and 229 controls. Relative risks were calculated for sisters of cases and

Table 13.10 Relative risk of breast cancer in relation to family history and laterality.[53]

	Premenopausal	*Perimenopausal*	*Postmenopausal*	*All*
No FH	1	1	1	1
FH-unilateral	2.7 (2.0–3.8)	1.5 (1.0–2.3)	2.5 (1.9–3.4)	2.3 (1.9–2.8)
FH-bilateral	1.5 (0.8–2.6)	0.7 (0.3–1.5)	2.4 (1.3–4.4)	1.6 (1.1–2.2)

Figures in parentheses are 95% confidence intervals.

controls and these are shown in Table 13.11. There were striking increases in relative risk among the sisters of women with bilateral breast cancer. This may of course be a reflection of the different racial mix of the Californian population.

Table 13.11 Relative risk (RR) of breast cancer in sisters of cases compared with age matched controls.

Patient	*Sister's RR*
Bilateral	
Age <40	10.5 (4.0–27.2)
Age 41–50	3.8 (1.6–9.3)
All	5.5 (2.5–12.0)
Unilateral	
Age <40	2.4 (0.5–10.9)
Age 41–50	0.9 (0.3–2.9)
All	1.1 (0.4–3.1)
Age 51–64	1.4 (0.5–3.6)
All	1.3 (0.6–3.0)

Figures in parentheses are 95% confidence intervals.

Goldstein et al applied segregation analysis to 200 families of patients with bilateral breast carcinoma.[55] Even when subdivided on a basis of menopausal status, the results suggested a mixed mode of transmission, that is, a major locus together with another genetic or environmental factor. An optimistic interpretation of this result would be that even for those women with a strong familial history of bilateral breast cancer, development of the disease is not inevitable.

Age and bilaterality

Apart from family history, the major risk for development of a subsequent contralateral breast cancer is young age at first diagnosis.[29,35] Storm and Jensen studied 56 237 breast-cancer cases from the Danish Cancer Registry and focused on 1840 who had bilateral disease. For patients who had their first cancer diagnosed before age 45, the relative risk was 5.5, which fell to 3.4 for those aged 45–54 and 2.1 for women aged over 55 years. Interestingly, when subdivided on a basis of whether they had received postoperative radiotherapy, the irradiated group had a diminished relative risk of contralateral disease.

Storm and Jensen calculated that one-quarter of women diagnosed before the age of 45 would develop a second primary breast cancer by the age of 75 years.[56] In part this is because of the greater number of years at risk, but also may arise because those who present with breast cancer at a young age have more unstable breast epithelium.

Prognosis

McCredie et al reported that the overall survival was none for patients with synchronous breast carcinoma, with a 10-year survival of only 40 per cent compared with 70 per cent for those with metachronous tumours.[29] However, in the synchronous group there was a high early mortality (probably due to inclusion of patients with metastatic disease), and then a plateau in the survival curve.

Fukami et al reported a similar survival for patients with unilateral and metachronous tumours, a better survival for those with synchronous disease and a dire prognosis for women with breast metastases.[41]

Michowitz et al reported a 5-year survival of 48 per cent after diagnosis of a metachronous tumour, and stated that the longer the interval between primary and secondary, the better the prognosis.[33] The delay between first and second primaries has been studied by Holmberg et al, who compared the survival of 67 bilateral cases and 1282 unilateral cases.[57] Overall, the 8-year survival was 69 per cent for the unilateral group and 53 per cent for bilateral cases. In a multivariate analysis this difference was not significant. In a second model, the interval between first and second tumours was examined. The hazard rate was highest for synchronous cases, and fell (non-significantly) with length of time between diagnosis of the two tumours. After allowance had been made for age, histology and nodal status, the interval between cancers became statistically significant. This could result from an innate aggressiveness of the early tumours derived from bilaterally transformed epithelium.

Treatment of bilateral breast cancer

For patients with synchronous breast cancers, the treatment will depend upon the clinical staging of the primary tumours. If both are technically operable, but one is greater than 5 cm and requires mastectomy, a bilateral simultaneous mastectomy should be performed unless the patient refuses this option. It is not usually going to be very helpful to carry out unilateral mastectomy and contralateral conservation, although a few patients may ask for this.

If both tumours are of a size that make them suitable for treatment by breast conservation, this can be safely performed, but careful planning of radiotherapy will be required to ensure that there is not an overlap of external beam irradiation across the midline. Patients with axillary nodal involvement will require adjuvant therapy, the nature of which will depend upon their menopausal status.

Women who develop a metachronous breast cancer will have treatment determined in part by the size of the second primary (provided that metastatic disease has been excluded), but also by the treatment used for the first primary and the patient's perception of the success of that therapy.

Prevention of bilateral breast cancer

Since the major risk factor for development of breast cancer is having had a prior mammary malignancy, all patients have to be regarded as at risk. They therefore form a very suitable group for studies of prevention. This approach has been adopted by the Milan group, who are testing the value of retinoids using Fenretinide, and a trial is now under way.[58] No results are yet available.

Studies using adjuvant chemotherapy or radiotherapy have suggested that these treatments neither diminish nor increase the risk of contralateral breast cancer. However, adjuvant studies of tamoxifen have shown a reduction in contralateral breast cancer among the treated groups.[59,60] This may yet prove to be a major benefit for this type of therapy. The late mortality from breast cancer results as much from new primary cancers as from the late emergence of metastatic disease.[61]

Prevention of second primary breast cancer would be an important step towards improving both the mortality and morbidity of patients with early breast cancer. A case could be made for testing the value of tamoxifen, not only as an agent to prevent contralateral breast cancer, but also for its possible effect on new second primary tumours in irradiated conserved breasts.

Medullary carcinoma

There was a time, before histopathology was born, when surgeons not only treated but also diagnosed breast cancer. They distinguished between two variants, the scirrhous (hard) tumours and the encephaloid (soft) masses. These latter tended to bulge when cut, had a softer texture and often appeared

to be better circumscribed. Geschickter described the histological appearance of such cancers which he called medullary.[62] These frequently possessed a large surrounding lymphoid infiltrate. He also suggested that the prognosis of medullary cancers was better than the more common infiltrating ductal carcinomas. Therein lies the interest of medullary lesions. Are they intrinsically more or less aggressive, and does the lymphatic infiltrate represent an immunological protective mechanism?

Pathology

The gross appearance of medullary carcinoma was described by Moore and Foote:[63]

'Relative softness and gross anatomical circumscription are the rule. The tumours appear more expansile than infiltrative in their local growth tendencies. On section the cut surfaces bulge, an appearance quite in contrast to the depressed cut surface of the ordinary scirrhous carcinoma. The tumours ordinarily are diffuse and homogeneous, gray and more moist and glistening. It is not uncommon to find scattered haemorrhages that may be old or recent.'

The microscopic findings are of a circumscribed growing edge, sometimes with surrounding compressed fibrous tissue. The tumour cells are arranged in cords with a loose connective tissue stroma. There are prominent mitotic figures and an infiltration of the surrounding stroma by small round cells comprising lymphocytes and plasma cells.

Ridolfi et al reviewed 192 cases of medullary carcinoma seen at the Memorial Hospital, New York, and subdivided them into typical and atypical variants.[64] The criteria used are given in Table 13.12. After 10 years of follow up, the survival of the typical medullary carcinomas group was significantly better than that of patients with non-medullary cancer. The atypical medullary group had an intermediate survival.

be an apparent disparity between the size of the tumour and the absence of clinical evidence of nodal involvement. Thus Black et al reported that 37 per cent of medullary cancers measured more than 4 cm in diameter. Of the patients with tumours 4.5–7 cm in diameter, only 33 per cent had axillary nodal metastasis.

Clinical aspects

The age of the patient at presentation is of no value in leading to a suspicion of medullary carcinoma. Although it was originally claimed that such cases were younger,[63] more recent larger studies have given an average age at presentation of 52 years,[64–6] which is similar to that of women with non-medullary cancers. Such cases are neither more nor less likely to give a family history of breast cancer, and the tumour can be present in any quadrant. Many patients may give a longer history of a painless breast lump, the texture of which is soft. There may

Imaging

Meyer et al reported the mammographic and ultrasonic characteristics of medullary carcinoma.[67] Radiologically the lesions appeared to be rounded, uniformly dense and to have lobulated margins. One-third displayed a partial or complete halo sign, a characteristic usually associated with benign breast lesions.

Ultrasound showed hypoechogenic lesions with an inhomogeneous texture. Occasional areas of cystic degeneration were identified and it was suggested that the radiologist should be able to suggest preoperatively that a medullary carcinoma might be present.

Table 13.12 Criteria for histological diagnosis of typical and atypical medullary carcinoma.[64]

	Typical	Atypical
Syncytial growth pattern	>75%	>75%
Completely circumscribed	Yes	No
Lymphatic infiltration	Moderate/marked	Mild/negligible
Nuclear grade	1/2	3
Microglandular features	No	Yes

Lymphoid stroma

Using immunohistochemistry, Hsu et al studied specimens for patients with medullary and non-medullary carcinomas.[68] The lymphoid infiltrate was shown to comprise predominantly plasma cells containing immunoglobulin A (IgA). The tumour cells themselves also stained positively for both IgA and secretory component (SC). In contrast, examination of non-medullary cancers revealed that the surrounding lymphoid cells were plasma cells containing immunoglobulin G (IgG). With non-medullary tumours there was no expression of either IgG or SC. Hsu et al suggested that this functional differentiation contributed to the better prognosis of medullary carcinomas.

Grading

Bloom et al applied their system of grading to a series of 1393 cancers treated at the Middlesex Hospital.[69] Included among these were 104 patients with medullary carcinoma. The comparative grades of the two groups are given in Table 13.13. Whereas only a quarter of non-medullary cancers were poorly differentiated (grade III), this group contained two-thirds of the medullary carcinomas. Bloom et al postulated that the lymphoid infiltrate was somehow restraining the aggressive nature of the medullary tumour, with a resultant improvement in prognosis. An alternative possibility is that the histological appearance of medullary cancers bears minimal relationship to their biological behaviour.

In parallel with the evidence of poorer differentiation of medullary lesions, it has also been reported that these lesions are more frequently hormone independent. A group of 22 patients with metastatic medullary carcinoma were treated at Roswell Park Memorial Institute.[70] Premenopausal patients treated by bilateral oöphorectomy (six) followed by adrenalectomy (three), showed no evidence of response. For the postmenopausal group, none of 13 responded to adrenelectomy nor was there any response to additive hormones.

Ponsky et al measured oestrogen receptor concentrations in 20 medullary carcinomas.[71] When a cut-off point of 10 fmol/mg was taken, these were negative in 15 (75 per cent). Of the positive results, most were marginal and the highest value was 29 fmol/mg. This strongly suggests a lack of endocrine sensitivity in medullary carcinoma.

Table 13.13 Tumour grade of medullary and non-medullary carcinoma.[69]

Grade	Medullary	Non-medullary
I	3 (3)	354 (27)
II	30 (29)	601 (47)
III	71 (68)	334 (26)

Percentages in parentheses.

Axillary nodal involvement

Despite the poor tumour grade and oestrogen receptor negativity, medullary carcinomas are less likely to metastasise to axillary lymph nodes than their non-medullary counterparts. The incidence of axillary nodal involvement in major series is given in Table 13.14.[2–5,8,11,12] Overall axillary nodal involvement occurred in only 38 per cent of cases of medullary carcinoma compared with 64 per cent of patients with

Table 13.14 Axillary nodal involvement in medullary carcinoma.

TMC		AMC		NMC	Ref
25/52	(42)	–		–	2
35/90	(39)	–		836/1307 (64)	8
27/85	(32)	–		–	11
13/57	(23)	24/79	(30)	–	3
59/143	(41)	–		–	12
28/62	(45)	–		–	4
12/26	(46)	12/23	(52)	30/46	5
196/515 (38)		36/102 (35)		866/1353 (64)	

TMC = typical medullary carcinoma; AMC = atypical medullary carcinoma; NMC = non-medullary carcinoma.
Percentages in parentheses.

Table 13.15 Survival after radical mastectomy for patients with medullary carcinoma.

Follow-up (years)	Category	Overall survival (%)	Reference
5	All	83	2
10	All	74	8
	N–	89	
	N+	63	
5	All	64	12
	N–	77	
	N+	55	
	<4 cm	82	
	>4 cm	60	
10	All	84	3
	N–	84	
	N+	84	
	<3 cm	94	
	>3 cm	54	
5	All	50	4
	N–	59	
	N+ (1–3)	53	
	N+ (>3)	18	
10	All	92	5

non-medullary tumours. Interestingly, the atypical medullary tumours metastasised less frequently than the typical medullary tumours.

Prognosis

Until recently, almost all patients with medullary carcinoma were treated by mastectomy, and no data are available to support or refute the safety of breast conservation for patients with this histological variant. Overall survival rates after mastectomy are given in Table 13.15.[63–6,69,73] Taken together, these do suggest that medullary cancers carry a better prognosis than non-medullary carcinomas. Bloom reported a 10-year survival of 89 per cent for patients with node-negative medullary tumours, compared with only 63 per cent for non-medullary tumours.[69] Even in those with nodal involvement, the medullary group fared better (63 versus 22 per cent). Maier et al showed that the prognosis of medullary cancers was related not only to axillary node status but also to tumour size.[73] When a cut-off point of 4 cm was taken, 82 per cent of those with smaller tumours survived 5 years, compared with 60 per cent of those with larger primaries.

Similar nodal and size effects were reported by Ridolfi et al.[64] After subdivision into typical and atypical variants, the 10-year survival of the former was 84 per cent, compared with 74 per cent for the latter. Black reported a lower 5-year survival of 50 per cent, which fell to 35 per cent at 10 years.

The survival of node-negative patients was 59 per cent and this fell to 18 per cent in the node-positive group who had metastases in more than three axillary nodes.

The most recent study from the Institut Gustave-Roussy has reported an excellent 10-year survival of 92 per cent for patients with medullary tumours, compared with 53 per cent for atypical lesions and 51 per cent for the group with non-medullary cancers. This impressive overall survival rate occurred despite 46 per cent of the medullary group having nodal involvement, but in none of the cases were there more than three nodes containing metastases. It was therefore argued that aggressive local treatment was adequate for patients with medullary cancer and that it was unnecessary to give adjuvant systemic therapy, even in the presence of histologically-confirmed metastases. This provocative suggestion requires testing.

These patients do have a good prognosis provided that they are treated adequately. Just because a patient has a medullary carcinoma this is not a reason for suboptimal local therapy. Larger (>4 cm) lesions will require a modified radical mastectomy. It is likely that women with smaller medullary cancer will be suitable for breast conservation, provided that adequate radiotherapy forms part of that treatment.

References

1 Paget J, On disease of the mammary areola preceding cancer of the mammary gland, *St Bartholomew's Hospital Reports* (1874) **10**:87–9.

2 Velpeau A, *A treatise on diseases of the breast and mammary region*, translated by H Mitchell (Sydenham Society: London 1856.)

3 Crocker HR, Paget's disease affecting the scrotum and penis, *Trans Pathol Soc Lond* (1889) **40**:187–91.

4 Kay S, Paget's disease of the nipple, *Surg Gynecol Obstet* (1966) **123**:1010–14.

5 Maier WP, Rosemond GP, Harasym EL et al, Paget's disease in the female breast, *Surg Gynecol Obstet* (1969) **128**:1253–63.

6 Rissanen PM, Holsti P, Paget's disease of the breast, *Oncology* (1969) **23**:209–16.

7 Nance FC, Deloach DH, Welsh RA et al, Paget's disease of the breast, *Ann Surg* (1970) **171**:864–74.

8 Ashikari R, Park K, Huvos AG et al, Paget's disease of the breast, *Cancer* (1970) **26**:680–5.

9 Kister SJ, Haagensen CD, Paget's disease of the breast, *Am J Surg* (1970) **119**:606–9.

10 Paone JF, Baker RR, Pathogenesis and treatment of Paget's disease of the breast, *Cancer* (1981) **48**:825–9.

11 Chaudary MA, Millis RR, Lane EB et al, Paget's disease of the nipple: a ten year review including clinical, pathological and immunohistochemical findings, *Breast Cancer Res Treat* (1986) **8**:139–46.

12 Darier J, Sur une nouvelle forme de psorospermose cutanee: la maladie de Paget du mamelon, *CR Soc Biol (Series 9)* (1889) **1**:294–7.

13 Orr JW, Parish DJ, The nature of the nipple changes in Paget's disease, *J Path Bacteriol* (1962) **84**:201–8.

14 Cheatle GL, Cutler M, Paget's disease of the nipple: review of the literature; clinical and microscopical study of 17 breasts by means of whole serial sections, *Arch Pathol* (1931) **12**:435–66.

15 Willis RA, *Pathology of tumours*, 4th edn. (Butterworth: London 1967.)

16 Muir R, The pathogenesis of Paget's disease of the nipple and associated lesions, *Br J Surg* (1935) **22**:728–37.

17 Inglis K, Paget's disease of the nipple with special reference to changes in the ducts, *Am J Pathol* (1946) **22**:1–33.

18 Sagebiel RW, Ultrastructural observations on epidermal cells in Paget's disease of the breast, *Am J Pathol* (1969) **57**:49–64.

19 Bussolati G, Pinch A, Mammary and extra-mammary Paget's disease, *Am J Pathol* (1975) **80**:117–24.

20 Nadji M, Morales AR, Girtanner RE et al, Paget's disease of the skin. A unifying concept of histogenesis, *Cancer* (1982) **50**:2203–6.

21 Vanstapel M-J, Gatter KC, De Wolf-Peters C et al, Immunohistochemical study of mammary and extra-mammary Paget's disease, *Histopathology* (1982) **8**:1013–23.

22 Ordonez NG, Awalt H, MacKay B, Mammary and extra-mammary Paget's disease. An immunocytochemical and ultrastructural study, *Cancer* (1987) **59**:1173–83.

23 Imam A, Yoshida SO, Taylor CR, Distinguishing tumour cells of mammary from extra-mammary Paget's disease using antibodies to two different glycoproteins from human milk-fat-globule membrane, *Br J Cancer* (1988) **58**:373–8.

24 Jones RE, Mammary Paget's disease without underlying carcinoma, *Am J Dermatol* (1985) **7**:361–5.

25 Culberson JD, Horn RC, Paget's disease of the nipple, *Arch Surg* (1956) **72**:224–7.

26 Ridenhour CE, Perez-Mesa C, Hori JM, Paget's disease of the nipple, *Cancer Bull* (1969) **21**:15–16.

27 Fourquet A, Campana F, Vielh P et al, Paget's disease of the nipple without detectable breast tumour: conservative management with radiation therapy, *Int J Radiat Oncol Biol Phys* (1987) **13**:1463–5.

28 Veronesi U, Rilke F, Salvadori B et al, Bilateral cancer of the breast. In: Severi L ed. *Multiple primary malignant tumours.* (Perugia Division of Cancer Research: Montluce 1974.)

29 McCredie JA, Inch WR, Alderson M, Consecutive primary carcinomas of the breast, *Cancer* (1975) **35**:1472–7.

30 Prior P, Waterhouse JAH, Incidence of bilateral tumours in a population-based series of breast cancer patients, *Br J Cancer* (1978) **37**:620–34.

31 Fukami A, Kasumi Hori M et al, Bilateral primary breast cancer treated at the Cancer Institute Hospital, Tokyo, *Prog Clin Biol Res* (1977) **12**:525–35.

32 Schell SR, Montague ED, Spanos WJ et al, Bilateral breast cancer in patients with initial Stage I and II disease, *Cancer* (1982) **50**:1191–4.

33 Michowitz M, Noy S, Lazebnik N et al, Bilateral breast cancer, *J Surg Oncol* (1985) **30**:109–12.

34 Smith EB, Primary bilateral breast cancer, *J Natl Med Assoc* (1986) **78**:1069–72.

35 Chaudary MA, Millis RR, Hoskins EO et al, Bilateral primary breast cancer: a prospective study of disease incidence, *Br J Surg* (1984) **71**:711–14.

36 McSweeney MB, Egan RL, Bilateral breast carcinoma, *Recent Results Cancer Res* (1984) **90**:41–8.

37 Tinnemans JGM, Wobbes T, Hendriks JHCL et al, The role of mammography in the detection of bilateral primary breast cancer, *World J Surg* (1988) **12**:382–8.

38 Leis HP, Mersheimer WL, Black NN et al, The second breast, *NY J Med* (1965) **62**:2460–8.

39 Urban JA, Papachristou D, Taylor J, Bilateral breast cancer. Biopsy of the opposite breast, *Cancer* (1977) **40**:1968–73.

40 Tulusan AH, Ronay G, Egger H et al, A contribution to the natural history of breast cancer. V. Bilateral primary breast cancer: Incidence, risks and diagnosis of simultaneous primary cancer in the opposite breast, *Arch Gynecol* (1985) **237**:85–91.

41 Ober KG, The opposite breast—a model that may help us to understand breast cancer, *Clin Oncol* (1982) **1**:401–10.

42 Lesser ML, Rosen PP, Kinne DW, Multicentricity and bilaterality in invasive breast carcinoma, *Surgery* (1982) **91**:234–40.

43 Anderson DE, A genetic study of human breast cancer, *J Natl Cancer Inst* (1972) **111**:301–8.

44 Harris RE, Lynch HT, Guirgis HA, Familial breast cancer: risk to the contralateral breast, *J Natl Cancer Inst* (1978) **60**:955–9.

45 Al-Jurf AS, Urdaneta LF, Jochimsen PR et al, Familial bilateral breast cancer, *J Surg Oncol* (1981) **17**:211–18.

46 Lynch HT, Albano WA, Layton MA et al, Breast cancer, genetics and age at first pregnancy, *J Med Genet* (1984) **21**:96–8.

47 Willis J, Shine M, Bilateral familial breast cancer, *Ir Med J* (1986) **79**:317–19.

48 Riley E, Swift M, A family with Peutz-Jeghers syndrome and bilateral breast cancer, *Cancer* (1980) **46**:815–17.

49 Trau H, Schewach-Millet M, Fisher BK et al, Peutz-Jeghers syndrome and bilateral breast carcinoma, *Cancer* (1982) **50**:788–92.

50 Sakamoto G, Sugano H, Kasumi F, Bilateral breast cancer and familial aggregations, *Prev Med* (1978) **7**:225–9.

51 Adami H-O, Hansen J, Jung B et al, Characteristics of familial breast cancer in Sweden, *Cancer* (1981) **48**:1688–95.

52 Chaudary MA, Millis RR, Bulbrook RD et al, Family history and bilateral breast cancer, *Breast Cancer Res Treat* (1985) **5**:201–5.

53 Sattin RW, Rubin GL, Webster LA et al, Family history and risk of breast cancer, *JAMA* (1985) **253**:1908–13.

54 Ottman R, Pike MC, King MC et al, Familial breast cancer in a population-based series, *Am J Epidemiol* (1986) **123**:15–21.

55 Goldstein AM, Haile RWC, Marazita MC et al, A genetic epidemiologic investigation of breast cancer in families with bilateral breast cancer. I. Segregation analysis, *J Natl Cancer Inst* (1987) **78**:911–18.

56 Storm HH, Jensen OM, Risk of contralateral breast cancer in Denmark 1943–1980, *Br J Cancer* (1986) **54**:483–97.

57 Holmberg L, Adami HO, Ekbom A et al, Prognosis in bilateral breast cancer. Effects of time interval between first and second primary tumours, *Br J Cancer* (1988) **58**:191–4.

58 Veronesi U, Costa A, Chemoprevention of contralateral breast cancer with the synthetic retinoid Fenretinide, *Cancer Invest* (1988) **6**:639–41.

59 Cuzick J, Baum M, Tamoxifen and contralateral breast cancer, *Lancet* (1985) **ii**:282.

60 Fornander T, Cedermark B, Mattson A et al, Adjuvant tamoxifen in early breast cancer: occurrence of new primary cancer, *Lancet* (1989) **i**:117–20.

61 Fentiman IS, Cuzick J, Millis RR et al, Which patients are cured of breast cancer? *Br Med J* (1984) **289**:1108–11.

62 Geschickter CF, *Diseases of the breast: diagnosis, pathology, treatment,* 2nd edn. (JB Lippincott: Philadelphia 1945) 565–75.

63 Moore OS, Foote FW, The relatively favourable prognosis of medullary carcinoma of the breast, *Cancer* (1949) **2**:635–42.

64 Ridolfi RL, Rosen PP, Port A et al, Medullary carcinoma of the breast. A clinicopathologic study with 10 year follow-up, *Cancer* (1977) **40**:1365–85.

65 Black CL, Morris DM, Goldman LI et al, The significance of lymph node involvement in patients with medullary carcinoma of the breast, *Surg Gynecol Obstet* (1983) **157**:497–9.

66 Rapin V, Contesso G, Mouriesse H et al, Medullary breast carcinoma. A re-evaluation of 95 cases of breast cancer with inflammatory stroma, *Cancer* (1988) **61**:2503–10.

67 Meyer, JE, Amin E, Lindfors KK et al, Medullary carcinoma of the breast: mammographic and US appearance, *Radiology* (1989) **170**:79–82.

68 Hsu S, Raine L, Nayak RN, Medullary carcinoma of breast: an immunohistochemical study of its lymphoid stroma, *Cancer* (1981) **48**:1368–76.

69 Bloom HJG, Richardson WW, Field, JR, Host resistance and survival in carcinoma of breast: a study of 104 cases of medullary carcinoma in a series of 1,411 cases of breast cancer followed for 20 years, *Br Med J* (1970) **3**:181–8.

70 Patel JK, Nemoto T, Dao TL, Is medullary carcinoma of the breast hormone dependent? *J Surg Oncol* (1983) **24**:290–1.

71 Ponsky JL, Gliga L, Reynolds S, Medullary carcinoma of the breast: an association with negative hormonal receptors, *J Surg Oncol* (1984) **25**:76–8.

72 Flores L, Arlen M, Elguezabal A, et al, Host tumour relationships in medullary carcinoma of the breast, *Surg Gynecol Obstet* (1974) **139**:683–8.

73 Maier WP, Rosemond GP, Goldman LI et al, A ten year study of medullary carcinoma of the breast, *Surg Gynecol Obstet* (1977) **144**:695–8.

CHAPTER 14

NON-EPITHELIAL CANCERS

I hate quotations. Tell me what you know.

Ralph Emerson

Sarcoma of the breast

These disparate mesenchymal tumours provide problems because of their rarity for both the pathologist who has to make the diagnosis and also for the surgeon who has to plan an effective scheme of management. What makes these cancers even more difficult to treat is their occasional occurrence in a younger group of women than would normally be expected to suffer from breast malignancy. Of necessity, information can only be gleaned from relatively small series and there is no guidance from controlled randomized trials to enable informed decisions to be made.

Phyllodes tumour

The change in nomenclature from 'cystosarcoma phyllodes' to 'phyllodes tumour' proposed by Azzopardi has at least meant that not all surgeons confronted with a diagnosis of sarcoma reach for their knives and indulge in unnecessarily aggressive surgery.[1] However, the term phyllodes tumour encompasses a spectrum ranging from tumours with very benign behaviour to others which are highly aggressive sarcomas which metastasise and kill patients.

Unfortunately, the histological appearance does not necessarily reflect the biological behaviour of the tumour, in particular its capacity to recur locally.

Distinction between fibroadenoma and phyllodes tumour

It is likely that many phyllodes tumours derive from fibroadenomas, sometimes as a result of the endocrine surges of puberty, pregnancy and lactation. Grossly, phyllodes are fleshy cellular tumours with leaf-like projections. Distinction between benign and malignant phyllodes tumours is not absolute. The features taken into account include mitotic activity (greater than 5 mitoses per 10 high power fields), stromal overgrowth, nuclear anaplasia and the margin of the tumour. An infiltrative margin is much more likely to be found in a malignant phyllodes tumour.

Presenting features

Patients with phyllodes tumours typically give a history of a painless breast lump present for some time, but which has recently undergone rapid increase in size. On examination the mass is usually well circumscribed, almost always measures greater than 4 cm in diameter, and may be associated with dilated veins in the overlying skin.

In younger women these tumours tend to be diagnosed as fibroadenomas and are treated by local excision, sometimes in the form of enucleation. In older women a phyllodes tumour may be mistaken for a medullary carcinoma. Neither mammography nor ultrasound can distinguish these lesions from either fibroadenomas or carcinomas.

Based on the histopathological features of stromal overgrowth, atypia, mitotic activity and tumour periphery the pathologist may be able to diagnose the lesion as being benign, borderline or malignant. Table 14.1 gives the breakdown of the larger series of cases of phyllodes tumours, and indicates that 50 per cent are described as benign.[2–10] This includes borderline cases which may make up 10–15 per cent of the benign group. The average age of those with benign lesions was 40 years, compared with 46 for those with malignant tumours.

Despite a benign diagnosis, local relapse of the tumour occurred in 20 per cent, but none developed distant metastases or died of disease. Local relapse of phyllodes was seen in 26 per cent of those diagnosed as malignant. Distant metastases developed in 20 per cent of this group and the majority died of the disease.

Table 14.1 Age and outcome of patients with benign and malignant phyllodes tumours.

No of cases	Benign	Mean age	Local recurrence	Death	Malignant	Mean age	Local recurrence	Death	Reference
17	12	–	6	0	5	–	4	1	2
26	12	48	2	0	14	48	4	4	3
42	23	43	5	1	19	45	0	3	4
40	23	32	3	0	17	52	0	3	5
20	10	37	0	0	10	38	5	3	6
32	23	30	0	0	9	42	2	1	7
25	15	48	4	0	10	51	6	4	8
45	28	42	10	0	17	48	5	4	9
48	35	40	7	0	13	46	4	1	10
295	181 (61%)	40	37	0	114 (39%)	46	30	24	

Treatment

Unless the pathologist is able to state unequivocally that the tumour is benign and has been completely excised, a further excision should always be considered. Almost all the relapses among the benign group in Table 14.1 were in patients treated by excision alone. Frond-like projections may easily be left at the biopsy site, particularly after enucleation of the tumour, and these will invariably lead to local relapse.

If the tumour shows atypical features a wider excision should be performed, and if this indicates that the phyllodes tumour has been incompletely re-excised a total mastectomy should be performed. There is little value in proceeding to wider excision in the event of a malignant histological report. These patients need a total mastectomy. Wide excision with radiotherapy has no role in this condition which is radio-resistant. Removal of axillary nodes is unnecessary.

For patients with malignant phyllodes tumours, despite local control with total mastectomy regrettably approximately one in five of patients will have blood-borne metastases and are likely to relapse with distant disease. No effective adjuvant therapy is available at present, and the long-term outlook has to be guarded. Although oestrogen and progesterone receptors have been reported within the stromal component of phyllodes tumours, there is no evidence that patients with these lesions show any significant response to endocrine therapy.[11,12] It is the stromal and not the epithelial elements which metastasise.

Liposarcoma

Although liposarcomas are the commonest soft-tissue cancers, they are rarely found within the breast. Ii et al reported a single

Table 14.2 Clinical features and outcome of patients with liposarcoma of the breast.

	Reference 13	*Reference 14*
No of cases	42	20
Mean age (years)	47	47
Male	1 (2%)	2 (10%)
Arising in phyllodes	12	7
Local relapse	5 (12%)	3 (15%)
Metastases	11 (26%)	3 (15%)

case and reviewed 42 from the literature.[13] Austin and Dupree presented results from the Armed Forces Institute of Pathology and these two studies are the largest recent series.[14] The clinical characteristics of cases in the two reviews are given in Table 14.2. The mean age of patients was 47 years, and approximately 30 per cent of these sarcomas arose from pre-existing phyllodes tumours or fibroadenomas.

Histologically, liposarcomas are characterized by the presence of heterogeneous cells, including myxoid cells containing intracytoplasmic lipid vacuoles. The stroma is rich in mucopolysaccharides and stains with Alcein blue. In addition, there is a rich network of blood capillary cells. It has been postulated that liposarcomas are a single histogenetic entity derived from perivascular mesenchymal cells.[15]

Enzinger and Weiss divided liposarcomas into four subtypes: well differentiated, myxoid, round cell and pleomorphic.[16]

In the series of Ii et al and Austin and Dupree, local relapse occurred in 13 per cent and distant metastases developed in 23 per cent, almost all of whom were reported to have died. The local treatment of such lesions is by wide excision with pathological confirmation of clear margins. Axillary nodal involvement only occurs after direct invasion of nodes and thus resection of nodes is unnecessary in the majority of cases.

Leiomyosarcoma

This particular tumour so rarely occurs in the breast that only 16 cases have been described, the majority of whom were cited by Gobardhan and Yamashina.[17,18] These are shown in Table 14.3. The average age at presentation was 52 years and four cases were male. The histological features include spindle cells with a mitotic rate of 5–15 per high power field, and frequent nuclear pleomorphism. At an ultrastructural level the tumour comprises thin mesenchymal cells within a basal lamina-like layer, many of which elaborate collagen. Yamashina has suggested that leiomyosarcoma, like liposarcoma, is derived from pluripotential mesenchymal stem cells.[18]

From the small number of available cases, dogmatic conclusions cannot be drawn. Local

Table 14.3 Reported cases of mammary leiomyosarcomas.

Age	Sex	Tumour size (cm)	Mitotic rate/10 HPF	Treatment	Result	Reference
35	F	19	?	RM	Local rec	18*
50	M	?	?	TM	?	18*
53	M	6	?	RM	?	18*
51	M	5	?	RM	Local rec	18*
77	F	8	?	TM	DF	18*
49	F	7	16	RM	DF	18*
40	F	4.5	?	TM	Local rec	18*
55	F	3	10	TM	DF	18*
53	M	4	15	RM	DF	18*
59	F	6	3	TM	Died	18*
24	F	1.5	14	Exc	Died	18*
56	F	2.5	21	RM	DF	18*
50	F	9	5	RM	DF	17
54	F	3	10	TM	DF	28
56	F	2	10	TM	DF	
62	F	2.5	15	TM	DF	18

*Cited by Yamashina.
HPF = High power field.
RM = Radical mastectomy.
TM = Total mastectomy.
Exc = Excision.
DF = Disease-free.
rec = Recurrence.

relapse occurred in three patients, all of whom were treated by radical mastectomy. Two patients died of metastatic disease.

Osteogenic sarcoma

This aggressive sarcoma is the most likely mesenchymal tumour of the breast to metastasise and kill patients. Until 1963, only 116 cases had been reported,[19] and a recent review was able to add only another 15 cases.[20] The average age of patients with osteogenic sarcoma of the breast is 63 years. Typically, patients complain of a breast lump which has recently increased in size.

Mutarrij and Feiner reported that of nine cases only two remained disease free. Three developed local recurrence and the majority, seven, had distant metastases in lung and bone and died of disease. Radiotherapy is of no value in local control and at high dosage chemotherapy is of no benefit. Unless wide local excision is performed, most of these tumours will relapse, and even in the absence of local relapse, systemic metastases are almost invariable.

Because of the presence of osteoid these lesions may be recognizable mammographically as masses with lobulated borders and fine, thread-like spiculations.[21] However, not all osteogenic sarcomas calcify and therefore they may be radiologically indistinguishable from giant fibroadenomas.[22] These lesions do exhibit some of the metabolic activities of bone, and therefore may take up the isotope on bone scintigraphy.[22–4]

Stromal cell sarcoma

The most common type of sarcoma of the breast is the lesion whose nomenclature induces most confusion and argument. Thus cases described by one pathologist as being fibrosarcomas may be called stromal cell sarcomas by another. The latter have been considered by some as breast-specific sarcomas. Is there any value in distinguishing between the various stromal subtypes in terms of treatment of prognosis?

In 1962 Berg et al reported a series of breast sarcomas.[25] After exclusion of lymphomas, malignant phyllodes tumours and angiosarcomas, there were 24 cases comprising tumours made up of spindle cells, without any epithelial component, which Berg called stromal cell sarcomas.

Curran and Dodge had previously divided breast sarcomas into three types: I, fibroadenoma with sarcomatous stroma; II, fibroadenoma almost totally replaced by sarcoma; and III, sarcoma without epithelial elements.[26] These type III sarcomas were the equivalent of stromal cell sarcomas.

Ludgate et al reported a series of 30 breast sarcomas, based on the Curran classification.[27] Of the 12 patients with type II sarcomas, only one died but there were 18 deaths out of 19 patients with type III lesions. The use of histological features such as stromal atypia, mitotic rate and metaplastic differentiation did not distinguish between cases with good and bad prognoses.

Callery et al reviewed 32 patients with breast sarcomas and recommended that classification should be based on tumour cell type and grade.[28] There were 10 high-grade sarcomas (5 fibrosarcoma, 3 malignant fibrous histiocytoma (MFH), 1 haemangiopericytoma, 1 leiomyosarcoma). Of these, one patient with an MFH relapsed and died. Four patients had intermediate grade sarcoma (2 fibrosarcoma, 1 MFH and 1 stromal sarcoma) and the patient with MFH relapsed and died. In the low-grade group of 11 (1 stromal sarcoma, 3 desmoid tumours, 2 fibrosarcomas, 2 dermatofibromas, 1 leiomyosarcoma, 1 liposarcoma, 1 MFH). Callery suggested that the title of stromal sarcoma should be reserved for the rare tumours whose origin could be traced to the perilobular or periductal stroma of the breast.

Christensen et al reported the Danish experience of breast sarcomas, which included 68 patients with a minimum follow up of 15 years.[29] Of these patients, 31 (46 per cent) had borderline or malignant phyllodes tumours and 22 (32 per cent) had stromal sarcomas. The majority (82 per cent) were treated by mastectomy. Local relapse occurred in 8 (36 per cent) and 10 (45 per cent) died of metastatic stromal sarcomas. Nine patients died from other causes so that only three (14 per cent) were alive without relapse.

Recently Terrier et al reviewed 33 patients with primary breast sarcomas, of whom 17 (52 per cent) had phyllodes tumours and 16 (48 per cent) had stromal sarcomas.[30] After 10 years the disease-free survival of the two groups was similar. The major determinant of relapse was tumour differentiation and mitotic activity. Terrier therefore questioned whether histological typing of breast sarcomas was a worthwhile exercise.

Angiosarcoma

In 1948, Stewart and Treves described the development of lymphangiosarcomas in six patients with long-standing gross arm oedema following primary treatment of breast cancer.[31] The Stewart-Treves syndrome is now agreed to be a very rare complication of long-standing lymphoedema and involves the development of a lymphangiosarcoma in the arm. That this is mesenchymal rather than metastatic from carcinoma has been confirmed by immunohistochemical studies.[32,33] Treatment is by forequarter amputation, but this may often be followed by the development of blood-borne metastases.[34]

As the combination of axillary surgery and irradiation is used less frequently, so gross lymphoedema resulting from treatment rather than relapse will become rare, as should the development of Stewart-Treves syndrome.

Primary angiosarcoma of the breast is a rare tumour, but because of its intimate relationship with blood vessels, blood-borne metastases are a common sequel. Some of these lesions appear to be of a benign nature histologically and closely resemble haemangiomas. It is therefore important that they be correctly classified in order to maximize the chance of disease control.

The largest series of angiosarcomas of the breast derives from the Memorial Sloan-Kettering Cancer Centre, in which Donnell et al reported the relationship of histopathology to outcome in 40 cases.[35] Until that review angiosarcomas had been regarded as having a universally dire prognosis.

Histologically, all patients had lesions involving the breast parenchyma, showing interanastomosing vascular channels lined by hyperchromatic endothelial cells. Patients were divided into three groups and the features of these are shown in Table 14.4. Of the 13 patients in group I, who had the more apparently benign angiosarcomas, 1 died of metastatic disease, compared with 29 per cent of those in group II and 78 per cent of patients in group III.

Merrino et al reviewed the slides of 15 patients with angiosarcoma on the Tumour Registrary of Connecticut.[36] Using similar criteria to those of Donnell, tumours were divided into groups I (well differentiated), II (moderately differentiated) and III (poorly differentiated). Of the five group I cases, one had relapsed and none had died. In group II (four cases) three died of disease and another had relapsed. In group III, three out of six patients had died of disease. These data suggest that the poor prognosis is borne almost equally by those with moderately and poorly differentiated angiosarcomas.

Rainwater et al reported the experience of the Mayo Clinic in a study which comprised

Table 14.4 Histological features and outcome of patients with angiosarcoma of the breast.[35]

	Group I	Group II	Group III
No of cases	13	7	20
Mean age	41	38	30
Endothelial tufting	Minimal	Present	Prominent
Papillary formation	Absent	Foci	Present
Solid and spindle cell foci	Absent	Absent/minimal	Present
Mitoses	Rare	Present	Numerous
Blood lakes	Absent	Absent	Absent
Necrosis	Absent	Absent	Present
Disease-free	10 (77%)	3 (43%)	2 (10%)
Died of disease	1 (8%)	2 (29%)	14 (78%)

20 patients with angiosarcoma, 10 of whom were originally diagnosed as having benign conditions.[37] Of the 20 patients all but one were females and the average age at presentation was 40 years. All had a breast lump, of which half were painful. The majority of patients were treated by mastectomy but, overall, only 30 per cent were alive at 5 years and only one patient survived 10 years.

Loosely based on the system described by Donnell, the series from the Mayo Clinic were divided into four groups ranging from well to poorly differentiated. However, there was little correlation between this four-grade system and prognosis; nor did tumour size appear to relate to outcome.

As with other sarcomas of the breast, neither radiotherapy nor chemotherapy appeared to be of benefit to patients. If local excision is non-curative these cases carry a dire prognosis.

Irrespective of histological type, the surgical management of operable breast sarcoma is a wide excision when feasible, and more frequently a total mastectomy. Patients with poorly differentiated sarcoma are more likely to relapse with metastatic disease, but no adjuvant therapies have been shown to have any benefit; nor does palliative treatment of advanced disease with systemic therapy appear to be of benefit.

The annual incidence of sarcoma of the breast in the USA would be less than one hundred cases. Unless structured protocols combining surgery and chemotherapy can be instituted, the treatment of breast sarcoma will continue to be empirical and haphazard.

Primary lymphoma of the breast

Primary breast lymphoma, as first evidence of disease without involvement of other sites is a very rare condition. Two of the larger series of cases, from the Memorial Hospital,

New York, and the MD Anderson in Houston, reported an incidence of 1–2 per 1000 breast malignancies.[38,39] Reviewing a series of 1269 patients with lymphoma, Rosenberg et al found that only four (0.3 per cent) presented with a breast lump.[40] Most reports have comprised only small numbers of cases, and many of the original publications are difficult to interpret because of changes in histological classification.

Most recent series have used the Rappaport system in which lymphomas are classified on the basis of their cytology and growth pattern.[41] Cytologically they are subdivided into lymphocytic well differentiated, lymphocytic poorly differentiated, mixed histiocytic/ lymphocytic, histiocytic and undifferentiated. The growth patterns are either diffuse or nodular.

The Kiel classification is more complex in its entirety, attempting to relate the malignant cells to their non-malignant counterpart and avoiding the questionable histiocytic terminology.[42] In essence, however, the Kiel system divides lymphomas into those of high grade and those of low grade, with multiple cell types in each main division.

Almost all the breast lymphomas reported have been of non-Hodgkins type; indeed many series have not included any cases of Hodgkins disease.

The diagnosis of primary breast lymphoma is almost never made clinically, but is the unexpected report on a lesion excised because it was thought to be a carcinoma. With such rarities it is best that the advice of an oncologist with experience in lymphomas is consulted in order to carry out appropriate staging and thus instigate appropriate local or systemic therapy.

Presentation

The mean age of patients presenting with breast lymphoma is 53 years so that they are in the age group in which a likely diagnosis of cancer would be made for any new breast lump.[39,42–7] Typically, solitary breast lymphomas are well circumscribed and may be fairly soft in texture so that they can be mistaken for medullary carcinomas. It has been suggested that some have a violaceous hue, but this is hardly pathognomic.[48] Suspicion may be aroused by the presence of more than one such lesion within the breast and there may be apparently disproportionate axillary nodal enlargement in relation to the size of the primary lesion.

A recent series indicated an increase in numbers of cases being diagnosed.[45] Dixon et al questioned whether this resulted from a true increase in incidence or because histopathologists, aided by immunohistochemistry, were more confident in making a diagnosis of lymphoma rather than a poorly differentiated carcinoma.

Histological subtypes

The larger series, which have used the Rappaport classification, are summarized in Table 14.5.[40,43–9] Lymphomas of the breast are no exception to the general rule that diffuse lesions are more common than nodular, and Hodgkin's disease is the least common. In the earlier series, despite apparent exclusion of metastatic disease, the majority of patients relapsed and died after mastectomy and radiotherapy. This underlines the need for more accurate staging and the frequent requirement for chemotherapy.

Staging

According to the Ann Arbor staging system, the majority of patients with primary breast lymphoma will be in Stages 1E and 11E, that

Table 14.5 Histological subtypes (Rappaport) in series of non-Hodgkins lymphoma of the breast.

No of cases	Mean	NML	NPDL	NHL	DHL	DML	DPDL	DWDL	UD	Reference
16	39	–	–	–	9	–	5	2	–	43
14	44	–	–	–	5	–	1	–	8	39
12	54	2	2	–	8	–	–	–	–	44
16	64	–	1	1	10	1	2	–	1	45
14	52	1	2	–	7	1	1	1	–	46
53	57	7	2	–	26	5	11	2	1	47
8	61	–	1	–	7	–	–	–		
133	53	10 (8%)	8 (6%)	1 (0.8%)	72 (54%)	7 (5%)	20 (15%)	5 (4%)	10 (8%)	

NML = Nodular mixed.
NPDL = Nodular poorly differentiated lymphocytic.
NHL = Nodular histiocytic.
DHL = Diffuse histiocytic.
DML = Diffuse mixed.
DPDL = Diffuse poorly differentiated lymphocytic.
DWDL = Diffuse well differentiated lymphocytic.
UD = Undifferentiated.

is having extranodal, with or without nodal, disease in one or more regions on the same side of the diaphragm.[50] A full history and clinical examination are of particular importance because they may reveal symptoms or signs of disease beyond the breast so that targetted investigations can be performed.

All patients with lymphoma will require basic tests, including full blood count, biochemical screen, chest X-ray scan and bone-marrow biopsy. In addition, CT scans of thorax and abdomen will be performed to assess the extent of disease elsewhere in the body. Only those patients with gastrointestinal or skeletal symptoms will need barium investigations, liver ultrasound or bone scintigraphy.

Treatment

The treatment of lymphoma of the breast is similar to that of patients with disease in other sites and is largely dependent upon the stage and histological type of the tumour. Patients with localized disease of low grade are usually treated with external radiotherapy. For those with localized high-grade lymphoma, first-line chemotherapy is used. This usually comprises CHOP (cyclophosphamide, adriamycin, vincristine and prednisone) or a variant thereof.[51] This can be backed up with adjuvant radiotherapy to sites of bulky residual disease.

Chemotherapy is the standard treatment for those with Stage III/IV disease, and the regimen used will depend upon the grade of the lymphoma. CHOP is used for high-grade lesions, whereas those with low-grade lymphoma are usually given chlorambucil.

Oncological expertise is required for the management of these patients. Attempts to treat lymphomas based on experience of breast cancer will not serve the best interests of the patient.

Hodgkin's disease

Such cases are exceedingly rare; up to 1966 only 16 cases had been recorded.[52] There has been only one series of any size derived from experience of treating 18 patients at MD Anderson Hospital.[53] All cases had Hodgkin's disease (HD) of nodular sclerosing subtype.

Of these 18 cases of HD involving the chest wall and breast, nine presented in this way and nine developed relapse of disease in these sites. All patients with HD involving the breast had involvement of nodes in either the neck or mediastinum, so that none could be said to have had solitary HD within the breast. All were treated with radiotherapy and/or chemotherapy. One-third died of the disease, whilst two-thirds were alive at the time of the report.

Plasmacytoma

There are several single case reports of plasmacytoma presenting as a solitary breast mass.[54–8] Such cases almost invariably progressed to develop multiple myeloma and required chemotherapy. Such extramedullary plasmacytomas, unless very bulky, do not produce monoclonal serum proteins, nor do patients exhibit Bence-Jones protein in their urine.

Cases presenting as solitary plasmacytomas should be treated with radiotherapy to the breast as primary therapy.[58]

References

1 Azzopardi JG, Problems in breast pathology. In: Bennington JL, consulting ed. *Major problems in pathology*, Vol 11, WB Saunders: Philadelphia 1979.)

2 Blichert-Toft M, Hansen JPH, Hansen OH et al, Clinical course of cystosarcoma phyllodes related to histologic appearance, *Surg Gynecol Obstet* (1975) **140**:929–32.

3 Hart WR, Bauer RC, Oberman HA, Cystosarcoma phyllodes, *Am J Clin Pathol* (1977) **70**:211–16.

4 Pietruszka M, Barnes L, Cystosarcoma phyllodes. A clinicopathologic analysis of 42 cases, *Cancer* (1978) **41**:1974–83.

5 Contarini O, Urdaneta LF, Hagan W et al, Cystosarcoma phyllodes of the breast: a new therapeutic proposal, *Am Surg* (1982) **48**:157–66.

6 Grigioni WF, Santini D, Grassigli A et al, A clinico-pathologic study of cystosarcoma phyllodes, *Arch Anat Cytol Pathol* (1982) **30**:303–6.

7 Chowdhury C, Chattopadhyay TK, Pramanik M et al, Cystosarcoma phyllodes—a clinicopathologic analysis of 32 cases, *Ind J Cancer* (1984) **21**:23–30.

8 Hines JR, Murid TM, Beal JM, Prognostic indicators in cystosarcoma phyllodes, *Am J Surg* (1987) **153**:276–80.

9 Inoshita S, Phyllodes tumour (cystosarcoma phyllodes) of the breast. A clinicopathologic study of 45 cases, *Acta Pathol Jpn* (1988) **38**:21–33.

10 Hart J, Layfield LJ, Trumbull WE et al, Practical aspects in the diagnosis and management of cystosarcoma phyllodes, *Arch Surg* (1988) **123**:1079–83.

11 Palshoft T, Blichert-Toft M, Daehnfeldt JL et al, Estradiol binding protein in cystosarcoma phyllodes of the breast, *Eur J Cancer* (1980) **16**:591–3.

12 Rao BR, Meyer JS, Fry CG, Most cystosarcoma phyllodes and fibroadenomas have progesterone receptor but lack estrogen receptor: stromal localisation of progesterone receptor, *Cancer* (1981) **47**:2016–21.

13 Ii K, Hizawa K, Okazaki K et al, Liposarcoma of the breast: fine structural and histochemical study of a case and review of 42 cases in the literature, *Tokushima J Exp Med* (1980) **27**:45–56.

14 Austin RM, Dupree WB, Liposarcoma of the breast: a clinicopathologic study of 28 cases, *Hum Pathol* (1986) **17**:906–13.

15 Kindblom LG, Save-Soderbergh J, The ultrastructure of liposarcoma. A study of 10 cases, *Acta Pathol Microbiol Scand Sect A* (1979) **87**:109–21.

16 Enzinger FM, Weiss SW, *Soft tissue tumours* (1983) (CV Mosby: St Louis, 1983) 242–80.

17 Gobardhan AB, Primary leiomyosarcoma of the breast, *Neth J Surg* (1984) **36**:116–18.

18 Yamashina M, Primary leiomyosarcoma in the breast, *Jpn J Clin Oncol* (1987) **17**:71–7.

19 Jernstrom P, Lindberg AL, Meland ON, Osteogenic sarcoma of the mammary gland, *Am J Clin Pathol* (1963) **40**:521–6.

20 Mufarrij AA, Feiner HD, Breast sarcoma with giant cells and osteoid, *Am J Surg Pathol* (1987) **11**:225–30.

21 Watt AC, Haggar AM, Krasicky GA, Extra osseus osteogenic sarcoma of the breast: mammographic and pathologic findings, *Radiology* (1984) **150**:34.

22 Achram M, Issa S, Rizk G, Osteogenic sarcoma of the breast: some radiological aspects, *Br J Radiol* (1985) **58**:264–5.

23 Thomas AMK, Nathan BE, Primary osteosarcoma of the breast, *Br J Radiol* (1984) **57**:762–3.

24 Savage AP, Sagor GP, Dovey P, Osteosarcoma of the breast: a case report with an unusual diagnostic feature, *Clin Oncol* (1984) **10**:295–8.

25 Berg JW, De Cosse JJ, Fracchia AA et al, Stromal sarcoma of the breast: a unified approach to connective tissue sarcomas other than cystosarcoma phyllodes, *Cancer* (1962) **15**:418–24.

26 Curran RC, Dodge OG, Sarcoma of breast with particular reference to its origin from fibroadenoma, *J Clin Pathol* (1962) **15**:1–16.

27 Ludgate CM, Anderson TJ, Langlands AO, Sarcoma of the female breast: report of a series of 30 cases, *Clin Oncol* (1977) **3**:97–103.

28 Callery CD, Rosen PP, Kinne DW, Sarcoma of the breast. A study of 32 patients with reappraisal of classification and therapy, *Ann Surg* (1985) **201**:527–32.

29 Christensen L, Schiodt T, Blichert-Toft M et al, Sarcomas of the breast: a clinicopathological study of 67 patients with long-term follow-up, *Eur J Surg Oncol* (1988) **14**:241–7.

30 Terrier P, Terrier-Lacombe MJ, Mouriesse H et al, Primary breast sarcoma: a review of 33 cases with immunohistochemistry and prognostic factors, *Breast Cancer Res Treat* (1989) **13**:39–48.

31 Stewart FW, Treves N, Lymphangiosarcoma in post-mastectomy lymphoedema, *Cancer* (1948) **1**:64–81.

32 Miettinen M, Lehto V-P, Virtanen I, Post-mastectomy angiosarcoma (Stewart-Treves Syndrome), *Am J Surg Pathol* (1983) **7**:329–39.

33 Setoyama M, Mera S, Nomoto S et al, A case of Stewart-Treves Syndrome, *J Dermatol* (1984) **11**:81–8.

34 Smith L, Buzdar AU, Rusch V et al, Post-mastectomy angiosarcoma: case report and review of the literature, *Tex Med* (1984) **80**:43–4.

35 Donnell RM, Rosen PP, Lieberman PH et al, Angiosarcoma and other vascular tumours of the breast, *Am J Surg Pathol* (1981) **5**:629–42.

36 Merrino MJ, Berman M, Carter D, Angiosarcoma of the breast, *Am J Surg Pathol* (1983) **7**:53–60.

37 Rainwater LM, Martin JK, Gaffey TA et al, Angiosarcoma of the breast, *Arch Surg* (1986) **121**:669–77.

38 DeCosse JJ, Berg JW, Fracchia AA et al, Primary lymphosarcoma of the breast. A review of 14 cases, *Cancer* (1962) **15**:1264–8.

39 Mambo NC, Burke JS, Butler JJ, Primary malignant lymphomas of the breast, *Cancer* (1977) **39**:2033–40.

40 Rosenberg SA, Diamond HD, Jaslowitz B et al, Lymphosarcoma: a review of 1269 cases, *Medicine (Baltimore)* (1961) **40**:31–84.

41 Rappaport H, *Atlas of tumour pathology*, Section III, Fascicle 8, Tumours of the haematopoetic system. (Armed Forces Institute of Pathology: Washington DC 1966) 49.

42 Gerard-Marchant R, Hamlin I, Lennert K et al, Classification of non-Hodgkins lymphomas, *Lancet* (1974) **ii**:1070–3.

43 Wiseman C, Liao KT, Primary lymphoma of the breast, *Cancer* (1972) **29**:1705–12.

44 Schaouten JT, Weese JL, Carbone PP, Lymphoma of the breast, *Ann Surg* (1981) **194**:749–53.

45 Liu FF, Clark RM, Primary lymphoma of the breast, *Clin Radiol* (1986) **37**:567–70.

46 Dixon JM, Lumsden AB, Krajewski A et al, Primary lymphoma of the breast, *Br J Surg* (1987) **74**:214–17.

47 Brustein S, Kimmel M, Lieberman PH et al, Malignant lymphoma of the breast, *Ann Surg* (1987) **205**:144–9.

48 Lamovec J, Jancar J, Primary lymphoma of the breast, *Cancer* (1987) **60**:3033–41.

49 Ti M, Elgnezabal A, Dosik H, Lymphosarcoma of the breast, *Am J Med Sci* (1975) **269**:409–13.

50 *Manual for staging of cancer.* (American Joint Committee for Cancer Staging and End Results Reporting: Chicago 1978).

51 Miller TP, Jones SE, Initial chemotherapy for clinically localised lymphomas of unfavourable histology, *Blood* (1983) **62**:413–18.

52 Lawler MR, Riddell DH, Hodgkins disease of the breast, *Arch Surg* (1966) **93**:331–4.

53 Meis JM, Butler JJ, Osborne BM, Hodgkins disease involving the breast and chest wall, *Cancer* (1986) **59**:1859–65.

54 Rosenberg B, Attie JN, Mandelbaum HL, Breast tumor as the presenting sign of multiple myeloma, *N Engl J Med* (1963) **269**:359–61.

55 Bassett WB, Weiss RB, Plasmacyomas of the breast: an unusual manifestation of multiple myeloma, *S Afr Med J* (1979) **72**:1492–4.

56 Bloomberg TJ, Glees JP, Williams JE, Bilateral breast lumps: an unusual feature of extramedullary plasmacytoma, *Br J Radiol* (1980) **53**:498–501.

57 Merino MJ, Plasmacytoma of the breast, *Arch Pathol Lab Med* (1984) **108**:676–8.

58 Kirshenbaum G, Rhone DP, Solitary extra medullary plasmacytoma of the breast with serum monoclonal protein: a case report and review of the literature, *Am J Clin Pathol* (1985) **83**:230–2.

CHAPTER 15

WHERE NEXT?

Now entertain conjecture of a time.

William Shakespeare

Prevention of breast cancer

Until the sequence of events has been identified which leads from normality to overt expression of malignancy, the eradication of breast cancer will remain an unattainable objective. However, while waiting for the molecular keys to the black box of mammary carcinogenesis, other approaches have to be considered, largely aimed at modulating the subsequent promotion of breast cancer by the endocrine system. As with responses to endocrine therapy in advanced and early breast cancer, it is likely that hormonal intervention might reduce but not abolish the incidence of breast cancer.

Evidence of endocrine involvement in the aetiology of breast cancer

The most compelling evidence of a hormonal involvement in breast cancer derives from age-incidence statistics of the disease. The age/incidence curves for Connecticut and Denmark are shown in Figure 15.1, and replotted on a semilogarithmic scale in Figure 15.2.[1] The most striking aspect of the transformed data is the inflexion at age 50 (Clemmesen's hook).[2] This implies that an

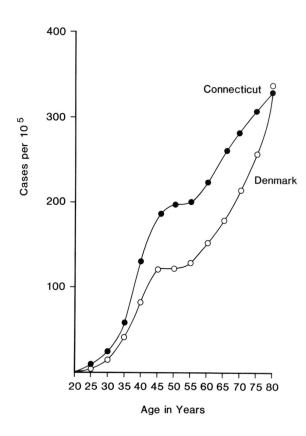

Figure 15.1   Age incidence curves for breast cancers in Connecticut and Denmark.

252

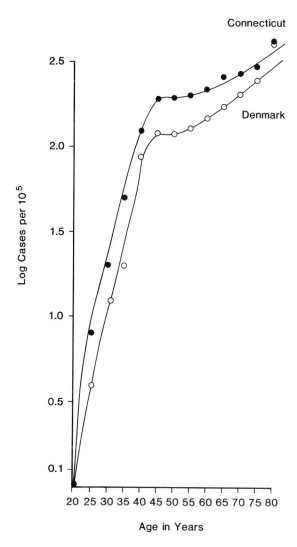

Figure 15.2 Age incidence curves for breast cancer in Connecticut and Denmark replotted on a semilogarithmic scale.

natural withdrawal of oestrogens leads to prevention of breast cancers which would otherwise have become evident but for the intervention of this major endocrine life event.

This protection by oestrogen suppression is supported by the work of Hirayama and Wynder who studied the relationship of early bilateral oöphorectomy to subsequent risk of breast cancer.[3] A case-control study was conducted using breast-cancer patients and controls attending a screening clinic. Overall, 14 per cent of the cases and 19 per cent of controls had undergone an artificial menopause. The relative risk of breast cancer in those undergoing bilateral oöphorectomy was 0.70, that is a 30 per cent reduction in incidence. When oöphorectomy was performed before the age of 37 (calculated as the lower age limit for natural menopause) the relative risk fell to 0.35. By definition, women treated by early hysterectomy and bilateral oöphorectomy have disease of the endometrium, myometrium or ovary and constitute an unusual subgroup and there may be alternative genetic or environmental explanations for their reduced risk of breast cancer. Nevertheless, these data have been used to suggest that 5 years of premenopausal ovarian suppression would lead to a 38 per cent reduction in breast cancer, with a 63 per cent reduction after 10 years, with 15 years of ovarian ablation leading to an 80 per cent reduction in risk.[4]

Without doubt, as a preventative measure, oöphorectomy is a non-starter. Primarily it would be unacceptable to the majority of women, not least because of the severe menopausal symptoms which would arise. Equally important in population terms, any reduction in mortality from breast cancer would almost certainly be nullified by increased deaths from cardiovascular disease and the complications of osteoporosis, arising directly from the withdrawal of ovarian steroid hormones.

Since any form of hormonal treatment will

event occurring at this age has a profound and prolonged inhibitory effect on the subsequent incidence of breast cancer. The most likely candidate is the menopause. Thus the be costly, and in order to minimize the development of side effects developing in normal women, it is necessary to identify a high-risk group and then target that cohort with the putative preventative therapy. This provides the major obstacle to the large-scale prevention of breast cancer. Not enough is known to be able to identify the one in 12 women who will develop breast cancer during their lifetime.

The Guernsey project

This was the first and certainly the most protracted study designed to assess prospectively putative risk factors for breast cancer with the objective of identifying a high-risk group with an abnormality that might be susceptible to change. The project arose as a result of work by Bulbrook and Hayward which had shown that it was possible to predict the response to adrenalectomy or hypophysectomy for patients with advanced breast cancer by measurement of urinary steroids.[5] It was found that those most likely to respond excreted more androgen (aetiocholanolone) than the non-responders. These data were used to construct a discriminant:

discriminant =
80 − 80[17 OHCS] + aetiocholanolone

17 hydroxycorticosteroids [17-OHCS] were measured in mg per 24 hours and aetiocholanolone in μg per 24 hours. Those with a positive discriminant were likely to respond.

Subsequent study of patients undergoing mastectomy for early breast cancer revealed that approximately half the cases had negative discriminants and these appeared to have a worse prognosis.[6] Thus low androgen excretion was related to more aggressive tumours and reduced likelihood of response

to endocrine therapy. It was postulated that this alteration in androgen metabolism might be aetiologically related. Were low levels of urinary aetiocholanolone the result of the malignant process or possibly a forerunner and therefore a marker of risk, which might be susceptible to modification?

To answer these questions the Guernsey project was set up to try and identify an endocrine risk marker in a normal population. Guernsey was chosen, not because of an increased incidence of breast cancer, but in order to study a relatively stable population (income tax is significantly lower than in Britain) which had a high standard of medical care and accurate population records.

In the first Guernsey study, 5000 volunteers were enrolled, aged 35–55, and a 24-hour urine specimen was collected from each. Aliquots were frozen and stored at −20°C. As breast cancers developed among the volunteers, so those individuals' pre-cancer urine specimens were examined, together with approximately 10 age-matched controls. The urine was assayed for 17-OHCS, androsterone and aetiocholanolone. After 27 volunteers had developed breast cancer and had been compared with 187 controls it was found that the excretion of aetiocholanolone was significantly lower in the breast-cancer cases.[7]

Thus there was hope that a high-risk group had been found. However, when assay results were available from 1445 women, Farewell conducted a multivariate analysis to determine risk factors.[8] Four emerged as significant: age at menarche, family history of breast cancer, age at first baby and aetiocholanolone (log of daily excretion). All four variables were additive so that a woman with four risk factors had a 0.27 (approximately 1 in 4) probability of developing breast cancer. However, such individuals were rare. When used on a population basis the risk factors were less useful, as is shown in Table 15.1. One risk factor was present in

Table 15.1 Common possession of risk factors by normal women and cancer cases.[8]

No of risk factors	Normal (%)	Cancer (%)
1	90	100
2	55	82
3	17	47
4	2	7

90 per cent of the entire population and 100 per cent of the breast-cancer cases. The best that could be achieved was with a combination of three risk factors, which delineated 17 per cent of the normal population and 47 per cent of the cases. Thus as an approximation, 20 per cent of the population could be identified who would develop 50 per cent of breast cancers. This is too large a group with insufficient specificity.

With advances in assay techniques it became possible to measure steroid hormones in blood, and the second Guernsey study collected both blood and urine from 5000 women. The result of this study was that cases of breast cancer displayed lower levels of adrenal androgens in their serum, compared with controls.[9] However, use of adrenal androgen as a risk indicator was insufficiently specific to be of clinical value.

The third Guernsey study was set up to extend the previous work and to determine whether there was a link between endocrine profile and the pattern of breast parenchyma on mammograms (Wolfe grade). During this study it became possible to measure the percentage of free oestradiol (free E_2) within the serum together with its major binding protein, sex hormone binding globulin (SHBG). In a case-control study it was found that the percentage free E_2 was a risk indicator.[10] Significantly higher percentages of free E_2 were present in women who went on to develop breast cancer. In parallel, such cases exhibited lower levels of SHBG.

At the same time, those whose mammograms were classified as Wolfe grades DY and P_2 encompassed 85 per cent of the cancers and 54 per cent of the controls, giving a relative risk of 1.6.[11] Thus the hypothesis was advanced that a high-risk group could be identified using a combination of factors.[12] It was proposed that the following could be used as selection criteria for a prevention study:

1 Nulliparity or late age at first baby (over 28 years)
2 Low-serum SHBG (below population median)
3 P_2/DY Wolfe grades
4 First-degree family history
5 Prior biopsy for benign breast disease

Using this combination it was postulated that a group with a 3–4 fold increase in risk could be delineated. Since such cases might have a 1 in 3/4 lifetime chance of developing breast cancer it was argued that they should be entered into a trial examining the efficacy of tamoxifen as a preventative agent. Not only would this drug block oestrogen receptors and counterbalance hyperoestrogenization, but it would also stimulate hepatic synthesis of SHBG, thereby binding more of the free oestradiol in plasma.

Tamoxifen as a preventative agent

There were two major obstacles which had to be overcome before such a trial could be run.

First, clinicians needed to be convinced that a high-risk group could actually be found, and second the medium- and long-term toxicity and acceptability of tamoxifen had to be determined. In relation to the problem of a high-risk group, a fourth Guernsey project is under way which is examining the constancy of risk factors such as Wolfe grade and SHBG. At present, the only risk factor which is ascertainable in any centre is family history, and this is likely to be the basis for the earliest trials of prevention. Complex multivariate analysis would be incompatible with the multicentre accrual which is necessary for any prevention trial with adequate statistical muscle.

In relation to the toxicity and acceptability, tamoxifen data are now available which show the low profile of side effects. Tamoxifen has been used experimentally to treat cyclical mastalgia and tested in clinical trials which have confirmed its efficacy and tolerability in premenopausal women.[13-15] However, there is a difference between symptomatic cases with mastalgia and asymptomatic at-risk women in terms of the level of long-term side effects that will be tolerable. Fears that tamoxifen would lead to bone demineralization have proved to be unfounded,[16,17] as have suspicions that tamoxifen would alter the lipoprotein profile and increase the risk of coronary heart disease.[18,19] Fortunately, in women tamoxifen appears to achieve a remarkable balance of oestrogen antagonism and agonism.

One major activity which is still in question is the effect of tamoxifen on the endometrium. In the Swedish adjuvant trial, within which patients were given long-term tamoxifen, there was a significantly increased number of cancers of the uterus and adnexae, 13 (1.3 per cent) in the tamoxifen-treated group compared with only 2 (0.2 per cent) in untreated controls.[20] This six-fold increase in risk occurred when patients were given 40 mg daily. In the Scottish adjuvant trial, in which treated patients were given 20 mg daily for 5 years, there was no difference between the number of endometrial cancers in the treated and control groups.[21] This preliminary data suggests that care should be exhibited when prescribing long-term tamoxifen to any woman with an intact uterus, who should be monitored by regular endometrial biopsies.

The Swedish study has provided strong supportive evidence for the preventative use of tamoxifen, since there was a significant reduction in new primary breast cancers among the treated group 18 (1.9 per cent) versus 32 (3.4 per cent). This was also suggested by data from the NATO trial where there were three cancers in the tamoxifen-treated group and 10 among the controls.[22] However, in the Scottish trial there were similar numbers of contralateral breast cancers in the treated and control groups, although very stringent criteria were used to define new primary cancers.

Pilot study of tamoxifen for prevention

Many of the outstanding questions concerning the feasibility, acceptability and compliance of a tamoxifen study have been satisfactorily answered in a recent report by Powles et al.[17] A high-risk group was delineated who had a first-degree family history of breast cancer and these were randomized to receive either tamoxifen or placebo on a lifelong basis. Results were reported once 200 cases had been entered into the trial. Eligible women were aged 35–65 and were drawn from a group attending a symptomatic breast clinic, and from others who were seen at a screening clinic at the Royal Marsden Hospital. At the start of the trial those with one first-degree relative were included, but midway this was changed to those with more than one affected first-degree relative.

Of a subset of 242 who attended the screening clinic and reported a family history, 75 (42 per cent) had more than one first-degree relative with the disease. Of those eligible, 29 (47 per cent) gave informed consent to enter the study. Similar side effects were reported by those receiving tamoxifen and placebo, except the former group more frequently reported hot flushes. Medication was stopped because of side effects in seven of those given tamoxifen and six receiving placebo.

Compliance with the assigned treatment at 12 months was very good, being 83 per cent in the tamoxifen group and 85 per cent in the control group. This is very encouraging with regards to the long-term acceptability of tamoxifen and it is unlikely that this could be improved upon. In parallel, tests were performed to examine objective toxicity. There was no effect on blood clotting nor on cholesterol levels, suggesting that tamoxifen in this dosage (20 mg daily) did not lead to an increased risk of thrombosis. In addition, no alteration in bone-mineral content was found; the use of single photon absorptiometry (SPA) suggested that tamoxifen did not produce demineralization.

For further discussion of tamoxifen treatment in the elderly see Chapter 11.

LHRH agonists

These agents, which reversibly suppress ovarian function, provide an opportunity to examine the effects of early menopause but without irrevocably ablating the ovaries. It is hoped that this lack of finality of ovarian suppression associated with LHRH agonists might make them more acceptable to women, particularly as they would also act as contraceptive agents. This has been proposed by Pike et al,[4] who suggest that because

of the known effects of oestrogen withdrawal on bone mineral and lipoprotein metabolism, it would be necessary to give replacement oestrogen.

One of the unquantified aspects of this type of approach to prevention is that it is not known whether there is one threshold for breast epithelial cell growth and another for bone protection and maintenance of premenopausal hepatic function. If not, this combination of LHRH and oestrogen replacement might represent an expensive and involved method to achieve no benefit in terms of breast-cancer risk.

Because of the effect of unopposed oestrogen on the endometrium, leading to increased risk of endometrial carcinoma, it would be necessary to give additional progestin, probably on an intermittent basis. This requires a pilot study.

Tamoxifen and progestins

It has been suggested that progestins may protect women against developing breast cancer.[23] Certainly there is a lot of experience of their administration to premenopausal women as an oral contraceptive, without major toxicity. In addition, there is evidence that they protect the endometrium against oestrogen-stimulated malignancy. Thus in order to overcome the collective *angst* concerning tamoxifen and the endometrium, it has been suggested that a factorial-design prevention trial could be considered.[24]

In this study, women at high risk, who would almost certainly be those with a strong family history of breast cancer, would receive one of four treatments, all of which could be formulated in identical tablets. Individuals would receive tamoxifen, progestin, both tamoxifen and progestin or placebo.

Prevention trials will require large numbers of women (5–10 000), simple design and ease of follow up since they will have to be multicentric in order to accrue adequate numbers of cases. The time is right. There are now no compelling arguments against such a study. The problem now has to be resolved in terms of cooperation and logistics.

Future moves for breast conservation

Now that the safety of breast conservation has been confirmed for patients with certain cancers, a clamour will arise to extend the indications to include larger and multifocal tumours. Whether this will prove to be in the best interests of such patients has yet to be determined. Rather than use what may be inadequate approaches to the salvage of women with larger tumours, it will be better to encourage earlier presentation—seemingly simple, but actually a task of Herculean proportions. Alternatively, through the education of clinicians rather than patients, it should be possible to increase the numbers of patients with suitable tumours who are actually treated by breast conservation.

A major obstacle blocking the wide use of breast conservation is the requirement for a prolonged course of external radiotherapy, which has been shown to be necessary in all successful trials. Failure to irradiate the breast, even after histological confirmation of complete excision, will lead to an unacceptably high rate of relapse within the breast, almost invariably at the original tumour site.

Along with the known risk of relapse within the original quadrant there is also the theoretical risk arising from multifocal infiltrating and non-infiltrating carcinoma. Review of specimens from 89 women treated by mastectomy in the Guy's component of the EORTC conservation study showed the presence of residual carcinoma at the biopsy site

in 15 (17 per cent). Multifocal carcinoma outside the original quadrant was present in 22 (25 per cent).

Of these cases, 16 (18 per cent) were non-infiltrating and only 6 (7 per cent) had multicentric infiltrating cancer. These results were from random sampling and percentages would be slightly higher if serial sections were taken. Nevertheless, the proportion was small. Of the cases with multifocal infiltrating cancer, two had axillary nodal involvement and would nowadays receive systemic adjuvant therapy. This in itself might act as treatment for multifocal disease, since local relapse rates are reduced. Thus only four (5 per cent) of patients had untreated infiltrating cancer. Thus 95 per cent of patients might have had unnecessary external irradiation.

For these reasons a different approach has been proposed. Why not increase the dose of interstitial irradiation and dispense with the external radiotherapy? This might affect the local control and cosmetic outcome, and would certainly simplify treatment. This type of approach would be suitable even for elderly patients. A pilot study has been conducted at Guy's in which 27 women with breast cancer have been treated with a high-dose iridium implant, without external radiotherapy. As part of this study the nature of the implant has been changed from a flexible to a rigid system using a template (Figure 15.2).

All patients were treated by tumourectomy and axillary clearance followed by a rigid implant. After-loading with iridium wires was used to give a tumour dose of 55 Gy. After a median follow up of only 22 months there have been no relapses and the cosmetic results were good/excellent in 85 per cent. Further follow up will be required to determine whether subsequent fibrosis and telangectases develop after high-dose implants and whether this adversely affects cosmesis. If these encouraging early results hold it is planned to conduct a trial to

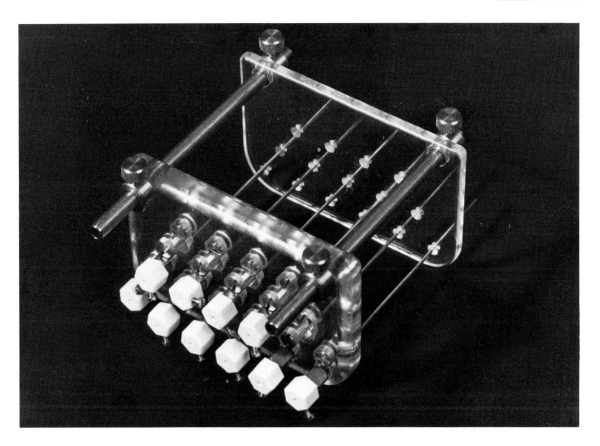

Figure 15.3   Template for high-dose iridium implants.

compare high dose with standard iridium implants in patients with early breast cancer.

Where iridium of presently available activity is used, the high-dose implant lasts for 5 days so that the potential exists for the patient to have definitive breast conservation treatment in less than 7 days. Not only might this technique obviate the need for external radiotherapy, it might also mean that the radiotherapist would not necessarily have to

be present in theatre to carry out the implant. A system could be devised whereby appropriate cases meeting pre-agreed criteria could have their primary treatment of axillary clearance, tumourectomy and implant carried out by the surgeon. The radiotherapist could then arrange for after-loading of the implant in an appropriately protected environment.

For the elderly, the unacceptability of

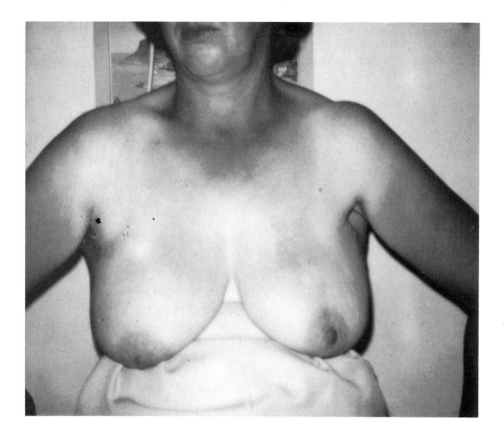

Figure 15.4   Patient treated 2.6 months previously by high-dose iridium implant.

mastectomy and the inadequacy of tamox-ifen could be circumvented by use of high-dose implants, provided that they can be shown to achieve good long-term control.

Adjuvant therapy

Meta-analysis of trials which had examined both endocrine and cytotoxic adjuvant therapies has resulted in universal acceptance that these treatments can reduce mortality from breast cancer.[25] The next phase of development will be a redefinition of the indications for such therapy. Thus other prognostic indicators will be sought in patients with node-negative disease and these will probably include tumour size, type, grade and S-phase fraction. Treatment of the premenopausal node-negative cases will be by chemotherapy, in the most part, but further studies will be needed to define the roles of tamoxifen and ovarian ablation with prednisolone and to determine whether success of adjuvant endocrine therapies bears any relationship to the receptor status of primary tumours.

Few would wish to give adjuvant chemotherapy to postmenopausal node-negative women, but undoubtedly the more hawkish medical oncologists will try. There will be increasing pressure to prescribe tamoxifen for all postmenopausal women with breast cancer, irrespective of nodal status, tumour type or grade. This should be resisted since it will mean the unnecessary treatment of a considerable number of women.

For patients with axillary nodal involvement there is a linear relationship between risk of relapse and number of nodes containing metastases.[26] Those with heavy nodal involvement, say >10 nodes, are at very high risk of dying from breast cancers. Based on successful results of treatment for other cancers, such as leukaemias and testicular tumours, attempts will be made to effect cures by means of more aggressive chemotherapy. This would include dose intensification, protected environments and bone-marrow transplantation. It is important to determine whether presently available chemotherapy can change the clinical course of patients at high risk of relapse, and the impact of aggressive adjuvant therapy on quality of life. The need to identify a high-risk group would mean a shift from axillary node sampling towards axillary clearance.

These various approaches are possible with existing drugs and are likely to lead to moderate but clinically important improvement. As the role of autocrine growth factors and their receptors becomes more clearly understood, so it may be possible to synthesize specific antagonists. Such agents might have a major impact as part of the primary treatment of breast cancer.

References

1 Moolgavkar SH, Stevens RG, Lee JAV, Effect of age on incidence of breast cancer in females, *J Natl Cancer Inst* (1979) **62**:493–501.

2 Clemmesen J, Statistical studies in malignant neoplasms. II. Basic tables. Denmark 1943–1957, *Acta Pathol Microbiol Scand* (1965) **174**:2–3.

3 Hirayama T, Wynder EL, A study of the epidemiology of cancer of the breast. II. The influence of hysterectomy, *Cancer* (1962) **15**:28–38.

4 Pike MC, Ross RK, Lobo RA et al, LHRH agonists and the prevention of breast and ovarian cancer, *Br J Cancer* (1989) **60**:142–5.

5 Bulbrook RD, Greenwood FC, Hayward JL, Selection of breast cancer patients for adrenalectomy or hypophysectomy by determination of urinary 17-hydroxycorticosteroids and aetiocholanolones, *Lancet* (1960) **i**:1154–7.

6 Bulbrook RD, Hayward JL, Spicer CC et al, Abnormal excretion of urinary steroids by women with early breast cancer, *Lancet* (1962) **ii**:1238–40.

7 Bulbrook RD, Hayward JL, Spicer CC, Relation between urinary androgen and corticoid excretion and subsequent breast cancer, *Lancet* (1971) **ii**:395–8.

8 Farewell VT, The combined effect of breast cancer risk factors, *Cancer* (1977) **40**:931–6.

9 Deshpande N, Hayward JL, Bulbrook RD, Plasma 17-hydroxycorticosteroids and 17-oxosteroids in patients with breast cancer and in normal women, *J Endocrinol* (1965) **32**:167–77.

10 Moore JW, Clark GMG, Bulbrook RD et al, Serum concentration of total and non-protein bound oestradiol in patients with breast cancer and in normal controls, *Int J Cancer* (1982) **29**:17–21.

11 Gravelle IH, Bulstrode JC, Bulbrook RD et al, A prospective study of mammographic parenchymal pattern and risk of breast cancer, *Br J Radiol* (1982) **55**:23–5.

12 Cuzick J, Bulbrook RD, Wang DY, The prevention of breast cancer, *Lancet* (1986) **i**:83–6.

13 Fentiman IS, Caleffi M, Brame K et al, Double blind controlled trial of tamoxifen therapy for mastalgia, *Lancet* (1986) **i**:287–8.

14 Powles TJ, Ford HT, Gazet JC, A randomised clinical trial to compare tamoxifen with dana-zol for treatment of benign mammary dyspla-sia, *Senologia* (1987) **2**:1–5.

15 Fentiman IS, Caleffi M, Hamed H et al, Dosage and duration of tamoxifen treatment for mastalgia: a controlled trial, *Br J Surg* (1988) **75**:845–6.

16 Fentiman IS, Caleffi M, Murby B et al, Dosage, duration and short-term effect on bone mineral content of tamoxifen treatment for mastalgia, *Br J Cancer* (1989) **60**:262–4.

17 Powles TJ, Hardy JR, Ashley SE et al, A pilot trial to evaluate the acute toxicity and feasibil-ity of tamoxifen for prevention of breast cancer, *Br J Cancer* (1989) **60**:126–9.

18 Rosner S, Wallgren A, Serum lipoproteins and proteins after breast cancer surgery and effects of tamoxifen, *Atherosclerosis* (1984) **52**:339–46.

19 Caleffi M, Fentiman IS, Clark GM et al, Effect of tamoxifen on oestrogen binding, lipid and lipoprotein concentrations and blood clotting parameters in premenopausal women with breast pain, *J Endocrinol* (1988) **119**:335–9.

20 Fornander T, Cedermark B, Mattsson A et al, Adjuvant tamoxifen in early breast cancer: occurrence of new primary cancers, *Lancet* (1989) **i**:117–19.

21 Stewart HJ, Knight GM, Tamoxifen and the uterus and endometrium, *Lancet* (1989) **i**:375–6.

22 Cuzick J, Baum M, Tamoxifen and contralater-al breast cancer, *Lancet* (1985) **ii**:282.

23 Gambrell RD, Proposal to decrease the risk and improve the prognosis of breast cancer, *Am J Obstet Gynecol* (1984) **150**:119–28.

24 Fentiman IS, Endocrine prevention of breast cancer, *Br J Cancer* (1989) **60**:12–14.

25 Early Breast Cancer Trialists' Collaborative Group, Effects of adjuvant tamoxifen and of cytotoxic therapy as mortality in early breast cancer, *N Engl J Med* (1988) **319**:1681–2.

26 Nemoto J, Vana J, Bedwani RN et al, Manage-ment and survival of female breast cancer: results of a national study by the American College of Surgeons, *Cancer* (1980) **45**:2917–21.

INDEX